Ultrastructure of Smooth Muscle

ELECTRON MICROSCOPY IN BIOLOGY AND MEDICINE

Current Topics in Ultrastructural Research

SERIES EDITOR: P.M. MOTTA

Already published in this series

Vol. 1 Motta, P.M. (ed.): Ultrastructure of Endocrine Cells and Tissues. ISBN: 0-89838-568-7.

Vol. 2 Van Blerkom, J. and Motta, P.M. (eds.): Ultrastructure of Reproduction: Gametogenesis, Fertilization, and Embryogenesis. ISBN: 0-89838-572-5.

Vol. 3 Ruggeri, A. and Motta, P.M. (eds.): Ultrastructure of the Connective Tissue Matrix. ISBN: 0-89838-600-4

Vol. 4 Motta, P.M. and Fujita, A. (eds.): Ultrastructure of the Digestive Tract. ISBN: 0-89838-893-7.

Vol. 5 Van Blerkom, J. and Motta, P.M. (eds.): Ultrastructure of Human Gametogenesis and Early Embryogenesis. ISBN: 0-89838-383-8

Vol. 6 Riva, A. and Motta, P.M. (eds.): Ultrastructure of the Expatraparietal Glands of the Digestive Tract. ISBN: 0-7923-0303-2.

Vol. 7 Bonucci, E. and Motta, P.M. (eds.): Ultrastructure of Skeletal Tissue. ISBN: 0-7923-0373-3.

Ultrastructure of Smooth Muscle

edited by

Pietro M. Motta, Ph.D., M.D.
Department of Anatomy
University of Rome "La Sapienza"
Rome, Italy

1990 **Kluwer Academic Publishers**
BOSTON DORDRECHT LONDON

Distributors

for North America:
Kluwer Academic Publishers
101 Philip Drive
Assinippi Park
Norwell, Massachusetts 02061 USA

Distributors
for all other countries:
Kluwer Academic Publishers Group
Distribution Centre
Post Office Box 322
3300 AH Dordrecht, THE NETHERLANDS

Library of Congress Cataloging-in-Publication Data

Ultrastructure of smooth muscle / edited by Pietro M. Motta.
p. cm. — (Electron microscopy in biology and medicine)
Includes bibliographical references.
ISBN-13:978-1-4612-8025-5 e-ISBN-13:978-1-4613-0683-2
DOI: 10.1007/978-1-4612-0683-2

1. Smooth muscle—Ultrastructure. I. Motta, Pietro M. II. Series.
[DNLM: 1. Muscle, Smooth—ultrastructure. W1 EL33E / WE 500 U47]
QP321.U48 1990
596'.01852—dc20
DNLM/DLC
for Library of Congress 89-20070
CIP

Preface

Recent advances in electron microscopy have opened up new dimensions and perspectives in the field of morphology, and these are presently being integrated with biochemical and physiopathological phenomena occurring in cells, tissues, and organs. Methods such as freeze-fracture, freeze-etching, scanning, and high-voltage electron microscopy have contributed immensely to this progress, as well as to the study of smooth muscle tissue and contractile cells in general.

The articles composing this book have been selected and edited with the purpose of updating and reviewing the most important aspects of smooth muscle cells as revealed by the integration of these submicroscopic techniques.

The chapters of this volume have been prepared by some of the most authoritative experts in the discipline. Therefore each article not only offers the reader a concise review of the specific topic, but also seeks to highlight areas that require further investigation.

Much of the volume is presented in an illustrative format so as to emphasize the remarkable results obtainable by the combination of the aforementioned methods, which allow a better appreciation of smooth muscle structure and ultrastructure.

This volume, like others in the series, is intended not only for researchers in the field, but also for graduate students of histology, embryology, anatomy, physiology, and pathology in both medical and veterinary colleges. My hope is that this book will prove to be a valuable academic resource to the audience of the world in this fascinating and expanding field.

I wish to express my gratitude to the authors who so kindly contributed to this book, not only for the quality of their chapters but also for their patience in responding to the often tedious and exacting editorial demands. In particular, my warm appreciation goes to Prof. Giorgio Gabella for his original suggestion to devote a volume of this series to smooth muscle tissue, and for his friendly and invaluable assistance in selecting appropriate topics and in seeking out some of the most distinguished experts in this sector to cover the various chapters of the volume.

I would like to extend special thanks to Dr. David Finn for having carefully checked the many manuscripts composing this book and to Dr. S.A. Nottola for her great help in preparing the index.

Finally, I would express my sincere thanks to Mr. Jeffrey K. Smith publisher and Mrs. Karen S. Cullen, editorial assistant, at Kluwer Academic Publishers for their kind and continuous help in the production of this volume.

Pietro M. Motta

Contents

Contributing authors

Aumüller, G., Department of Anatomy and Cell Biology, Philipps University, D-3550 Marburg, Federal Republic of Germany

Bagby, R.M., Department of Zoology, University of Tennessee, Knoxville, TN 37996-0810, USA

Campbell, G.R., Department of Anatomy, University of Melbourne, Parkville, Victoria, 3052 Australia

Campbell, J.H., Baker Medical Research Institute, Commercial Road, Prahran, Victoria, 3181 Australia Australia

De Shan, Z., Department of Anatomy and Embryology, The Third Military Medical School, Chonching, China

Dixon, J.S., Department of Cell & Structural Biology, University of Manchester, Stopford Building, Oxford Road, Manchester M 13 9PT, England

Familiari, G., Department of Human Anatomy, Faculty of Medicine, University of Rome "La Sapienza", Via A. Borelli, 50, 00161 Rome, Italy

Fujii, S., Department of Obstetrics & Gynecology, Kumamoto University, Medical School, Kumamoto City, 860, Japan

Fujiwara, T., Laboratory Animal Center, Ehime University, School of Medicine, Shigenobu, Ehime 791–02, Japan

Gabella, G., Department of Anatomy and Developmental Biology, University College London, Gower Street, London WC1E 6BT, England

Gosling, J.A., Department of Anatomy, The Chinese University of Hong Kong, Shatin, N.T., Hong Kong

Inoué, T., Department of Anatomy, Tottori University, School of Medicine, Yonago, 683, Japan

Kaidoh, T., Department of Anatomy, Ehime University, School of Medicine, Shigenobu, Ehime 791–02, Japan

Katabuchi, H., Department of Obstetrics & Gynecology, Kumamoto University, Medical School, Kumamoto City, 860, Japan

Konishi, I., Department of Obstetrics & Gynecology, Kumamoto University, Medical School, Kumamoto City, 860, Japan

Motta, P.M., Department of Human Anatomy, Faculty of Medicine, University of Rome "La Sapienza", Via A. Borelli, 50, 00161 Rome, Italy

Muglia, U., Department of Veterinary Anatomy, Faculty of Veterinary Medicine, University of Messina, Via S. Cecilia, 30, 90100 Messina, Italy

Nakashiro, S., Department of Anatomy, Ehime University, School of Medicine, Shigenobu, Ehime 791–02, Japan

Okamura, H., Department of Obstetrics & Gynecology, Kumamoto University, Medical School, Kumamoto City, 860, Japan

Todd, M.E., Department of Anatomy, The University of British Columbia, 2177 Wesbrook Mall, Vancouver, B.C. V6T 1W5, Canada

Uehara, Y., Department of Anatomy, Ehime University, School of Medicine, Shigenobu, Ehime 791–02, Japan

Vizza, E., Department of Human Anatomy, Faculty of Medicine, University of Rome "La Sapienza", Via A. Borelli, 50, 00161 Rome, Italy

Ultrastructure of Smooth Muscle

CHAPTER 1

General aspects of the fine structure of smooth muscles

GIORGIO GABELLA

1. Introduction

Smooth muscle is a tissue that is found in almost every organ of the body. It is a major component of the walls of hollow organs (Table 1). Its ability to contract therefore serves varied functions in organs enormously different in size, speed of contraction, and nature of their contents, and this variability is reflected in all aspects of the muscle fine structure. Some features are common to virtually all smooth muscles: the muscle cells are minute in size, uninucleated, packed with actin and myosin filaments; the cell membrane forms caveolae but not T-tubules, and a substantial amount of it bears attachment of filaments; there is no obvious lateral register between filaments, hence no cross-striation; there are innumerable cell-to-cell junctions and cell-to-stroma junctions; the cells (and the muscle as a whole) can undergo extreme changes in length and girth; the stroma is well developed and is a major load-bearing element; and there is no connetive tissue sheath or perymisum. A common structural theme is very much in evidence in smooth muscles of all vertebrates, but characteristic individual features, specific to one muscle and clearly or presumably related to its functional specializations, are equally common. An exhaustive description of a smooth muscle includes morphological parameters that are best analyzed when grouped into a range of structural levels. This introductory chapter will briefly describe 1) the architecture of smooth musculature, that is, histological features such as the extent of the muscle, its insertions (when they exist), its boundaries, and the three-dimensional arrangement of muscle cells into layers, cords, and bundles; 2) the various cell types and the extracellular materials making up a smooth muscle; 3) the fine structure of smooth muscle cells; and 4) the presence and spatial distribution of chemical markers of muscle cells, such as proteins associated with muscle filaments.

2. Architecture of smooth musculature

Some smooth muscles have the form of cords or bands, usually with a straight course and with muscle cells running approximately parallel to the long axis. Examples are the taeniae of the large intestine, or the expansor secundariorum of the wing of birds, or muscles found in the peritoneum, such as the suspensor of the duodenum or the anococcygeus, or the arrectores pilorum. More often, smooth musculature is in the form of sheets that form layers in the walls of hollow organs. In the intestine, in each of the two muscle layers the cells run parallel to each other and parallel to the serosal surface, and at right angle to the cells of the adjacent muscle layer. The geometrical order of this structure is very high, is acquired in the early stages of development, and is maintained even in the hypertrophic growth. The arrangement is possibly required because of the relative scarcity of intramuscular connective tissue in the gut and because of the characteristic structure of the submucosa, onto which the mechanical activity of the muscle coat is discharged. In other hollow

Table 1-1. Distribution of the main smooth muscles

□ Muscle coats of the uterine tubes, biliary pathways, ureter, vas deferens	□ Intrinsic ocular muscles: ciliary muscle, sphincter and dilator pupillae
□ Taeniae of colon and caecum	□ Muscle of nictitating membrane
□ Muscle coats of the intestinal wall	□ Superior (Müller's) and inferior tarsal muscles
□ Muscle in the media of blood vessels	□ Costo-uterine muscle
□ Muscle of the urinary bladder	□ Expansor secundariorum
□ Muscle of the gallbladder	□ Suspensor of the duodenum
□ Myometrium	□ Anococcygeus, rectococcygeus
□ Muscle in cardiac valves	□ Tracheal muscle
□ Muscle in capsule of spleen, kidney, testis	□ Arrectores pilorum
□ Muscularis mucosae of the gut	□ Bronchial musculature
□ Muscle of the mesotubarium superius	□ Muscle of the amnion
	□ Myoepithelial cells
	□ Myofibroblasts

viscera the boundaries and orientations of muscle layers are less clear, and the musculature is an assembly of bundles rather than a discrete sheet. In the vas deferens, the two muscle layers are not always clearly separated: the bundles of muscle cells within each layer do not run circularly and longitudinally, but in concentric helices of very small (inner layer) and very large (outer layer) pitch. The diameter of the vas deferens increases from the epididymal end to the urethral end, and the muscle coat shows a parallel increase in thickness; the arrangement of the muscle bundles also becomes progressively less regular (1).

In blood vessels, the three-dimensional arrangement of muscle cells varies with the diameter of the vessel and the thickness of the wall (2). In large elastic arteries, the media consists of up to 60–70 concentric lamellar units, each made of a monolayer of muscle cells, separated by abundant elastic material. The predominant orientation of the muscle cells is cirumferential, but the arrangement is less uniform and less orderly than in the intestine, probably on account of the much larger amount of intercellular connective tissue in the media, onto which the mechanical activity of each muscle lamella or bundle is directly discharged. There is an even greater variability in the layout of the musculature in the media of muscular arteries. While the predominant orientation is circumferential, there are bundles running obliquely or spirally or helically, and occasionally there are also large bundles of longitudinal musculature. In arterioles, muscle cells usually form a single layer in the media and are wound circularly or in helices of small pitch; a single muscle cell can form many turns around the small lumen.

3. Cell types and extracellular materials

A smooth muscle is more than an assembly of muscle cells: it is in fact a *tissue*, and it is composed of several types of cell and of characteristic material in the extracellular space. The tissue is usually compact, and in a visceral muscle there can be as many as 190,000 muscle cells per gram of tissue. The cell density is dictated not only by the size of muscle cells but also by the extent of the extracellular space. The extracellular space can be measured by morphometry or by the use of impermeant tracers, but the results are often difficult to assess. In visceral muscles, the extracellular space usually represents 15%–30% of the tissue. In vascular muscles there is greater variation, since the extracellular space can occupy nearly two thirds of the volume of the media in large arteries, whereas in small muscular arteries the cells are as tightly packed as in a visceral muscle. So, for example in the rat, an extracellular space of 50% to 60% is found in the media of the aorta and one of 15% to 20% in the distal renal artery (3); a similar reduction of the amount of extracellular space from the ascending aorta to the muscular arteries is common to all species. In veins, there is in general a greater amount of extracellular material than in arteries (4); however, in the portal vein the muscle cells, which are arranged in an inner circular layer and an outer longitudinal layer, are as tightly packed as in a visceral muscle (5).

The extracellular (or intercellular) spaces are occupied by the so-called ground substance, of poorly known chemical composition, and by fibrillar material, mainly collagen and elastic fibers, which together constitute the stroma. The collagen content, determined by measuring the concentration of hydroxyproline in the tissue, varies from one muscle to another. In the guinea pig the collagen concentration in mg/g of wet tissue is about 32 in the taenia coli, 36 in the myometrium, and 78 in the aorta; by comparison, it is about 6 in the myocardium, 9 in skeletal muscles, and 197 in tendons (6). The collagen content of muscle is accounted for by the collagen fibrils and the basal laminae; the latter are as extensive as the cell surfaces and represent, therefore, a large component of the tissue. Some collagen fibrils and many microfibrils of 10 nm diameter run close to a basal lamina and probably provide mechanical links between muscle cells and stroma. Some microfibrils are identified as fibronectin, others are associated with elastic fibers. The elastic fibers are individual cylindrical cables of very variable size and indefinite length (Fig. 1-1); they usually branch extensively and can form continuous laminae or fenestrated sheets (7). The elastic material is composed, as in other tissues, of amorphous bands surrounded by microfibrils 11 nm in diameter (7, 8). Microfibrils are often interposed between elastic fibers and the surface of muscle cells (Fig. 1-2).

Most of the material in the extracellular space is probably synthesized by the muscle cells themselves, as shown by studies of freshly isolated muscle cells (9), muscle cells in culture (10), developing myometrium and aorta (11), and hypertrophic intestinal muscle cells (12). Smooth muscle cells are therefore endowed with the ability to synthesize both the intracellular contractile apparatus and part at least of the extracellular stroma.

A special situation is found in the rare smooth muscles that possess one or two insertion tendons. One such muscle is the anococcygeus muscle, well developed in the rat, a kind of sling that loops around the rectum and is inserted to the ventral surface of the coccyx. Prominent tendons are found in the gizzard (muscular stomach) of birds. The tendons are structurally similar to those of skeletal muscles, and at the myotendon junction the smooth muscle cells are anchored to the collagen fibrils through structural specializations that include tunnel-like invaginations of the cell membrane and an increased number of dense bands.

Other cell types found in smooth muscles are interstitial cells of Cajal, common within the musculature of the gut, and fibroblasts (Fig. 1-3). There are also endothelial cells of intramuscular blood vessels, usually capillaries, and mast cells; the frequency of the latter cell type varies between animal species, and they are usually common in the musculature of airways. Lastly, an important cell type found within smooth muscles is the nerve elements, axons of autonomic ganglion neurons and sensory ganglia, and their supporting Schwann cells.

4. Smooth muscle cells

Smooth muscle cells are minute in size; in the intestine of the guinea pig they measure about 3500 μm^3, and in other tissue, especially in blood vessels, they are even smaller. This volume correspond to that of a monocyte (a sphere of 19 μm diameter). The differences in muscle cell size between different animal species are relatively small. An exception is the muscle cells of the stomach of *Amphibia*, which can reach a volume of 30,000 μm^3 or more; the largest muscle cells are found in the stomach wall of *Amphiuma*, where they measure up to 12 μm in diameter and 1.5 mm in length (13). Finally, the volume of muscle cells not only changes during development, but is also altered with atrophy and hypertrophy in mature individuals.

By contrast, the cell surface (at 5000 μm^2 in the guinea pig intestine) is very extensive, and there is about 1.5 μm^2 of cell surface for every cubic micron of cell volume, a ratio that is the same as that found in human red blood cells (14). A high surface-to-volume ratio is characteristic of all smooth muscle cells. It has been calculated that one gram of taenia coli contains nearly 1 m^2 of cell membrane. The actual amount of cell membrane is greatly increased by the presence of caveolae.

Caveolae are flask-shaped invaginations of the cell membrane; their density ranges between 20 and 35 per μm^2 and they are confined to the domains of the cell membrane not occupied by dense bands. They measure about 70 nm across and 120 nm in length; their size and number are not changed when their muscle contracts or is stretched. The basal lamina does not penetrate into the caveolae but passes over their necks (the width of the narrowest part of the neck is about 35 nm) without change in appearance. The cavity

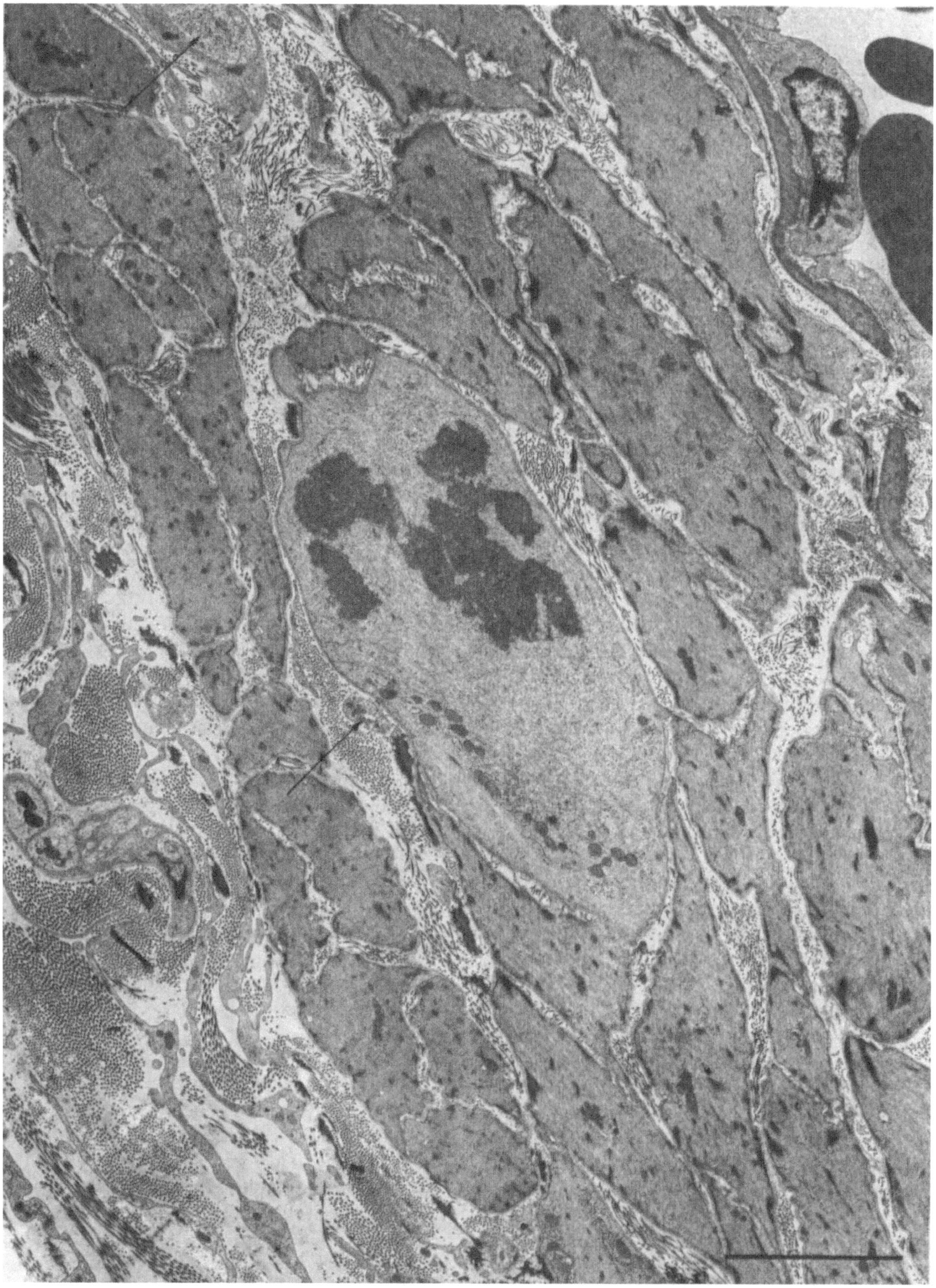

Figure 1-1. Section through a small mesenteric artery of an adult (about five-month-old) guinea pig. In the top right corner is the lumen with red blood cells, outlined by an endothelium lying over a prominent inner elastic lamella. The muscle cells of the media show many dense bodies and dense bands, and they are surrounded by collagen fibrils and elastic fibers. The muscle cell in the center is undergoing mitotic division, and shows chromosomes. In the bottom left corner is the adventitia, made of collagen and elastic fibers, fibroblast processes, and nerve bundles. Some nerve fibres (arrows) lie within the media. Calibration bar: 5 μm.

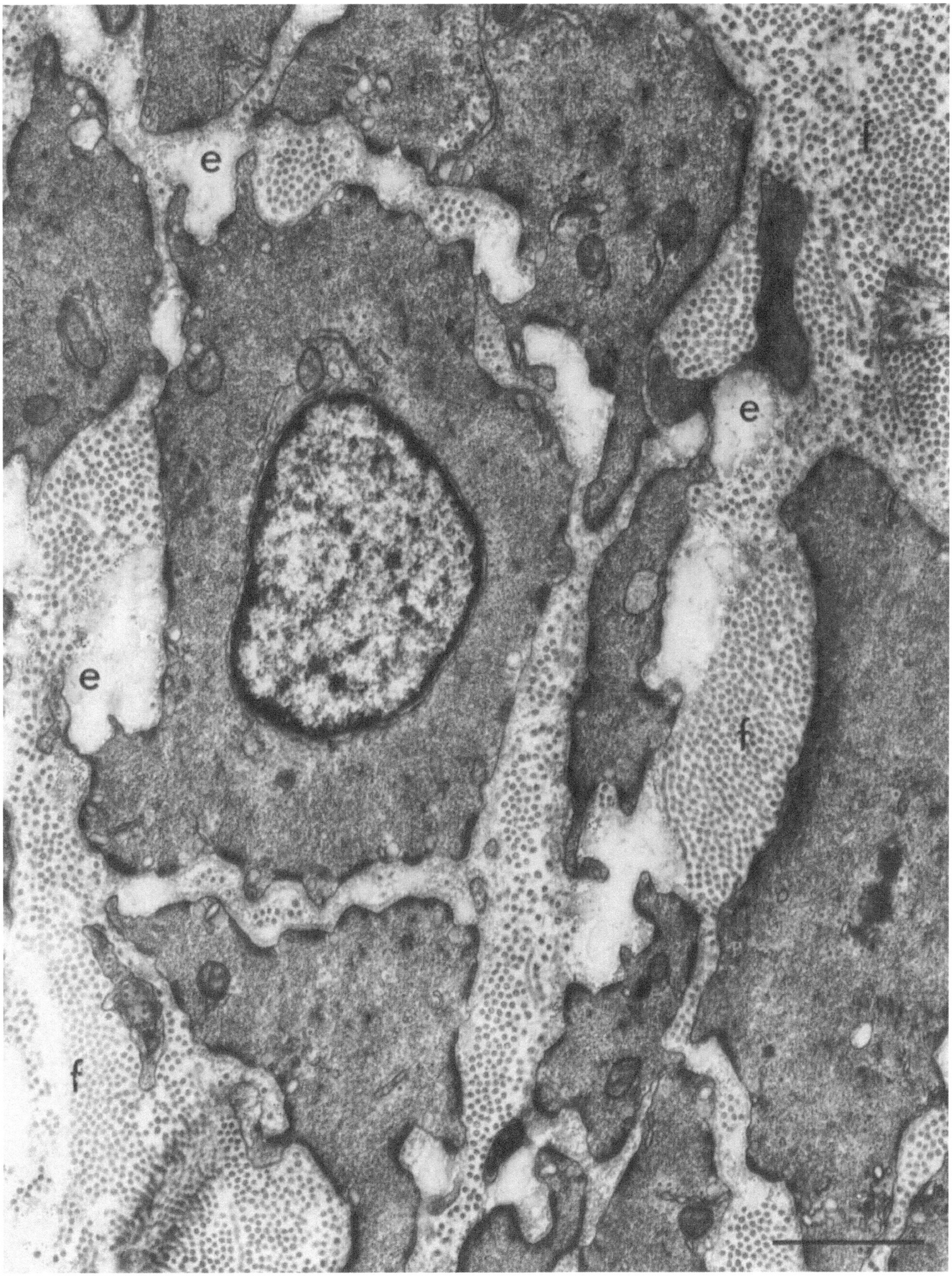

Figure 1-2. Transverse section of the taenia coli of a rabbit, showing several muscle cell profiles, one of which is nucleated. The print is slightly overexposed to bring out the material around the cell. Note the extent of the extracellular space and the large number of elastic fibers (e) and collagen fibrils (f). Most of the elastic fibers run close to the cell membrane of a muscle cell and at the point of contact there is probably a mechanical link between the two structures. Calibration bar: 1 μm.

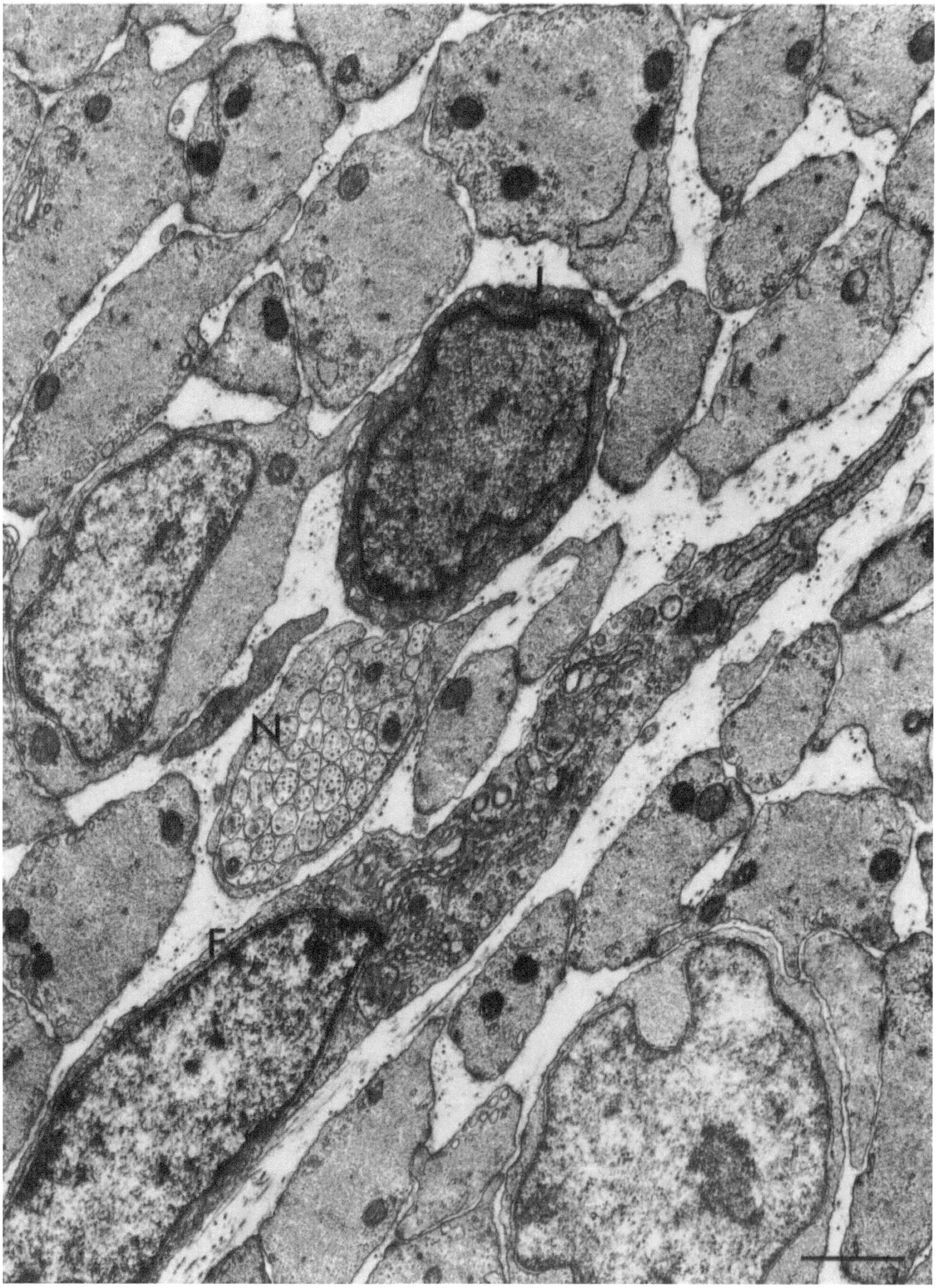
N
F

of a caveola is accessible to extracellular space tracers, but the caveolae are stable structures that are not rapidly internalized into cytoplasmic vesicles (unlike true micropinocytotic vesicles). Caveolae are also found in other cell types, such as endothelial cells, cardiac and skeletal fibers, and cells lining pulmonary alveoli — that is, in general, in cells that are exposed to frequent stretching. Their significance in any of these cell types is still a matter of conjecture. Those of smooth muscle cells are characterized not only by their linear distribution but also by the presence of a ring of intramembrane particles around the opening.

Between the rows of caveolae, the cell membrane is occupied by dense bands (or membrane-bound dense bodies) that receive attachment of the contractile apparatus (Fig. 1-4). The bands of electron-dense material are 30–40 nm thick (considerably more in some vascular muscle cells) and are penetrated at the inner surface by bundles of actin filaments, which probably terminate there, and by intermediate filaments; the outer aspect of the dense bands firmly adheres to the cell membrane. Half or more of the cell surface may be occupied by dense bands. Other strongly electrondense structures are found in the sarcoplasm and are the dense bodies, closely associated with the contractile apparatus.

Another feature of the cell membrane is the specialized cell junctions. Two types of junction are well recognized and are of well-established functional significance. The gap junction or nexus of smooth muscle is similar in structure to gap junctions of other tissues. A gap of 2–3 nm separates the apposed membranes. The junction itself is made of aggregates of connexons, each of which provides a hydrophilic channel directly connecting the cytoplasm of the two muscle cells and allowing exchange of ions and small molecules. Nexuses are common in some smooth muscles and rare or absent in others, and their distribution does not seem to correlate well with the occurrence of electrical coupling in various smooth muscles. Another type of junction is the intermediate junction (or attachment plaque), which consists of two dense bands matching each other in adjacent cells, with an intercelular gap of 40–60 nm occupied by a band of electron-dense material. These junctions, being connected with bundles of myofilaments in each of the two cells, provide mechanical coupling between muscle cells.

Among the cytoplasmic organelles, the sarcoplasmic reticulum is usually well represented in smooth muscle cells in the form of flat cisternae or small tubules sometimes arranged in a labyrinthine pattern. In visceral muscle cells the smooth reticulum predominates over the rough reticulum, and together they occupy about 2% of the cell volume. In some cells large cisternae of reticulum lie immediately beneath the cell membrane, separated by a gap of only about 10 nm, which is traversed by regularly spaced electron densities (15); this arrangement suggests the occurrence of *peripheral couplings* between cell membrane and reticulum, such as those observed in cardiac muscle (16). The granular and some of the smooth reticulum (the distinction between the two is not always clear-cut, since there are intermediate forms) are probably involved in synthetic processes (for example, those of membranes and extracellular materials). Granular reticulum is better developed in muscle cells of elastic arteries. Histochemical studies have shown that the smooth sarcoplasmic reticulum is the main site for calcium storage and release (17, 18, 19), and electron probe analysis on vascular muscle cells has directly localized calcium within the reticulum (20, 21). The influx of calcium through the cell membrane is the main source of calcium for activation of the contractile apparatus; however, a relatively modest source of calcium is also provided by an intracellular store, the reticulum. Other common organelles include mithochondria (4%–9%) and a small number of lysosomes, centrioles, and multivescicular bodies; microtubules are always present.

←

Figure 1-3. Section through the musculature of the gizzard of a 20-day-old chick embryo. The muscle cells are more differentiated than in Figure C; the cell profiles are more regular, and there are fewer mitochondria, less sarcoplasmic reticulum, and a greater amount of myofilaments. Dense bands and caveolae are more numerous, but still much less than in mature muscles. A nerve bundle (N), a fibroblast (F), and an interstitial cell (J) are clearly recognizable. Calibration bar: 1 μm.

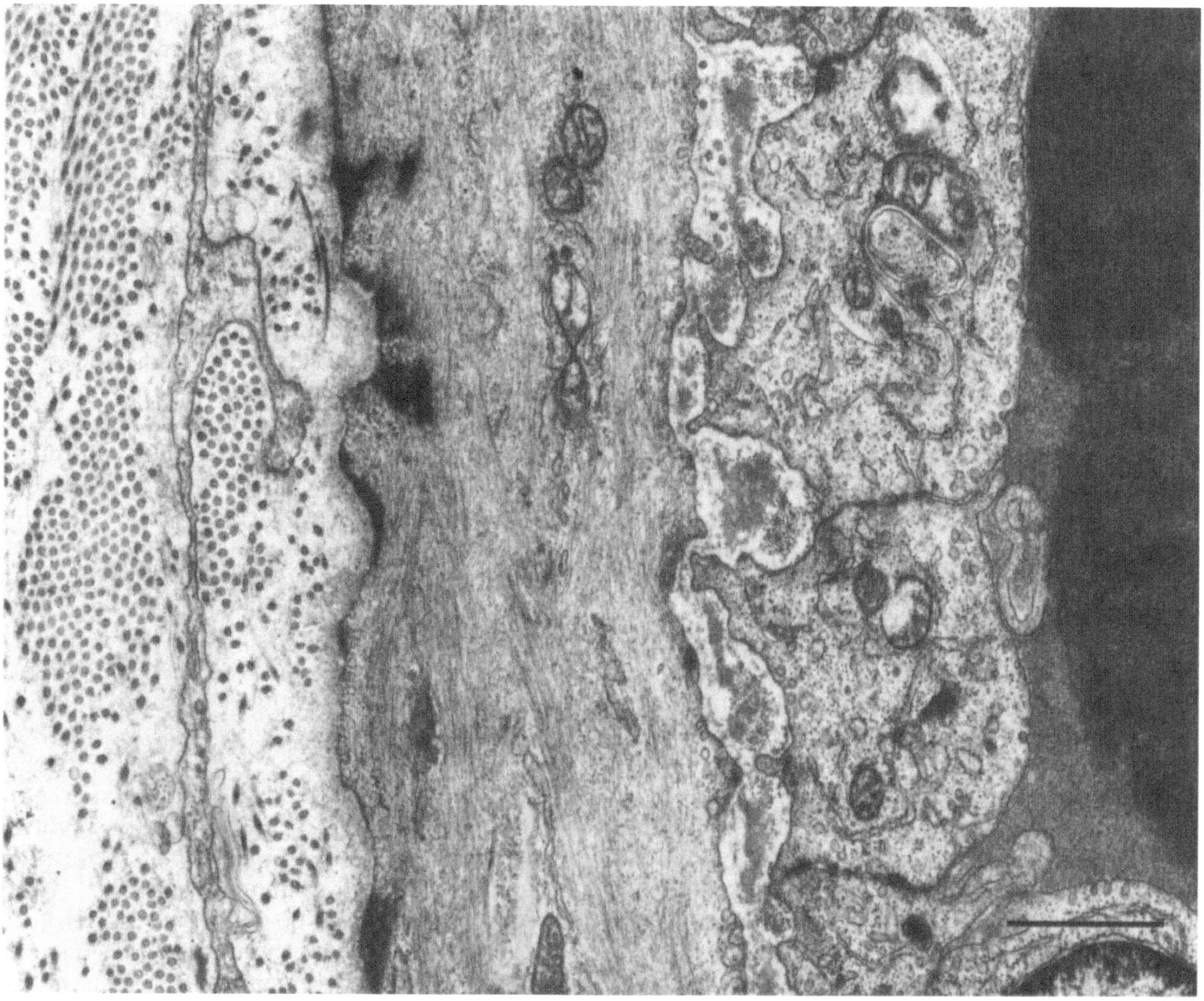

Figure 1-4. Transverse section of an arteriole in the wall of the colon of a pig. In the middle is a muscle cell in longitudinal section. To the right are red blood cells (in the lumen of the vessel) adjacent to a layer of endothelial cells (intima). To the left is the adventitia with many collagen fibrils and a fibroblast process. Between the endothelium and the muscle cells are elastic fibers and collagen, and processes from the two cell types project towards each other. The muscle cell displays mitochondria, sarcoplasmic reticulum, caveolae, dense bands, and myofilaments. Characteristically, the dense bands are more numerous and more extensive on the membrane at the abluminal side of the cell than on the lumenal side, an arrangement that is found when muscle cells are coiled around the lumen of a vessel of small caliber. Calibration bar: 1 μm.

4.1. Filaments

Three main types of filament are found in muscle cells (Fig. 1-5). Thin filaments measure 6–8 nm in diameter, are uniform in appearance in various preparations and different muscles, and are readily preserved for electron microscopy after glutaraldehyde fixation. The length of the individual filaments is not established; it differs in the models proposed by different authors from less than one micron to several microns (22, 23). Actin filaments, gathered in rosettes or in bundles, penetrate into dense bands and dense bodies (24, 25, 26). The thin filaments are formed by two coiled strands of actin molecules, and their chemical nature can be recognized by virtue of their specific binding to heavy meromyosin (decorated filaments). Actin is a 42,000 Dalton protein, and although there are several types of it, its structure in smooth muscles varies only mini-

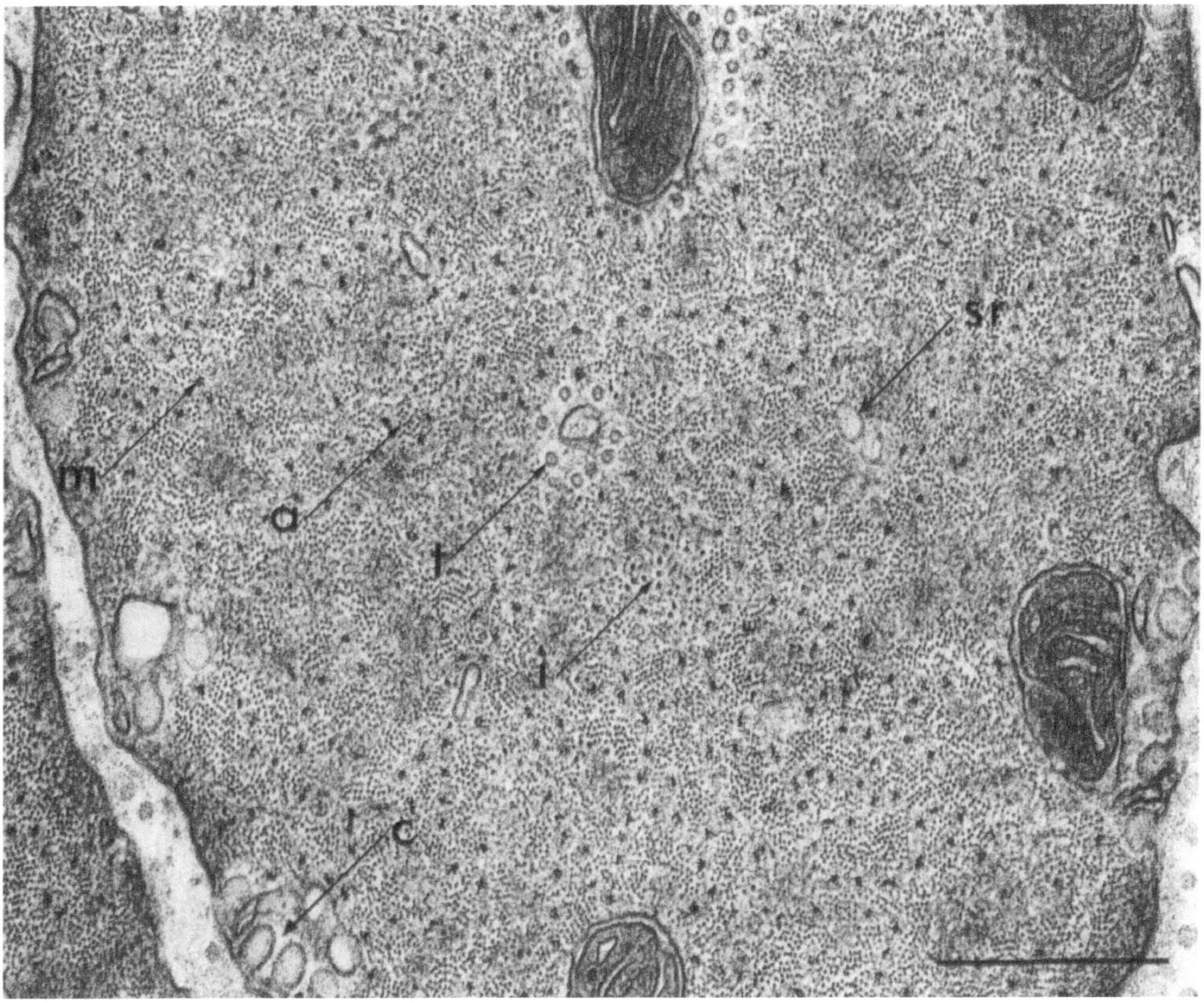

Figure 1-5. Muscle cell of the taenia coli of a guinea pig in transverse section. Mitochondria can be seen near the edges and a dense band at the lower right corner. a: actin filaments; c: caveolae; i: intermediate filaments; m: myosin filaments; sr: sarcoplasmic reticulum; t:microtubules. Calibration bar: 0.5 μm.

mally from that of other cell types or in different animal species (27). More than one type of it is present in any tissue. The full sequence of amino acid has been worked out for the predominant type of actin in the chicken gizzard and the bovine aorta (28).

Thick filaments (myosin) measure 14–16 nm in diameter. They are rather difficult to preserve for microscopy, and with some preparative procedures they aggregate side by side and give rise to ribbons. In vascular muscle cells, myosin filaments measure 2.2 μm in length (25). The myosin molecules, of about 470,000 molecular weight (MW), are similar in shape to those obtained from skeletal muscle (29), but the way they are assembled into filaments is substantially different and not completely clear. According to a well-known model, smooth muscle myosin filaments are made of bipolar building units, most likely antiparallel dimers (22, 30). On the basis of optical diffraction analysis, it has been proposed that such dimers are arranged in a six-stranded helix of 72 nm repeat. The absence of a central bare zone, the finding that the terminal portions of in vitro myosin filaments are devoid of projections (or cross-bridges), and the occurrence of a 14.4 nm continuous repeat are all accounted for by this model (22, 30). Differences between myosin from smooth and striated muscles include not only the way the myosin molecules are assembled into thick filaments but also their amino acid composition and type of light chains. There are also chemical differences between myosins from different smooth muscles or from different animal species.

Intermediate filaments measure 10 nm in diameter and are of indeterminate length. They have a sharp outline after positive staining and after negative staining (8, 31), and are formed by four filamentous subunits of 3.5 nm diameter (31). In most smooth muscle, intermediate filaments are of the desmin type, a 50,000 MW protein (32), and the chicken gizzard is the main source of desmin for immunofluorescence and biochemical studies. However, in intermediate filaments of vascular muscle cells, vimentin, a 52,000 MW protein (32), is often the predominant intermediate filament protein (33, 34). Intermediate filaments of the myoepithelial cells are of the keratin type (35).

5. Morphodynamics of smooth muscle

While the illustrations of smooth muscles found in this book provide perforce static views of tissues, cells, and organelles, smooth muscle is a very dynamic structure (36). In contraction the muscle shortens, it hardens, it flattens, and it elongates. A brief description of the morphology of contracting smooth muscles follows. In smooth as in all other types of muscle, two contrasting modes of contraction are the isometric type (development of tension and hardening without change in length) and the isotonic type (shortening and bulging out). The muscle in isometric contraction is able to generate an amount of force comparable to that produced by skeletal muscles that have a much higher myosin content (hence a larger number of potential cross-bridges) (37), whereas in isotonic conditions the muscle can shorten, in certain cases, to as little as one fifth of its resting length. Moreover, muscles can undergo passive changes in shape such as those imposed, for example, by active contraction of adjacent muscles. Some of these changes will be briefly described as passive contraction.

5.1. Structural apparatus for force generation

The generation of force, which leads to the development of tension and shortening, occurs by the interaction between actin and myosin filaments and is triggered by a rise in calcium concentration. An ad hoc version of the sliding-filament mechanism that has been proposed for skeletal muscle (38) is believed to be at work in smooth muscle too. Among its characteristic features is a myosin-linked calcium-regulatory system (27), a maximum rate of (unloaded) shortening of about 0.1 muscle lengths per second (39, 40), and probably the formation of attached, noncycling cross-bridges (latch bridges) that allow maintenance of force at low energy cost (41, 42). In all smooth muscles, the myosin content and the molar ratio of myosin to actin are low by comparison with those of striated muscles (27), whereas the amount of force generated per unit sectional area of muscle is comparable in the two tissues (43).

The spatial arrangement of the three types of filament in mucle cells is not yet understood, partly because the preservation of filaments, especially myosin, and their distribution are very sensitive to the preparative procedures currently used. Estimates of the ratio of actin filaments to myosin filaments (i.e., the ratio between the number of filament intersections in transversely sectioned cells) in visceral muscles are 8:1 to 15:1, a range of values that probably includes variability between different muscles. The weight ratio of actin to myosin in visceral muscle cells is about 2.0, while in vascular muscle cells it is 2.7–3.4, values much higher than those of skeletal muscle fibers (about 0.35) (44), clearly indicating that actin represents a relatively higher proportion of the contractile apparatus in smooth muscle than in skeletal muscle. Actin filaments are arranged either as rosettes around thick filaments or as bundles (or cables) with an orderly packing and a latticelike appearance. Bundles of actin filaments branch and merge, thus forming a network spreading along the length of the cell. Actin bundles penetrate into dense bodies and into both ends of dense bands, and the individual filaments show a distinct polarity: when decorated with S-1 myosin subfragments, the resulting arrowheads point away from the dense body or the dense band into which the filaments are inserted (45), and arrangement similar to that found in actin filaments inserted into the Z-lines in skeletal muscles or into the cell membrane in microvilli. Dense bodies and dense bands contain alpha-actinin, a 100,000 MW protein originally isolated from Z-bands of skeletal muscles, where it acts as a cross-linker and a spacer between actin filaments. Dense bands are distributed over the entire cell length, and occupy 50% or more of the cell surface. This suggests that the pull generated by the contractile apparatus is not transmitted from one end of the cell to the other, but rather is discharged over the entire cell surface.

The myofilaments run longitudinally and parallel to each other. According to some models of smooth muscle contraction, however, they form a small angle with the long axis of the cell (see 23). Serial section studies and immunofluorescence studies have suggested the occurrence of some compartmentalization of myofilaments into discrete contractile units that might be regarded as a kind of myofibril or a minisarcomere (22, 25).

Intermediate filaments run in more irregular directions than myofilaments. They are seen penetrating into some of the dense bands and lying along the dense bodies and encircling them, usually without penetrating into them (25, 26). Intermediate filaments are probably attached to the dense bodies and link dense bodies together and to the membrane-bound dense bands, thus forming a supporting framework or cytoskeleton inside a muscle cell. Microtubules are also common in smooth muscle cells, and they too probably have a cytoskeletal role.

The major components of the stroma are collagen fibrils, elastic fibers and lamellae, and the so-called ground substance. The high collagen content of smooth muscles supports the idea that their stroma serves a mechanical role in the transmission of force and could perhaps be regarded as constituting intracellular microtendons. The force generated by the contractile apparatus and distributed to the cell surface is then partly transmitted through cell-to-cell junctions to adjacent cells and partly brought to bear on the collagen fibrils surrounding an individual muscle cell and from these to progressively larger components of the stroma, such as intramuscular septa (and from these to supporting structures such as the submucosa of the intestine and the adventitia of blood vessels). The minute changes in shape of individual muscle cells or the minute tensions generated are transmitted and added to each other until they become a macroscopic event involving the entire wall of an organ.

5.2. *Isometric contraction*

In an isometric contraction, a smooth muscle virtually does not change in length. Within the muscle, however, this type of contraction is accompanied by structural changes, including small changes in length of the contracting cells to take up any slack present either in the contractile apparatus or in the stroma; however, the longitudinal displacement of the muscle components is very small compared with that occurring in isotonic contraction.

A distinctive ultrastructural feature of the isometrically contracted muscle is a checkered appearance of the muscle cell sectional surface; this is due to the presence in the muscle cell profiles of several sharply out-lined areas of the cytoplasm that are devoid of myofilaments and are therefore of lighter appearance in the electron microscope (Fig. 1-6). These areas lie mostly at the periphery of the cell, beneath the cell membrane, sometimes arranged in a regular array around the perimeter of the cell, and often causing small protrusions of the cell profile. Areas of similar appearance form a cone, tens of microns in length, at either side of the nucleus: these large conical domains of nonfilamentous cytoplasm are centrally placed in the proximity of the nucleus (as is the nucleus itself), but often become eccentric along their course and may reach the cell membrane. The nonfilamentous domains are sharply outlined and contain mitochondria, ribosomes, glycogenlike granules, cisternae of smooth and rough endoplasmic reticulum, Golgi apparatus, a few filaments, and many microtubules. The myofilaments, which occupy the rest of the cell, have a higher packing density than in the muscle cell at rest, and they appear perfectly longitudinally arranged. According to Gillis et al. (46), in the rat anococcygeus muscle the myofilament packing density is in-

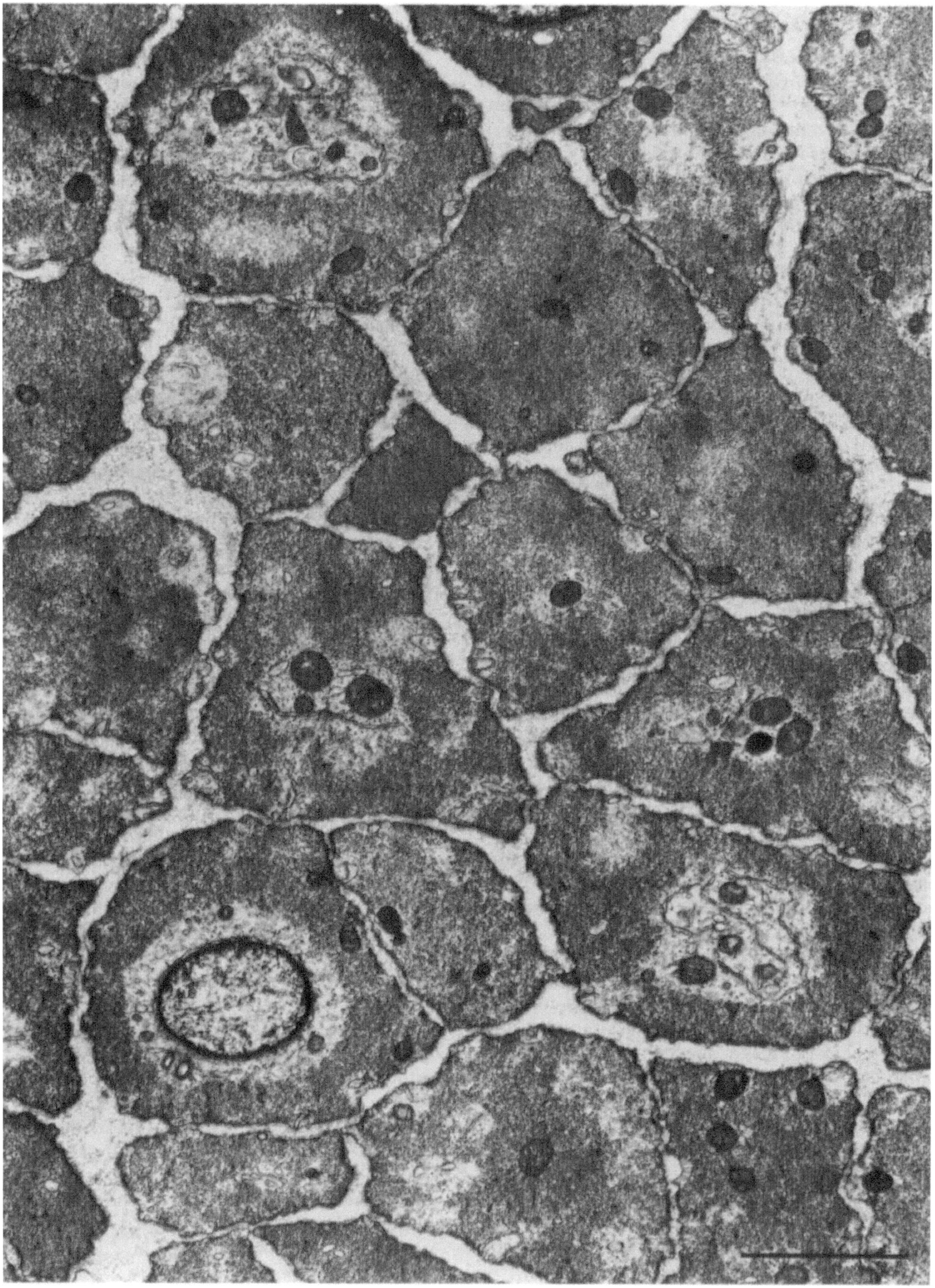

creased by a factor of two during isometric contraction, and in this preparation the contracted muscle cells are of a smaller volume than when at rest.

5.3. *Isotonic contraction*

Smooth muscles can contract very extensively. In certain conditions, their contracted length can be less than one fifth the resting length, and upon relaxation the muscle reverts to its original length. The extent of shortening is limited by structural constraints in the wall of the organ, such as the presence of adjacent layers of muscle or connective tissue, or the presence of incompressible materials, in the lumen of the organ for example, or in other parts of the wall. While it shortens, the muscle increases its lateral dimensions, its width and thickness, while its volume remains approximately the same, and the increase in cross-sectional area is about equal to the decrease in length. The same is true of the individual muscle cells undergoing isotonic contraction (43). The size of the muscle cell profiles is much increased; in the case of the taenia coli, one can count about 18,000 muscle cell profiles per square millimeter in a contracted muscle strip, as opposed to about 90,000 in a strip at rest. The long axis of the contracted muscle cells is no longer parallel to the length of the muscle but deviates appreciably from it, a change more apparent in muscles containing many intramuscular septa. Moreover, the cells are no longer straight and virtually parallel to one another (as they are in the muscle at rest) but rather are somewhat contorted; a torsion of their long axis gives them the shape of irregular and long-pitched helices (43). These changes in shape are in part imposed by the stroma and by the surrounding muscle cells; however, Warshaw et al. (47) have observed a corkscrewlike shortening of single isolated muscle cells, and have discussed this observation in terms of a possible helical arrangement of the cytoskeleton and of the contractile apparatus.

During isotonic contraction the cell surface is thrown into myriad projections that are mainly laminar and run at an angle to the cell length; the projections bear mainly caveolae, whereas the dense bands are mainly located in the regions of the membrane that have expanded least and appear therefore invaginated (Fig. 1-7). Other projections of the cell membrane in contracted cells, more irregular and less numerous, are bulbous and connected to the cell body through a short peduncle; they develop rapidly at the onset of the contraction and disappear slowly during relaxation. Similar projections are seen on a greater scale and cover the entire cell surface in single muscle cells contracting in isolation in a fluid medium (48).

While in the muscle at rest the collagen fibrils surrounding the muscle cells run about longitudinally, or at a small angle to the axis of the muscle cells, in the shortened muscle the fibrils are wound around the cells and run obliquely or almost transversely to their long axis (43). The experimental observations in visceral and vascular muscles support a theoretical model (49) according to which collagen provides a mechanism for binding cells together and for transmitting the tension generated by the myofilaments in directions up to 90° away from the direction of the myofilaments.

Similarly, in the intramuscular septa the collagen fibrils run obliquely to the length of the muscle; when the muscle shortens the septae also shorten, their depth increases, and the collagen fibrils increase the angle they form with the long axis of the muscle. In smooth muscles, because of the arrangement of collagen (and of cell junctions), a mechanical advantage is obtained by both the cell shortening and the cell flattening; indeed, given the tightly knit three-dimensional mesh of the muscle stroma, any change in muscle cell shape probably contributes to the mechanical performance of the tissue.

5.4. *Passive contraction*

Within a strip of muscle, especially when it is set up and stimulated in vitro, there are often some muscle cells that fail to be activated and are

←

Figure 1-6. Transverse section through the taenia coli of a guinea pig. The taenia was set up in an organ bath and stimulated with carbachol to contract isometrically. In each muscle cell profile, there are areas devoid of myofilaments and occupied by organelles or by amorphous material. The cell outlines are slightly more corrugated than in the cells fixed at rest. Calibration bar: 2 μm.

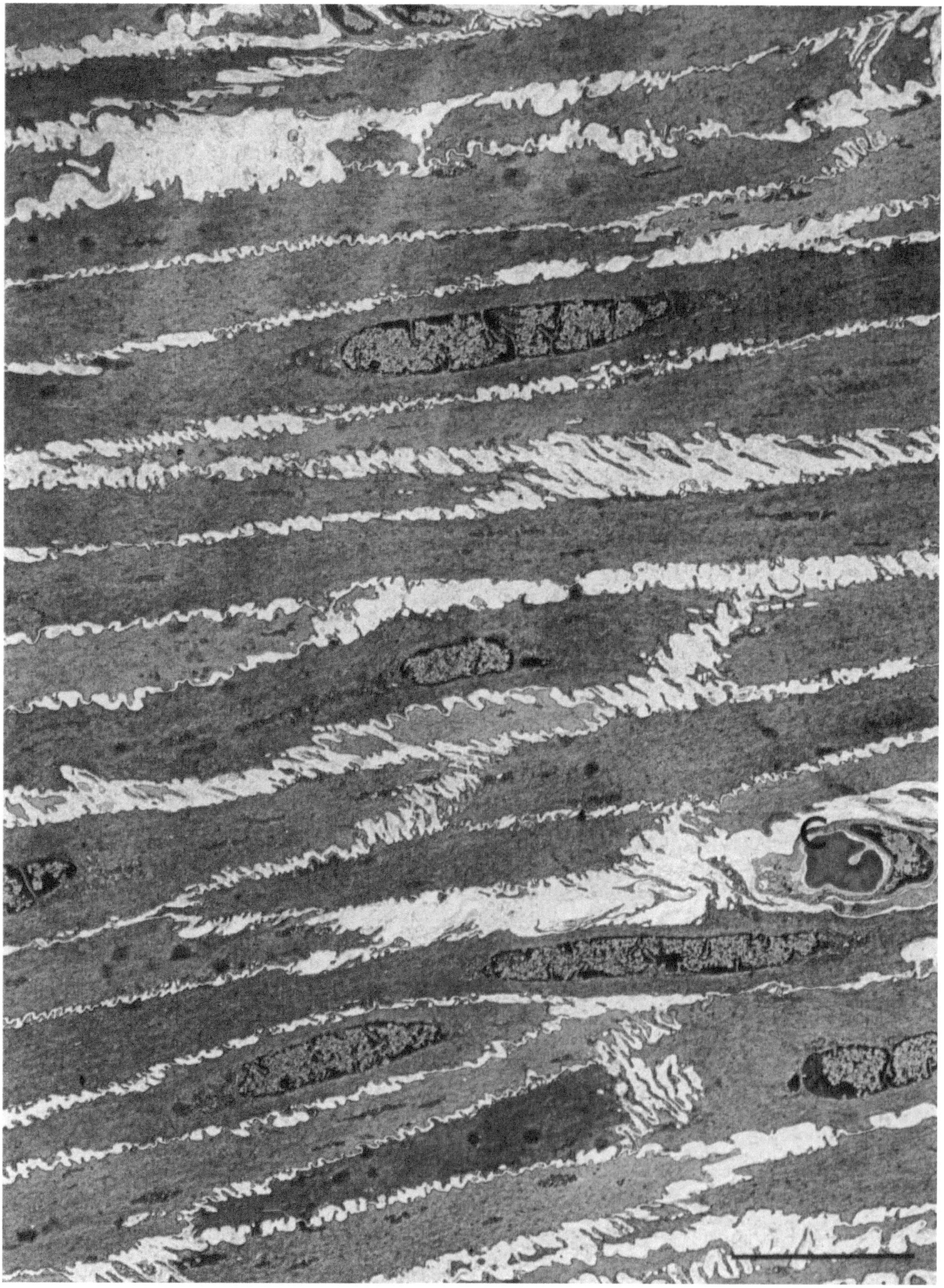

shortened passively by the action of the adjacent contracting cells. The passively contracted cells appear regularly coiled and their surface is devoid of evaginations (43). Cells have been found that are passively contracted over a portion of their length and actively contracted over the remaining part.

There are also passive changes in the shape of the muscle cells that occur by the effect of contraction in adjacent muscles. A contraction of the longitudinal muscle of the intestine shortens the gut and compresses sideways the muscle cells of the circular layer, which thus acquire an elliptical profile; when the circular muscle contracts in its turn, the shortening and flattening of the muscle cells produces a lateral expansion of the muscle so that the gut elongates and the longitudinal muscle cells grow thinner and longer.

The profile of muscle cells can change markedly depending on forces imposed by nearby tissues; the profiles can be approximately circular or very flat. The arrangement of the cytoskeleton and of the contractile material is such that these passive changes in shape are possible, are fully reversible, and do not seem to affect the ability of the cells to contract in their turn.

6. Other dynamic aspects

Other structural changes in smooth muscle occur on a longer time scale, and are usually directional and often irreversible — the changes that occur during development, with hypertrophy in adult subjects, and with aging.

6.1. Development of smooth muscles

Embryologically, the majority of smooth muscles derive from mesenchymal cells, and the mesenchyme derives from the mesoderm or — for example, in the head and neck and in parts of the heart — from the neural crest (50, 51). The muscle cells in the iris and the myoepithelial cells are of ectodermal origin. Growth and differentiation of visceral and vascular muscle cells have been studied extensively in tissue culture (52). However, the development that takes place in vitro does not invariably reproduce processes occurring during normal development in situ, especially because it is usually preceded by a more or less complete dedifferentiation of the transplanted cells.

In the primordium of a smooth muscle in situ, the cells divide repeatedly and are indistinguishable from fibroblasts. The cells then elongate, and actin filaments appear in the cytoplasm, accompanied by dense bodies (53, 54, 55, 56). Myosin filaments, caveolae, dense bands, and a basal lamina appear at a later stage. Characteristically, there are variations in the time of onset and rate of differentiation in different smooth muscles of the body. In the chick embryo, the musculature is more mature in the gizzard than in the small intestine, but less than in large blood vessels; the musculature of the amnion of the 11-day-old chick embryo is very similar to a mature muscle (57, 58), whereas the musculature of the ureter and vas deferens of the rat and mouse differentiate only after birth (54, 56). In the mammalian intestine, the circular musculature develops earlier than the longitudinal musculature (59, 60).

A muscle in which the embryological development has been studied in detail is the gizzard of the chicken (36, 55, 60, 61) (Fig. 1-8). By immunofluorescence, actin and myosin are detected in precursor cells on day 5 and day 7, respectively, and in each case the corresponding filaments are recognized by electron microscopy about two days later (55, 62, 63, 64). Spontaneous but not well-coordinated contractions are observed from the eighth day of incubation (65). At ten days the cells are still immature, but most of the distinctive features of muscle cells are already present; the muscle cells are clearly distinguishable from adjacent interstitial cells and from fibroblasts, and nerve bundles and capillaries begin to penetrate the muscle bundles. At this stage the muscle cells

←

Figure 1-7. Longitudinal section of the taenia coli of a guinea pig. The taenia was set up in an organ bath and stimulated with carbachol to contract isotonically under a load of one gram. Note that the cells do not run exactly parallel to each other and that their surface is thrown into many laminar folds that partly interdigitate. The nuclei show deep crenations. C is an intramuscular capillary. Calibration bar: 10 μm.

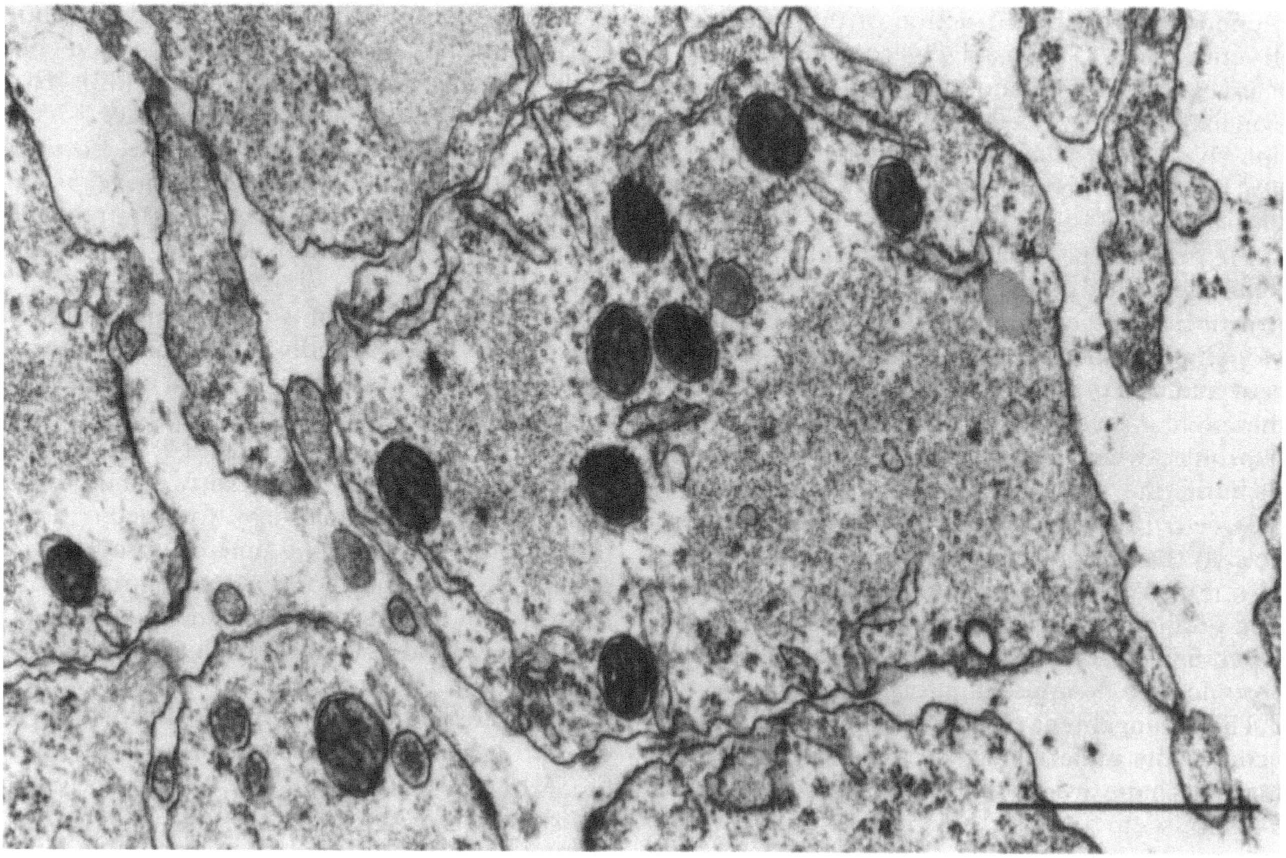

Figure 1-8. Section through the musculature of the gizzard of a 14-day-old chick embryo. At this embryonic stage, muscle cells are rich in mitochondria and sarcoplasmic reticulum and myofilaments occupy about half of the cell volume. The cell profile is irregular and the cell membrane has few caveolae and few dense bands. Collagen fibrils begin to appear in the intercellular space. Calibration bar: 1 μm.

contain bundles of myofilaments (actin filaments, myosin filaments, and dense bodies) loosely associated with one another and with intermediate filaments. Myofilaments occupy between 25% and 50% of the cell and are mainly found in its central portion. Only later in the embryonic development, when the number of myofilament bundles increases, do a vast number of dense bands appear; they provide extensive attachment of myofilaments to the cell membrane. This observation suggests that myofilament formation and alignment is not a process initiated or directed by the cell membrane, and that only late in development do the bundles of myofilaments become inserted over the full extent of the cell membrane. From the early stages of development, endoplasmic reticulum and mitochondria are well developed; mitochondria actually decrease slightly in spatial density during development. In contrast, caveolae and dense bands appear later, and so do gap junctions (66). The stroma is initially very scanty and it develops progressively, being in part at least produced by the muscle cells themselves.

In addition to an increase in muscle cell size (by about a factor of four in the chicken gizzard from the tenth day in ovo to adulthood), there is a vast increase in muscle cell number. The increase in cell number is not due to a late differentiation of immature cells, but occurs by mitosis of the existing muscle cells. Mitoses are found at all stages of muscle development, usually with a peak in late embryonic life (on the 17th to 19th day in ovo in the chick embryo gizzard); the dividing cells are not undifferentiated cells but are muscle cells with a high degree of differentiation. Characteristically, smooth muscle cells undergo mitotic division at a stage when they are already packed with myofilaments and connected by junctions to the neighoring cells. The process of division affects the middle portion of the cell, which takes up an ovoid shape and eventually divides. In contrast, the remaining portions of the cell do not differ in appearance from the surrounding muscle cells, in their organelles, filament content, and membrane specializations, including cell junctions.

Generally speaking, the growth and differentiation of muscle cells within a smooth muscle proceeds uniformly for the entire population of cells and there are no undifferentiated cells left behind in the tissue for later development (Fig. 1-3).

6.2. *Hypertrophy of smooth muscle*

Little is known about chemical turnover and cell replacement in smooth muscles of adult individuals, when the growth of the organ has come to a halt or has become almost insignificant. Muscle cells in mitotic division and muscle cells in degeneration can be found in adult visceral muscles, but only quite rarely (Fig. 1-1). The visceral musculature is therefore probably a rather stable tissue and the turnover of muscle cells must be extremely slow. However, a study of the muscle of the gizzard has shown a relatively high turnover of noncollagen protein (67). The synthesis rate of about 12% per day is considerably lower than that of most nonchicken muscle tissues (68), but it compares with rates of 14% for cardiac muscle and 17% and 7% in slow and fast skeletal muscle, respectively, of the same species (67). The collagen degradation in the intestine of the rat is extremely slow, even during development (69). A small amount of collagen is continuously being produced in smooth muscle, and one of the characteristic features of this tissue in aging subjects is an increase in the number of collagen fibrils running between the muscle cells.

The potential for growth is not exhausted in the mature musculature and can be manfested when increased functional demands are imposed upon an organ; these conditions occur naturally or experimentally, and when they are of a chronic nature they induce a hypertrophic response within the muscle. Among the best-known examples are the myometrium during pregnancy (70, 71), the ureter and bile duct when affected by calculi, blood vessels in certain forms of hypertension (72), and the urinary bladder when outflow is impaired, for example, as a consequence of motor denervation or prostatic enlargement (73, 74, 75, 76). A particularly extensive hypertrophy can be obtained in the urinary bladder (Figs. 1-9 and 1-10). In the intestine, hypertrophy occurs on the oral side of a partial obstruction, due for example to an intraluminal outgrowth or to an experimental stenosis. Accumulation of ingesta and consequent dilatation of the lumen and distension of the wall accompany the development of muscle hypertrophy. The muscle coat increases markedly in thickness, due both to an increase in muscle cell size and to an increase in muscle cell number (12). The mitoses are found in muscle cells which in all other respects are fully differentiated. Mitoses in mature muscle cells are also found in other hypertrophic visceral and vascular muscles and in smooth muscle in the vicinity of surgical cuts (77, 78). In the hypertrophic intestine, the enlarged muscle cells have permanent corrugations and invaginations of the cell surface, which provide additional sites for insertion of filaments and metabolic exchanges; nevertheless, as a consequence of the massive increase in cell volume, the surface-to-volume ratio is much lower in hypertrophic muscle cells than in controls. The number of mitochondria per cell increases but their volume density is markedly reduced. The hypertrophic muscle cell has a great deal more contractile material than the control muscle cell; intermediate filaments increase more than the myofilaments (12), and they come to occupy large areas of the cell (Fig. 1-11). In hypertrophic vascular muscle cells of the rabbit portal vein, intermediate filaments increase by more than three times as much as actin filaments (79). Myosin filaments increase much less (12) or not at all (79). The hypertrophic process involves synthesis of new extracellular material, probably by the muscle cells themselves, and formation of new intramuscular blood vessels. The intramuscular nerves become more widely dispersed and their arborization pattern is somewhat altered. In the hypertrophic intestine there is also a very extensive growth in size of the intramural nerve cells, but no change in their numbers.

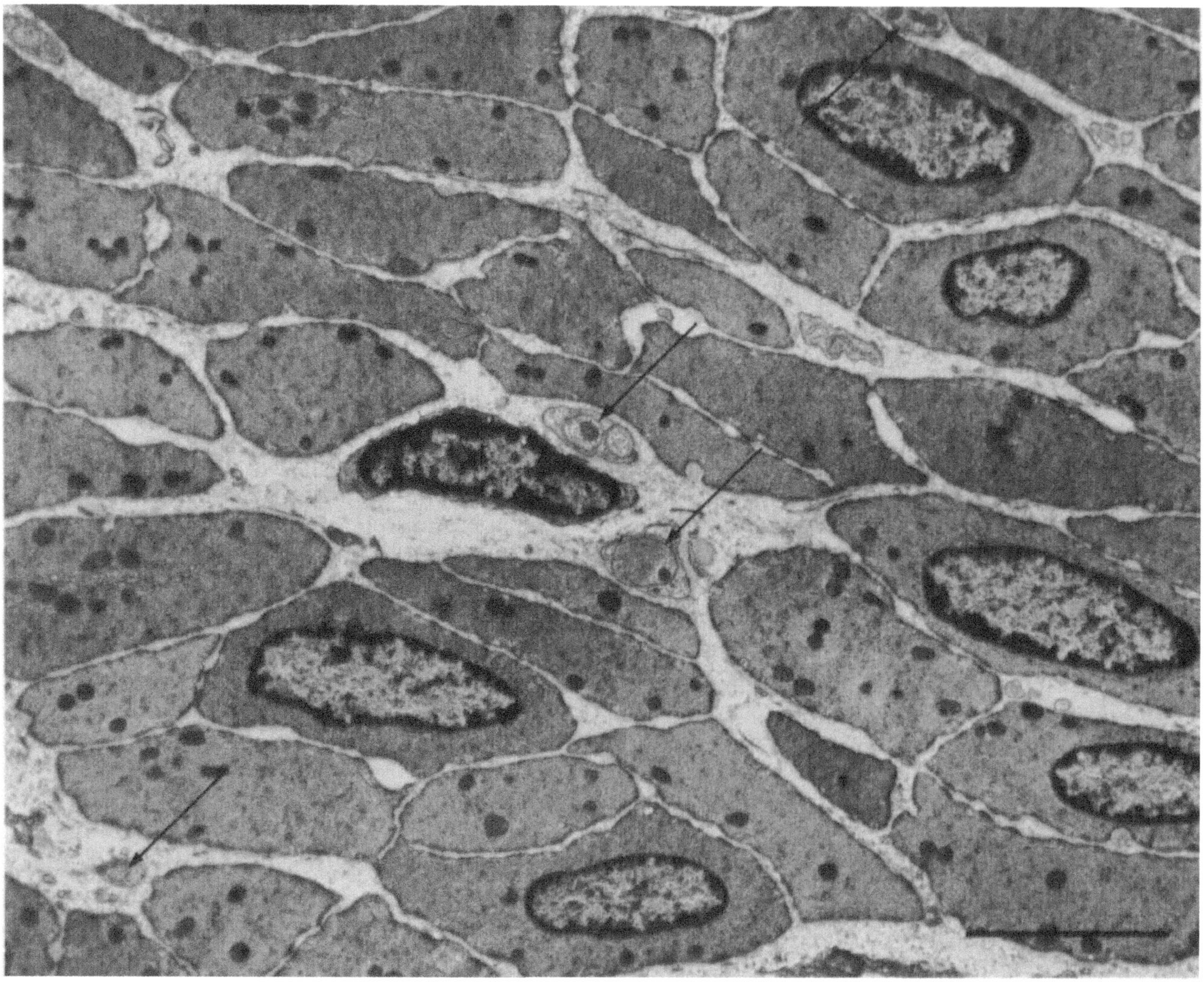

Figure 1-9. Section through the detrusor muscle of the urinary bladder of a rat. There are numerous single nerve fibers (arrows) or small bundles of fibers between the muscle cells. Calibration bar: 3 μm.

7. Conclusions

This brief survey of smooth muscle fine structure has stressed the complexity of smooth muscle morphology at various levels of structural organization — from the histology of the muscle layers and septa to the arrangement of the molecules of the contractile apparatus. There is a common structural plan in all smooth muscles, and from this plan arise the structual specializations and adaptations of the muscles of so many different organs. Each muscle thus has acquired a characteristic set of structural features through which its functional specialization is expressed. Smooth muscle is a highly dynamic tissue, both in the short term, when it contracts and relaxes, and in the long term, when it grows and develops and when it changes its structure in response to changed functional demands, such as when it atrophies or hypertrophies. It is, therefore, a difficult and challenging task to capture these dynamic aspects through static preparations of the tissue and through static micrographs. In spite of these difficulties, morphology is a most powerful tool for understandings how smooth muscle works.

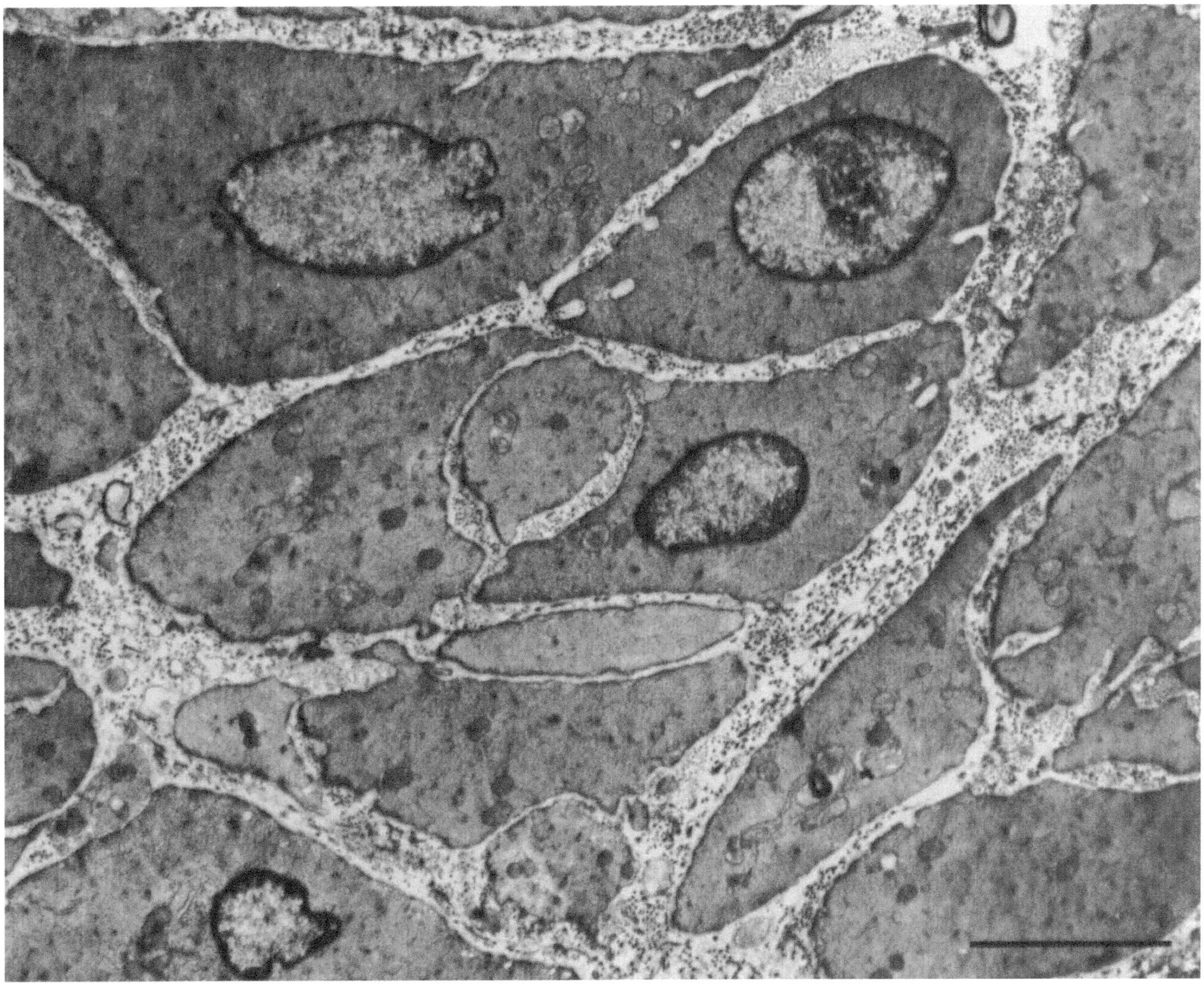

Figure 1–10. Section through the detrusor muscle of the urinary bladder in a rat with experimental bladder hypertrophy. Compare with Figure 1-1, which is at the same magnification, and note the large increase in cell size, the greater amount of intramuscular collagen, and the deep invaginations of the cell surface in some muscle cells. Nerve fibers can be seen. (From an unpublished investigation by Gabella and Uvelius.) Calibration bar: 3 μm.

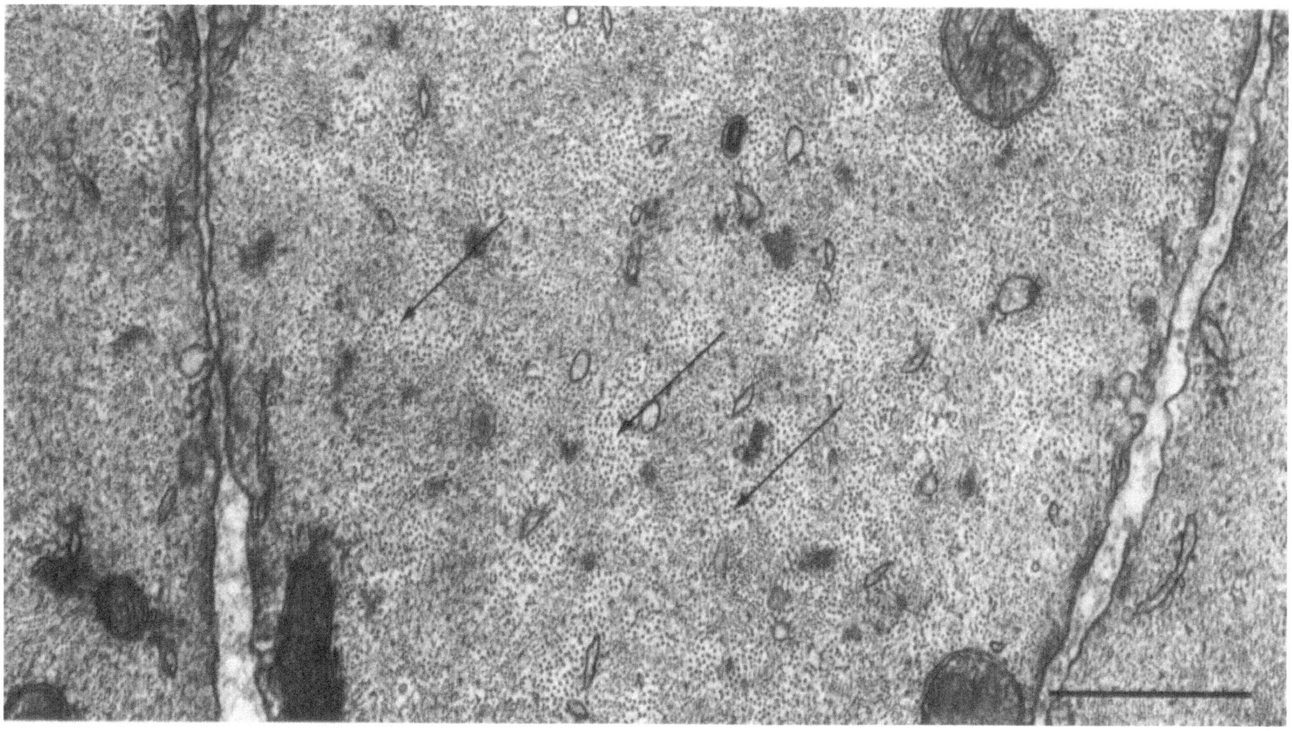

Figure 1-11. Transverse section of muscle cell of the circular layer of the rat ileum, in condition of hypertrophy on the oral side of an experimental stenosis. In addition to actin and myosin filaments, dense bodies, and mitochondria, note the numerous bundles of intermediate filaments (arrows) and the abundance of sarcoplasmic reticulum. Calibration bar: 0.5 μm.

References

1. Anton PG, Duncan ME, McGrath JC: An analysis of the anatomical basis for the mechanical response to motor nerve stimulation in the rat vas deferens. *J Physiol (Lond)* 273: 23–43, 1977.
2. Rhodin JA: Architecture of the vessel wall. In: Handbook of Physiology, Section 2, vol II. DF Bohr, AP Somlyo, HV Sparks Jr (eds), Bethesda, MD: American Physiological Society, p 1–31, 1980.
3. Osborne-Pellegrin MJ: Some ultrastructural characteristics of the renal artery and abdominal aorta in the rat. *J Anat (Lond)* 125: 641–652, 1978.
4. von Kügelgen A: Weitere Mitteilungen über den Wandbau der grossen Venen des Menschen unter besonderer Berücksichtigung ihrer Kollagenstrukturen. *Z Zellforsch Mikr Anat* 44: 121–174, 1956.
5. Ts'ao C-H, Glagov S, Kelsey BF: Structure of mammalian portal vein. Postnatal establishment of two mutually perpendicular medial muscle zones in the rat. *Anat Rec* 171: 457–470, 1971.
6. Gabella G: Structure of smooth muscle. In: Smooth Muscle, An Assessment of Current Knowledge. E Bülbring, AF Brading, AW Jones, T Tomita p 1–46, (eds) London: Edward Arnold, 1981.
7. Wolinsky H, Glagov S: Structural basis for the static mechanical properties of the aortic media. *Circ Res* 14: 400–413, 1964.
8. Somlyo AV: Ultrastructure of vascular smooth muscle. In: Handbook of Physiology. The Cardiovascular System. Vascular Smooth Muscle. DF Bohr, AP Somlyo, HV Sparks Jr (eds), Bethesda, MD: American Physiological Society, p 33–67, 1980.
9. Jones PA, Scott-Burden T, Gevers W: Glycoprotein, elastin, and collagen secretion by rat smooth muscle cells. *Proc Natl Acad Sci USA* 76: 353–357, 1979.
10. Ross R: The smooth muscle cell. II. Growth of smooth muscle in culture and formation of elastic fibers. *J Cell Biol* 50: 172–186, 1971.
11. Ross R, Klebanoff SJ: The smooth muscle cell. I. In vivo synthesis of connective tissue proteins. *J Cell Biol* 50: 159–171, 1971.
12. Gabella G: Muscle hypertrophy in the partially obstructed intestine. In: Hypertrophic Response in Smooth Muscle. CL Seidel, NW Weisbrodt (eds), Boca Raton, FL: CRC Press, p 45–76, 1987.
13. Heidlage JF Anderson NC Jr: Ultrastructure and morphometry of the stomach muscle in *Amphiuma tridactylum. Cell Tissue Res* 236: 393–397, 1984.
14. Linderkamp O, Meiselman HJ: Geometric, osmotic, and membrane mechanical properties of density-separated human red cells. *Blood* 59: 1121–1127, 1982.
15. Devine CE, Somlyo AV, Somlyo AP: Sarcoplasmic reticulum and excitation–contraction coupling in mammalian smooth muscles. *J Cell Biol* 52: 690–718, 1972.
16. Fawcett DW, McNutt NS: The ultrastructure of the cat myocardium. I. Ventricular papillary muscle. *J Cell Biol* 42: 1–45, 1969.

17. Jonas L, Zelch U: The subcellular calcium distribution in the smooth muscle cells of the pig coronary artery. *Exp Cell Res* 89: 352–358, 1974.
18. Popescu LM, Diculescu I: Calcium in smooth muscle sarcoplasmic reticulum in situ. *J Cell Biol* 67: 911–918, 1975.
19. Heumann HG: The subcellular localization of calcium in vertebrate smooth muscle: Calcium-containing and calcium-accumulating structures in muscle cells of mouse intestine. *Cell Tissue Res* 169: 221–231, 1976.
20. Somlyo AP, Somlyo AV, Devine CE, Peters PD, Hall TA: Electron microscopy and electron probe analysis of mitochondrial calcium accumulation in smooth muscle. *J Cell Biol* 61: 723–742, 1974.
21. Somlyo AP, Somlyo AV, Shuman H: Electron probe analysis of vascular smooth muscle. J Cell Biol 81: 316–335, 1979.
22. Small JV, Sobieszek A: The contractile apparatus of smooth muscle. *Int Rev Cytol* 64: 241–306, 1977.
23. Bagby RM: Organization of contractile/cytoskeletal elements. In: Biochemistry of Smooth Muscle. NL Stephens (ed), Boca Rato, Fl: CRC, p 1–84, 1983.
24. Pease DC, Molinari S: Electron microscopy of muscular arteries; pial vessels of the cat and monkey. *J Ultrastruct Res* 3: 447–468, 1960.
25. Ashton FT, Somlyo AV, Somlyo AV: The contractile apparatus of vascular smooth muscle: Intermediate high voltage stereo electron microscopy. *J Mol Biol* 98: 17–29, 1975.
26. Cooke P: A filamentous cytoskeleton in vertebrate smooth muscle fibers. *J Cell Biol* 68: 539–556, 1976.
27. Hartshorne DJ, Gorecka A: Biochemistry of the contractile proteins of smooth muscle. In: Handbook of Physiology. The Cardiovascular System. Vascular Smooth Muscle. DF Bohr, AP Somlyo, HV Sparks Jr (eds), Bethesda, MD: American Physiological Society, p 93–120, 1980.
28. Vandekerckhove J, Weber K: The complete amino acid sequence of actins from bovine aorta, bovine heart, bovine fast skeletal muscle, and rabbit slow skeletal muscle. *Differentiation* 14: 123–133, 1979.
29. Elliot A, Offer G, Burridge K: Electron microscopy of myosin molecules from muscle and non-muscle sources. *Proc R Soc Lond B* 193: 45–53, 1976.
30. Hinssen H, D'Haese J, Small JV, Sobieszek A: Mode of filament assembly of myosin from muscle and non-muscle cells. *J Ultrastruct Res* 64: 282–302, 1978.
31. Small JV, Sobieszek A: Studies on the function and composition of the 10 nm (100 A) filaments of vertebrate smooth muscle. *J Cell Sci* 23: 243–268, 1977.
32. Lazarides E: Intermediate filaments: A chemically heterogeneous, developmentally regulated class of proteins. *Annu Rev Biochem* 51: 219–250, 1982.
33. Gabbiani G, Schmid E, Winter S, Chaponnier C, De-Chastonay C, Vandekerckhove J, Weber K, Franke WW: Vascular smooth muscle cells differ from other smooth muscle cells: predominance of vimentin filaments and a specific alpha-type actin. *Proc Nat Acad Sci USA* 78: 298–302, 1981.
34. Frank ED, Warren L: Aortic smooth muscle cells contain vimentin instead of desmin. *Proc Natl Acad Sci USA* 78: 3020–3024, 1981.
35. Franke WW, Schmid E, Freudenstein C, Appelhaus B, Osborn M, Weber K, Keenan TW: Intermediate-sized filaments of the prekeratin type in myoepithelial cells. *J Cell Biol* 84: 633–654, 1980.
36. Gabella G: Dynamic aspects of the morphology of the intestinal muscle coat. In: Cellular Physiology and Clinical Studies of Gastrointestinal Smooth Muscle. JH Szurszewki (ed), Amsterdam: Elsevier, p 5–31, 1987.
37. Murphy RA, Driska SP, Cohen DM: Variations in actin to myosin ratios and cellular force generation in vertebrate smooth muscles. In: Excitation–Contraction Coupling in Smooth Muscle. R Casteels, T Godfrains, JC Rüegg (ed), Amsterdam: Elseviers/North Holland, p 417–424, 1977.
38. Huxley AF: Review lecture. Muscular contraction. *J Physiol (Lond)* 243: 1–43, 1974.
39. Johansson B: Mechanics of vascular smooth muscle contraction. *Experientia* 31: 1377–1386, 1975.
40. Dobrin PB: Mechanical properties of arteries. *Physiol Rev* 58: 397–460, 1978.
41. Siegman MJ, Butler TM, Mooers SU, Dvies RE: Calcium-dependent resistance to stretch and stress relaxation in resting smooth muscle. *Am J Physiol* 231: 1501–1508, 1976.
42. Dillon PF, Aksoy MO, Driska SP, Murphy RA: Myosin phosphorylation and the cross-bridge cycle in arterial smooth muscle. *Science* 211: 495–497, 1981.
43. Gabella G: Structural apparatus for force transmission in smooth muscles. *Physiol Rev* 64: 455–477, 1984.
44. Murphy RA, Driska SP, Cohen DM: Variation in actin to myosin ratios and cellular force generation in vertebrate smooth muscles. In: Excitation–Contraction Coupling in Smooth Muscle. R Casteels, T Godfraind, C Rüegg (eds), Amsterdam: Elsevier/North Holland, p 417–424, 1977.
45. Bond M, Somlyo AV: Dense bodies and actin polarity in vertebrate smooth muscle. *J Cell Biol* 95: 403–413, 1982.
46. Gillis JM, Cao ML, Godfraind-De Becker A: Density of myosin filaments in the rat anococcygeus muscle, at rest and in contraction. II. *J Muscle Res Cell Motil* 9: 18–28, 1988.
47. Warshaw DM, McBride WJ, Work SS: Corkscrew-like shortening in single smooth muscle cells. *Science* 236: 1457–1459, 1987.
48. Fay FS, Delise CM: Contraction of isolated smooth-muscle cells — structural changes. *Proc Natl Acad Sci USA* 70: 641–645, 1973.
49. Mullins GL, Guntheroth WG: A collagen net hypothesis for force transference of smooth muscle. *Nature (Lond)* 206: 592–594, 1965.
50. Le Lièvre CS, Le Douarin NM: Mesenchyme derivatives of the neural crest: Analysis of chimeric quail and chick embryos. *J Embryol Exp Morphol* 34: 125–154, 1975.
51. Kirby ML, Gale TF, Stewart DE: Neural crest cells contribute to aorticopulmonary septation. *Science* 220: 1059–1061, 1983.
52. Chamley-Campbell J, Campbell GR, Ross R: The smooth muscle cell in culture. *Physiol Rev* 59: 1–61, 1979.
53. Yamamoto I: An electron microscope study on development of uterine smooth muscle. *J Electron Microsc* 10:

145–160, 1961.
54. Leeson TS, Leeson GR: The rat ureter. Fine structural changes during its development. *Acta Anat* 62: 60–79, 1965.
55. Bennett T, Cobb JLS: Studies on the avian gizzard: the development of the gizzard and its innervation. *Z Zellforsch* 98: 599–621, 1969.
56. Yamauchi A, Burnstock G: Post-natal development of smooth muscle cells in the mouse vas deferens. A fine structural study. *J Anat* 104: 1–15, 1969.
57. Pierce ME: The amnion of the chick as an independent effector. *J Exp Zool* 65: 443–473, 1933.
58. Evans DHL, Evans EM: The membrane relationships of smooth muscles: an electron microscope study. *J Anat (Lond)* 98: 37–46, 1964.
59. Gershon MD, Sherman P, Gintzler AR: An ultrastructural analysis of the developing enteric nervous system of the guinea-pig small intestine. *J Neurocytol* 10: 271–296, 1981.
60. Bailey CG, Bagby RM, Kreyling MC: Morphogensis of the contractile system in embryonic chick gizzard smooth muscle cells. (Abstr.) J Cell Biol 99: 29a, 1984.
61. Gabella G: Development of smooth muscle: an ultrastructural study of the gizzard of the chick embryo. In Anat Embryol 180: 213–226, 1989.
62. Hirai S, Hirabayashi T: Developmental changes of protein constituents in chicken gizzards. *Dev Biol* 97: 483–493, 1983.
63. Hirai S, Hirabayashi T: Development of myofibrils in the gizzard of chicken embryos. Intracellular distribution of structural proteins and development of contractility. *Cell Tissue Res* 243: 487–493, 1986.
64. Stuewer D, Gröschel-Stewart U: Expression of immunoreactive myosin and myoglobin in the developing chicken gizzard. *Roux's Arch Dev Biol* 194: 417–424, 1985.
65. Donahoe JR, Bowen JM: Analysis of the spontaneous motility of the avian embryonic gizzard. *Am J Vet Res* 33: 1835–1848, 1972.
66. La Mantia J, Shafiq SA: Developmental changes in the plasma membrane of gizzard smooth muscle of the chicken. A freeze-fracture study. *J Anat (Lond)* 134: 243–353, 1982.
67. Laurent GJ, Sparrow MP, Bates PC, Millard DJ: Turnover of muscle protein in the fowl (Gallus domesticus). *Biochem J* 176: 393–405, 1978.
68. Waterlow JC: Protein turnover with special reference to man. *QJ Exp Physiol* 69: 409–438, 1984.
69. Klein L, ChandraRajan J: Collagen degradation in rat skin but not in intestine during rapid growth: effect on collagen types I and III from skin. *Proc Natl Acad Sci USA* 74: 1436–1439, 1977.
70. Dessouky DA: Ultrastructural observations of the human uterine smooth muscle cells during gestation. *Am J Obstet Gynecol* 125: 1099–1107, 1976.
71. Dessouky DA: Electron microscopic studies of the myometrium of the guinea-pig. The smooth muscle cell of the myometrium before and during pregnancy. *Am J Obstet Gynecol* 100: 30–41, 1968.
72. Wiener J, Loud AV, Giacomelli F, Anversa P: Morphometric analysis of hypertension-induced hypertrophy of rat thoracic aorta. *Am J Pathol* 88: 619–634, 1977.
73. Carpenter FG: Histological changes in parasympathetically denervated feline bladder. *Am J Physiol* 166: 692–698, 1951.
74. Peterson CM, Goss RJ, Atryzek V: Hypertrophy of the rat urinary bladder following reduction of its functional volume. *J Exp Zool* 187: 121–126, 1973.
75. Goss RJ, Liang MD, Weisholtz SJ, Peltzer TJ: The physiological basis of urinary bladder hypertrophy. *Proc Soc Exp Biol Med* 142: 1332–1335, 1973.
76. Brent L, Stephens FD: The response of smooth muscle cells in the rabbit urinary bladder to outflow obstruction. *Invest Urol* 12: 494–502, 1975.
77. Jurukova Z, Atanassova E: Smooth muscle cell regeneration in repair of gastric anastomosis in the dog. *Res Exp Med* 162: 299–312, 1974.
78. McGeachie J: Smooth muscle regeneration: a review and experimental study. *Monogr Dev Biol* vol. 9.
79. Berner PF, Somlyo AV, Somlyo AP: Hypertrophy-induced increase of intermediate filaments in vascular smooth muscle. *J Cell Biol* 88: 96–101, 1981.

Author's address:
Prof. Giorgio Gabella
Department of Anatomy and Developmental Biology
University College London
Gower Street
London WC1E 6BT
England

CHAPTER 2

Ultrastructure, cytochemistry, and organization of myofilaments in vertebrate smooth muscle cells

ROLAND M. BAGBY

1. Introduction

1.1. Problems with paradigms

"For now we see through a glass darkly ... " (80).

This familiar quotation from the apostle Paul's letter to the Corinthians was used to describe man's present poor knowledge of spiritual things in contrast to some future time when all truth will be revealed. It could also be used to describe our present poor understanding of the organization of the myofilaments within vertebrate smooth muscle cells. The quotation seems particularly descriptive to an author who has spent hours in a dimly lit room peering through heavily leaded glass at the faintly glowing fluorescent screen of an electron microscope, hoping to see an image which would reveal how the myofilaments of smooth muscle cells are organized to produce force and/or shortening appropriate to their function. But the glass within these microscopes is far clearer than another "glass" through which we peer just as hopefully. This "glass" is the paradigm that influences us to see only what we expect to see. The ultrastructure of the myofilaments and their organization into sarcomeres and myofibrils in vertebrate striated muscles constitute a paradigm that has had a great influence on the direction of research into smooth muscle cell organization. We have often used striated muscle as the standard to which we expected smooth muscles to conform. This misuse of a paradigm has led to some inappropriate techniques being applied and to disappointments when the expected structural organization did not emerge clearly. Truly, we now see through a paradigm darkly.

It is time to realize that there are structural features of smooth muscles that are quite unlike those in striated muscles and that new techniques better suited to their peculiarities must be applied if we are to understand how smooth muscles are organized. For example, in the striated vertebrate skeletal muscles, where the contractile units are mostly parallel to the axis of gigantic fibers, it is quite simple to see entire contractile units in an ultrathin section. In smooth muscle tissue, where not all cell axes are parallel (35, 122) and where the contractile units within cells are often not parallel to each other and may follow a nonplanar path (4–7, 20, 26–28, 30, 31, 38, 62, 94–97, 100, 109), it is almost impossible to obtain ultrathin sections that contain an entire contractile unit. Thick sections give a better statistical probability of viewing entire contractile units or even entire filaments (2), but the correct sectioning plane is difficult to predict even so. An assumption of the vertebrate skeletal muscle paradigm has been that thick filaments and thin filaments in smooth muscles have the same biochemical makeup as in vertebrate striated muscles. Although many biochemical and immunochemical differences between the striated muscles and smooth muscle myosins and actins have been recognized (9, 21, 22, 46–48, 54, 74, 75, 97, 100, 101) and the biochemical reactions controlling contraction have been shown to be different (1, 61, 77, 84, 101,

103), it has taken a long time for immunocytochemical techniques to be applied to vertebrate smooth muscle ultrastructure to identify the protein makeup of the structural components of the contractile system. These relatively new immunocytochemical findings, which are considered extensively in this chapter (Section 3), should finally convince us to abandon the vertebrate skeletal muscle paradigm as a general model for all muscles (including smooth muscles) and restrict its use to comparisons and contrasts with other muscle types.

There is another emerging paradigm being applied to smooth muscle whose use can also lead to a distorted view of smooth muscle cell organization. This is the paradigm of the cultured nonmuscle cell. Immunochemically, the contractile proteins of smooth muscle cells often have more in common with nonmuscle cells than with skeletal muscles (46, 49). Indeed, since chicken gizzard provides the purest, most easily obtainable source of large amounts of smooth muscle proteins, it has been used repeatedly as a source for purified proteins used as antigens for inducing antibodies that cross-react with both smooth muscle and nonmuscle cells in many cases (15, 29, 42, 43, 89, 127), but often not with striated muscle cells (46, 48, 75). Since immunocytochemical localizations are most easily performed with thin monolayers of cultured cells, the cultured cell has been the subject of most immunocytochemical studies. The cultured nonmuscle cell has stress fibers that contain many of the same kinds of proteins seen in the myofibrils of striated muscles (14–16, 29, 32, 44, 47, 60, 64, 68, 88, 89, 93, 124, 127). These stress fibers often display "striations" similar in some respects to the striations in skeletal muscle myofibrils (15, 29, 44, 64, 68, 88, 89, 127). Cultured smooth muscle cells may show an overall structural organization similar to cultured nonmuscle cells, but we must always keep in mind that *in situ* spindle-shaped smooth muscle cells can undergo large changes in length and have a length-influenced ability to produce force (7, 19, 77) that the cultured muscle cell and the in situ nonmuscle cell cannot mimic. Therefore, although smooth muscle cells are immunochemically similar to nonmuscle cells, the organization of smooth muscle cell contractile proteins within *in situ* cells cannot be based on what is seen in flattened monolayers of cultured cells, even cultured smooth muscle cells.

A final paradigm whose use should be restricted is the one imposed by the loose classification *smooth muscle*. In some classifications of muscle, all muscles whose cells are without obvious cross-striations are termed smooth muscles whether they are found in vertebrates or invertebrates. Apart from the absurdity of the implied logic that muscles that are different from cross-striated muscle in one respect are similar to each other in every other respect, there is plenty of evidence to show there is great diversity among the muscles not classified as cross-striated (83), including the obliquely striated muscles in several phyla (69, 86) and the paramyosin muscles of molluscs (104).

1.2. Phylogenetic boundaries of this chapter

It is somewhat presumptuous to expect that all vertebrate smooth muscles have the same organization, but there are many more similarities between individual vertebrate smooth muscles than between vertebrate smooth muscles and invertebrate nonstriated muscles, as one might have expected from the much closer phylogenic relationships among the vertebrates. Should phylogenetic relationships be accepted as a major factor for classifying the structural organizations of nonstriated muscles? Based on the relative structural homogeneity among vertebrate smooth muscles investigated thus far (for reviews, see 4, 5, 18, 36, 37, 38, 100, 106) and a striking similarity between the organization of vertebrate smooth muscles and that in nonstriated muscles of the ascidians (114, 115), a protochordate group that is more closely related to the vertebrates than most other invertebrate groups, it appears that the phylogenetic argument for classification of nonstriated muscles has great validity and provides the justification for further comparative studies of protochordate muscle organization. In the meantime, the classification *vertebrate smooth muscle* seems to be justified and will serve as the boundary for this chapter.

1.3. Aim of this chapter

The aim of this chapter is to look as objectively as possible at the relevant data from vertebrate smooth muscles while realizing that much of it was gathered by investigators, including this author, who were influenced by one or more paradigms. By looking at the data, if not with new eyes then at least through new glasses, the hope is that models of organization for the contractile machinery will emerge that provide better explanations of how structure relates to function in vertebrate smooth muscles.

1.4. Chapter organization

The first task will be to identify the contractile components of smooth muscle. Although ultrastructural characteristics alone have usually been used to distinguish contractile from cytoskeletal components, this approach operates under the assumption that the striated muscle paradigm is entirely valid for smooth muscles, an assumption that should not be made. Another way of distinguishing contractile components is by their biochemical makeup. This assumes that a particular protein has the same function regardless of the cell in which it is found. This assumption has been found to be reasonably accurate, and with the advent of immunocytochemistry and other types of protein-specific cytochemistry being applied to ultrastructural studies, it provides an additional criterion for determining the function of an ultrastructural entity. Because the ultrastructural evidence was gathered first, it will be considered first, but final identification of a component as contractile or cytoskeletal will be based on cytochemical as well as ultrastructural data.

The ultimate aim of any cellular organization study is to show the whole cell and how different regions of the cell have different distributions of the structural/cytochemical components. The whole-cell approach, utilizing isolated smooth muscle cells to study the cellular distribution and organization of the contractile proteins (3–7, 9, 10, 20, 26–28, 30, 31, 62, 95–98, 100, 126), has contributed greatly to our present understanding of the smooth muscle contractile system (for reviews considering isolated smooth muscle cells and their impact on concepts of organization, see 4, 5, 26, 100). The conclusions drawn from whole-cell studies, many of which utilized immunocytochemistry, were often at odds with conclusions drawn from thin sections, making those who studied the ultrastructure of smooth muscles with thin sections feel veguely uncomfortable. Immunocytochemistry has only recently been applied to ultrathin sections of smooth muscle viewed both with the light and electron microscopes. It is hoped that these studies, which bridge the gap between whole cells and thin sections, will be able to reconcile former apparent discrepancies. Some aspects of organization are still best seen in whole cells, however, and the reader is asked to have patience with the few low-resolution studies presented in this chapter for that purpose.

Finally, the effects of relative length changes and state of contraction on ultrastructure will also be considered as important indicators of organization of the contractile system and its mechanical relationship to the cytoskeleton.

2. Structural components of the contractile system

2.1. Structural identification of contractile components

The smooth muscle cell has a roughly fusiform shape, with the cell nucleus and Golgi bodies, rough endoplasmic reticulum, and a concentration of mitochondria at either pole of the nucleus, forming an axial ellipsoid mass in the middle region of the cell. This central axial region of the cell is clearly vegetative/nutritive. The two distal regions of the cell and, to a varying extent, the peripheral areas of the middle region are packed with filaments, indicating their contractile function. But are *all* filaments in the contractile regions contractile, or are some cytoskeletal? Fig. 2-1 shows a longitudinal section of guinea pig taenia coli, a favorite tissue for smooth muscle physiologists and cell biologists. This section is typical of the structure of distal regions of cells of many other smooth muscle tissues, except that this section has a more truly longitudinal orientation and better preservation of structural detail than most. Two types of filaments can be identified: the occasional thick filament with projecting bridges, and the other filaments, most of which are probably thin filaments, but some of which could be intermediate filaments, a type that was

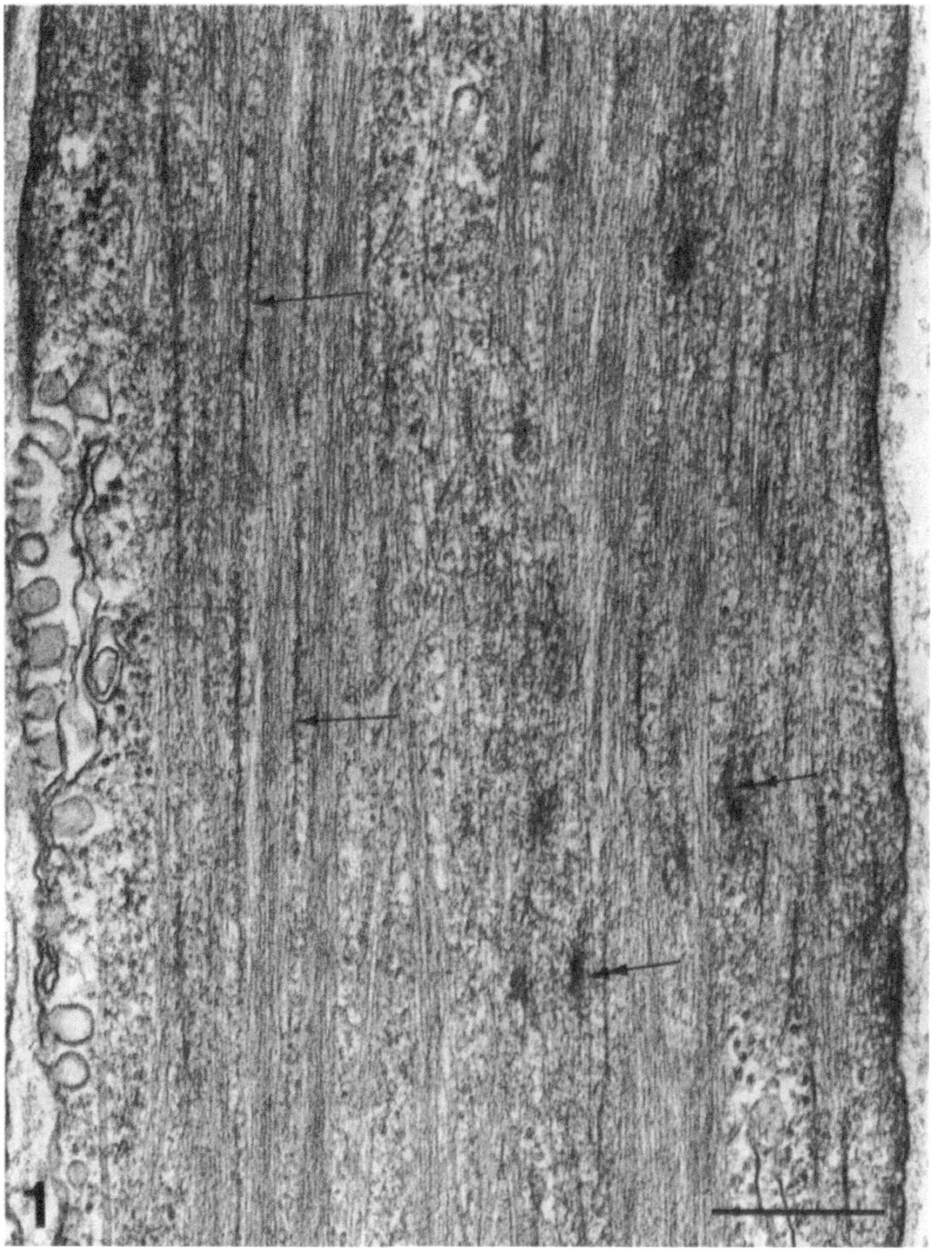

Figure 2-1. Longitudinal section of guinea pig taenia coli. Thick filaments (arrows) are easily identified by their larger diameter and projecting cross-bridges. Thin filaments are mostly in bundles. Intermediate filaments are also present but are often difficult to distinguish from thin filaments in longitudinal sections. Caveolar plasmalemmal areas are seen on the left cell border while an MADB (membrane-associated dense body) area is shown along the right cell border. CDBs (cytoplasmic dense bodies) are scattered through the cytoplasm (double arrows). X 42,000. Calibration bar represents 0.5 μm. (Reprinted from Cooke, 1983 (18) by permission of the author and Plenum Publishing Co.)

discovered in vertebrate smooth muscles (119) and that is much more abundant than in skeletal muscles.

Because of the uncertainty in identifying thin filaments by structural characteristics in longitudinal sections (except by cytochemical means discussed later), transverse sections are preferred by most investigators for determining filament types, their distributions, and their ratios. Figures 2-2 and 2-3 show typical transverse sections of

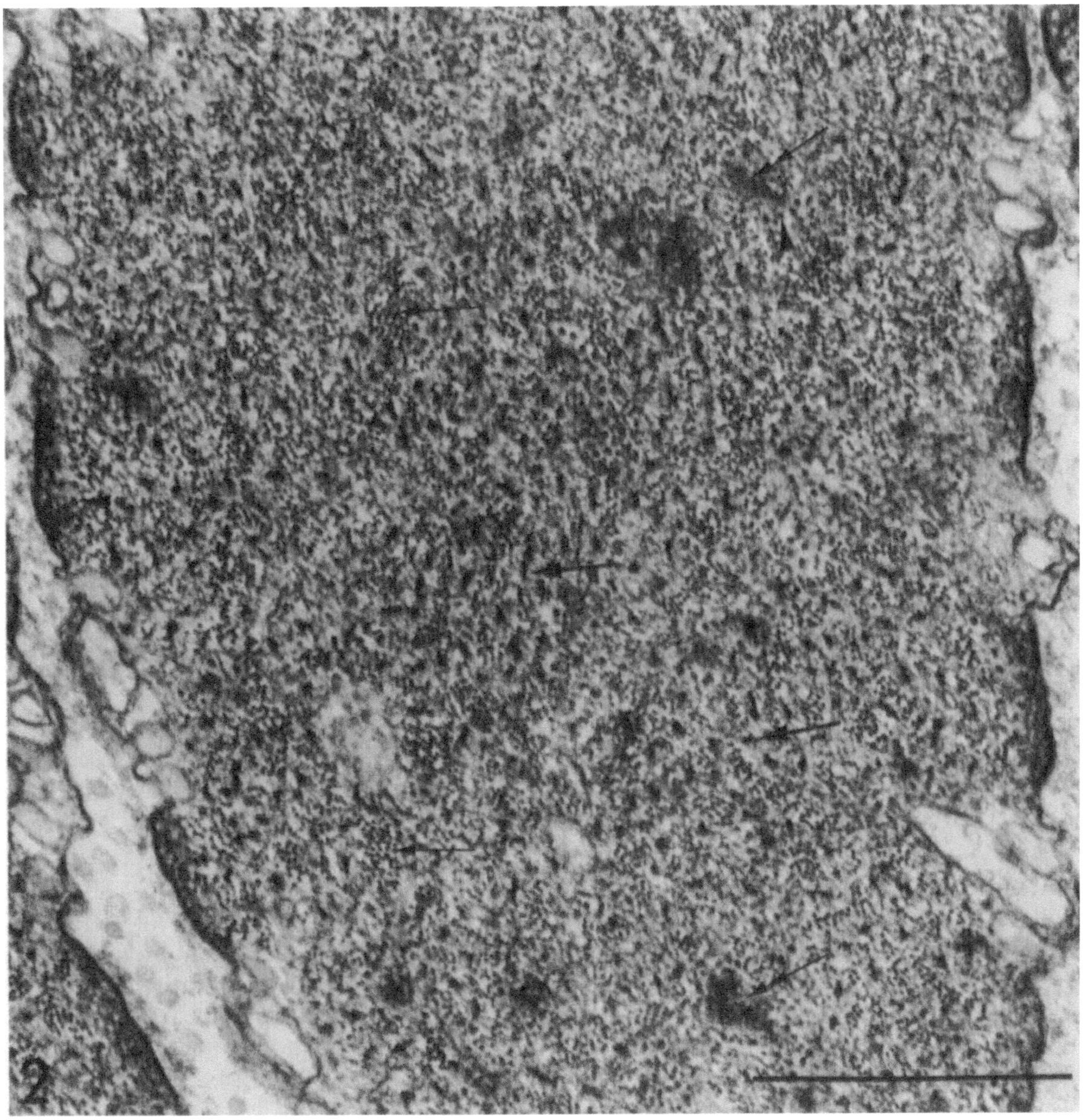

Figure 2-2. Typical transverse section of guinea pig taenia coli in a relaxed state at .56L_o. MADB areas alternate with caveolar plasmalemmal areas around the cell border. CDBs (double arrows) are distributed evenly throughout the cytoplasm. Thick filaments (large arrows) and thin filaments (small arrows) are distributed fairly evenly, but there are occasional areas where thin filaments are in bundles. Intermediate filaments (arrowheads) are usually found around CDBs or next to MADBs. X 84,000. Calibration bar represents 0.5 μm. (Reprinted from Bagby and Corey-Kreyling, 1984 (7), p. 61, by courtesy of Marcel Dekker, Inc.)

smooth muscles from guinea pig taenia coli and *Bufo marinus* stomach, respectively. In Figure 2-2, one sees irregular profiles of thick filaments, identified by having the largest cross-sectional profile (≥ 12 nm in thickness) among the filaments; much more numerous thin filaments, having more uniformly round cross-sectional shapes and diameters of 6–8 nm; and the less numerous intermediate filaments (IFs) with very dense, sharply defined profiles and extremely uniform diameters of 10 nm, leading to their often being termed 10 nm or 100A° filaments. Figure 2-3 shows only two types of filaments: very numerous thin filaments, and ribbon-shaped thick filaments. IFs are infrequently seen in *Bufo marinus* stomach muscle (20) (Bagby, unpublished data).

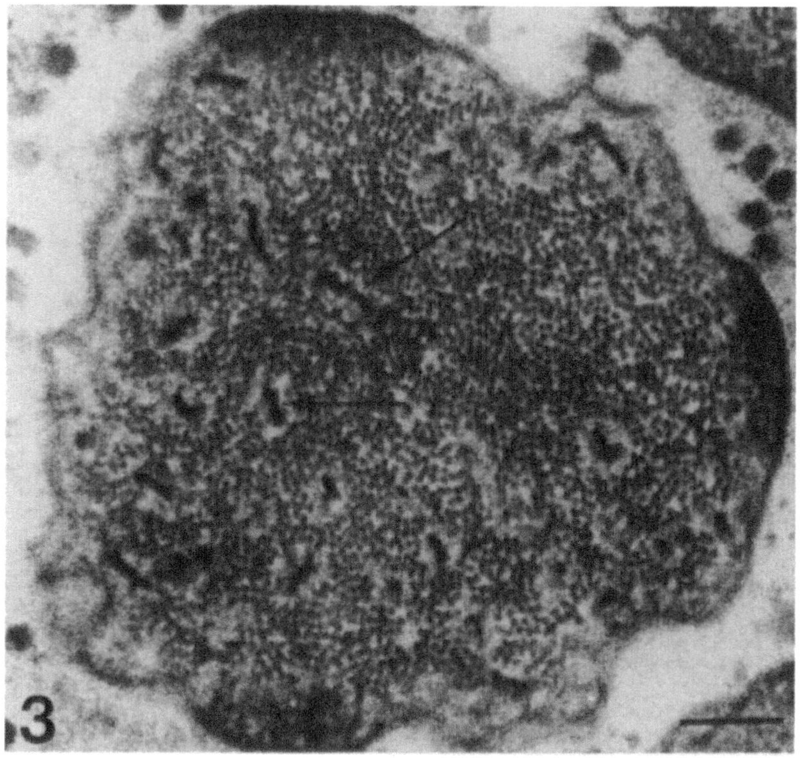

Figure 2-3. Transverse section of *Bufo marinus* stomach muscle fixed in a relaxed state at 1.6 L_o. Thick filaments (arrows) have mostly ribbon-shaped cross-sectioned profiles. Thin filaments are densely packed. Intermediate filaments are absent. Three MADB areas alternate with non-MADB areas around the periphery. At this level of the cell, which is near the terminal portion, CDBs are rare. X 119,000. Calibration bar represents 0.1 μm. (Micrograph by Roland Bagby and Margaret C. Kreyling.)

No contractile system in a muscle cell can function without points of attachment to transmit force to the plasma membrane. The plasmalemma shows a division into two types of areas. One type, with longitudinal rows of invaginated vesicles called caveolae, is not categorized as part of the contractile system. The other type of plasmalemmal area has dense, thickened basement membranes, and the two areas usually alternate around the circumference of the cell (see Figs. 2-2, 2-3). These latter areas have a length much greater than their width in many smooth muscles, leading to their designation as "dense bands" by Gabella (34–40). A more generic term, membrane-associated dense bodies (MADBs), will be used in this chapter, since it is not certain that all MADBs are band-shaped. However, regardless of morphology, MADBs are universally regarded as terminal attachments points for the contractile system (for reviews, see 4, 5, 18, 36–38, 100, 106), and they will be considered in detail in subsequent sections.

Cytoplasmic dense bodies (CDBs) share many points of morphology with MADBs, except for *not* being part of a basement membrane structure, and they are likewise tentatively considered part of the contractile system based on their associations with thin filaments (2, 4, 5, 11, 106, 107, 110, 118). However, as will be seen in a later section (Section 3.3), being associated with thin filaments may not be a sufficient criterion for considering CDBs to be part of the contractile system. Both MADBs and CDBs associate also with IFs (2, 4, 5, 11, 17, 18, 19, 97, 99, 100, 118). Since IFs have no biochemical role in the contractile process and may or may not participate in transmission of force from contractile components to the plasmalemma (for a discussion of the evidence, see 4), they are always categorized as cytoskeletal rather than contractile, leaving open the question of whether CDBs and MADBs should be considered contractile or cytoskeletal or both. Immunocytochemical studies (Section 3.3) shed new light on this issue. The remainder of the chapter will deal with the ultrastructure (Section 2), cytochemistry and immunocytochemistry (Section 3), and functional organization (Section 4) of the tentatively identified components of the contractile system. Thick filaments, thin filaments, CDBs, and MADBs will be considered in detail, since they either are part of the contractile system or may possibly be attachment sites for the contractile system, but IF structure and composition will not be emphasized, since IFs appear to be strictly cytoskeletal (for recent reviews on the roles of the intermediate filaments, see 4, 5, 18, 38, 101, 106).

2.2. *Ultrastructure of thick filaments*

The thick filament has been a controversial structure since it was first seen in vertebrate smooth muscles. The main controversy, whether thick filaments existed in *living* muscles, was mostly laid to rest due to consistent and very effective fixation of thick filaments in both relaxed and contracted muscles by the Somlyos and their associates in the 1970s (2, 107, 109, 112). However, the controversy has been reopened by *in vitro* studies that show that myosin with unphosphorylated regulatory light chains has a shape that should prevent it from forming filaments, and yet in the relaxed state of smooth muscle this light chain is unphosphorylated. Furthermore, MgATP disassembles unphosphorylated myosin filaments under approximately physiological conditions (see Smith et al. (103) for a review of the evidence). It is possible, however, that other proteins or other factors in the cell maintain thick filaments even in the unphosphorylated state.

Another early controversy arose due to the report by Small and coworkers that thick filaments were "ribbon-shaped', with cross-bridges on opposite faces (72, 102) instead of helically arranged around a "rod-shaped" filament, as one would expect from the striated muscle paradigm (57, 58). Somlyo and coworkers (109, 112) showed convincingly that "unphysiological" conditions such as hypertonic fixatives and extreme stretch during fixation led to a predominance of ribbon-shaped thick filaments, while "physiological" conditions led to more rod-shaped profiles in transverse sections. At that time, *rod-shaped* was interpreted to mean *striated muscle type*, and since striated muscle thick filaments have helically arranged cross-bridges of opposite polarity on either end of the filament with the opposite polarity bridges separated by a bridgeless region, the central bare zone (57, 58), it was assumed that these filaments possessed that structure also. Somlyo et al. (111) recently described chevron structures on thin filaments due to ~45° attached rigor cross-bridges from neighboring myosin filaments. On at least one of the thick filaments there was a chevron pattern, indicating that polarity on either edge of the filament was the same, consistent with a bipolar thick filament. The filament could not be followed far enough to tell if the chevron structure reversed polarity at the other end. However, there were and are some data that fit a ribbon-shaped filament better than a bipolar one. Synthetic thick filaments grown from myosin of several smooth muscles or from nonmuscle myosins to lengths approaching the 2.2 μm length of in situ filaments (2) showed morphology consistent with that of the ribbon-shaped filaments (21, 54, 91). Only in the smallest aggregates, where filaments were only slightly longer than a tail-to-tail dimer, could the morphology be interpreted as bipolar (54, 91). In most models derived from synthetic filaments of myosin and from ribbon-shaped filaments, myosin tail-to-tail dimers are obliquely aligned with the filament axis such that flat filaments with two faces result, with each face bearing the myosin heads, and the polarity of all myosin heads on one face is the same and is opposite to that of the myosin heads on the opposite face (21, 72, 102). The terms *face-polar* or *side-polar* are used distinguish them from the Huxley model for striated muscle, bipolar thick filaments (57, 58). Bagby and coworkers showed that thick filaments in smooth muscles of the toad *Bufo marinus* were even more labile than in mammalian smooth muscles and that ribbons were the commonest type seen, with the ratio between ribbon and rod structures being dependent upon calcium concentration, ATP level, and state of contraction, in addition to the degree of stretch (7, 8, 30). Figure 2-3 shows a cross-section of a cell from *Bufo marinus* stomach under conditions that led to predomimantly ribbon-shaped thick filaments. A definitive experiment is reported by Small and Sobieszek (100), who isolated thick

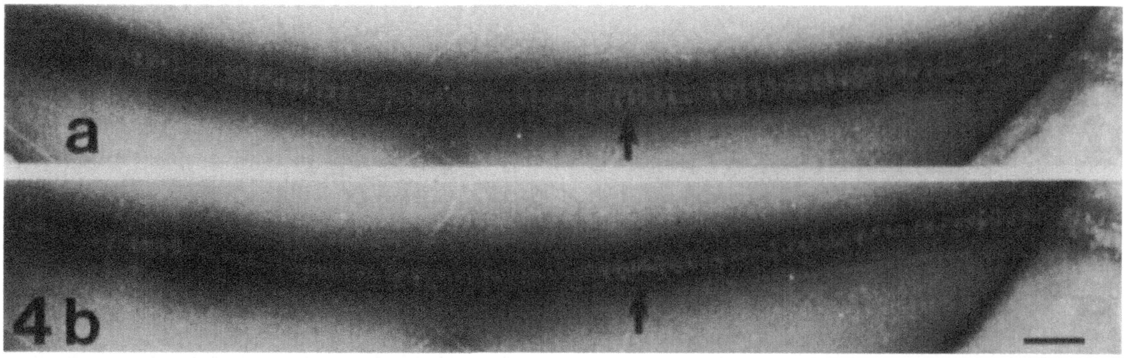

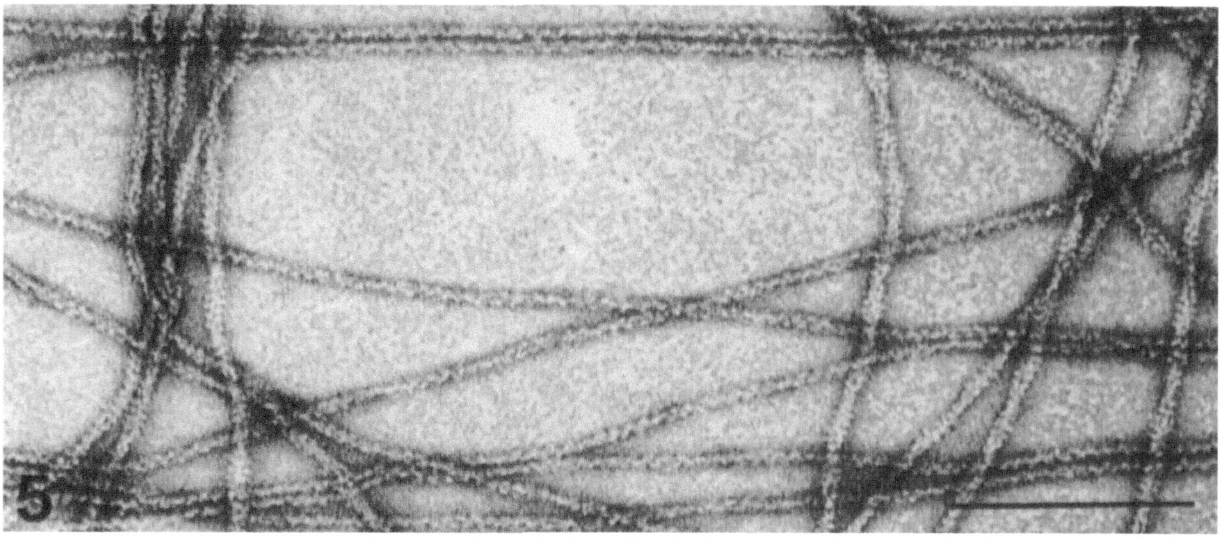

Figure 2-4. Thick filaments isolated from *Bufo marinus* stomach muscle and negatively stained. In (a) the filament has a 14.5 nm periodicity across a broad surface. When the viewing stage was tilted, the same filament area (arrows) shows an edge-on view (b) revealing features of a side-polar filament, with bridges having a 14.5 nm period projecting from each face. X 69,000. Calibration bar represents 0.1 μm. (Reprinted from Cooke, et al., 1987 (20), by permission of the author and Alan R. Liss, Inc.)
Figure 2-5. Thin filaments isolated from chicken gizzard. The double helical array of actin monomers is self-evident. X 295,000. Calibration bar represents 0.1 μm. (By permission of Dr. Catherine Moody and Dr. William Lehman.)

filaments from fixed guinea pig taenia coli tissue, which, when embedded and cross sectioned, showed rod-shaped profiles. The isolated filaments, however, showed no central bare zone and had the same uninterrupted axial 14.4 nm repeating period as the side-polar filament (21, 72, 102). Hinssen et al. (54) proposed a "row-polar" thick filament that had a rod shape, with no central bare zone and possibly helically arranged bridges, as a sort of compromise structure, but new evidence (20) favors the side-polar filament.

It now seems that any helical structure seen in isolated thick filaments could be due to random twisting of a ribbon-shaped filament (a filament with a square or rectangular-shaped profile in cross section, with bridges only on two opposite faces). Convincing evidence for this opinion is seen in Figure 2-4, taken from studies by Cooke and coworkers (20) of thick filaments isolated from *Bufo marinus* stomach and viewed with a tilting stage. The same region of the filament viewed at one tilt angle shows clearly an edge view of a "ribbon" with bridges projecting from opposite faces, while at another tilt angle the filament shows only a 14.5 nm axial repeat period, which could be produced by a face-view that looked like a rod-shaped filament. They also reported seeing random twists of the filaments, which could lead to the "helical" bridges seen by Somlyo et al. (107) or to the bridges seeming to surround some of the synthetic filaments prepared from smooth muscle and nonmuscle myosins (54).

As was pointed out in an earlier review (4), it does not seem possible that bipolar rod-shaped thick filaments having a central bare zone can aggregate laterally (due to stretch or hypertonic solutions) into side-polar ribbon-shaped filaments that display no central bare zone. Therefore, this author strongly suggests that we abandon the bipolar model for smooth muscle thick filaments. This recommendation is not made lightly, because side-polar (face-polar) thick filaments have implications for a quite differently functioning contractile unit (see models by Hinssen (54) and Gröschel-Stewart and Drenckham (49)) than that which exists in vertebrate skeletal muscles.

2.3. *Ultrastructure of thin filaments*

The thin filament is by far the most abundant contractile component of smooth muscles and apparently is a rather stable component with most fixation protocols, compared to the more labile thick filament. The thin filaments of smooth muscles were shown to be ultrastructurally indistinguishable from those of all other muscles (52), and the basic structural model based on thin filaments of striated muscles (57, 58) still seems adequate to explain the structures seen in vertebrate smooth muscles, despite some striking differences in protein constituents (see 33, 70, 73, 74, 99, 101, 105). The presence and localization of these other proteins are discussed in the next section (Section 3.3). Figure 2-5 shows the ultrastructure of isolated native thin filaments from chicken gizzard. The prodominant feature shown is two strands of actin wrapped around each other in a double helix. Within each actin strand, the individual actin subunits may sometimes be seen. The presence of actin was confirmed quite early, since the ultrastructure of the isolated smooth muscle thin filament was identical to that of synthetic actin filaments and to that of striated muscle thin filaments (52). The characteristic double strand is not easily seen in longitudinal sections, and thin filaments are most easily identified in thin sections by their diameter of 6–8 nm, seen especially clearly in transverse sections (Figs. 2-2, 2-3).

The clarity of thin filament profiles in transverse sections seems to be improved considerably by the inclusion of tannic acid in the aldehyde primary fixative and/or by en bloc staining in aqueous uranyl acetate prior to dehydrating fixed tissues (Bagby, unpublished data), treatments that were introduced and used routinely by Somlyo's group (2, 11, 106–109), although they claim no improvement in viewing filaments (2). The rather indiscriminate use of these agents has probably contributed to the broad range of diameters (6–8 nm) reported for thin filaments. In our laboratory, we have noted that tannic acid increases the diameter of thin filaments as well as the clarity of their profiles, and the change in both characteristics has at times made it more difficult to distinguish thin filaments from intermediate filaments (Bagby, unpublished observations).

There are also treatments that tend to diminish the stability of thin (and thick) filaments during fixation, such as lowering the calcium ion concentration of prefixation and primary fixation solutions with EGTA or EDTA (17, 19, 25). Apparently the loss of thick and thin filaments due to low calcium is pH-dependent, since lowering pH to 6.5 led to both thick and thin filaments being preserved (97, 100), while similar low calcium treatment at pH 7.4 did not (17, 19, 25).

2.4. *Ultrastructure of MADBs (membrane-associated dense bodies)*

MADBs are easily identified in either longitudinal or transverse sections as areas where the plasmalemma is free of caveolae and where the basement membrane is considerably thickened by the presence of both fibrous and amorphous components (see Fig. 2-1–2-3). In some cases, the MADB may extend for some distance into the cytoplasm, even displaying fingerlike projections (37, 79, 94), but in most cases the thickened area is confined to within 100 nm of the plasmalemma. The most commonly reported morphology is bands that run roughly longitudinal to the cell axis in most tissues (2, 4, 18, 34, 36–39, 98, 106, 107), whose widths are less than one micrometer, and whose lengths are indeterminate but may be close to the length of the cell (see Section 3.4 for cytochemically identified dense-band structures in isolated cells). In arteriolar smooth muscle cells, the bands may run transversely (94).

Both thin filaments (2, 17, 19, 27, 30, 31, 37–40, 50, 62, 73, 79, 81, 90, 94, 96, 99–101, 106, 107, 109,

110, 118, 121) and intermediate filaments (17, 19, 37–40, 73, 99–101, 110, 116) associate with the cytoplasmic surface of the MADBs, and the penetration of filaments into the body of the MADB accounts in part for the fibrous component observed. Profiles of filaments having the same diameter as thin filaments are sometimes seen within the body of the MADBs (2, 38, 106, 107), whereas intermediate filaments seem to be restricted to lateral associations on the cytoplasmic surfaces (11, 106, 107, 110, 116). There are additional fibrous components, whose ultrastructure appears to be different from that either of thin filaments or of intermediate filaments, and there are also amorphous components that add to the density of MADBs and tend to obscure the profiles of all fibrous components (2, 7, 17–20, 30, 36–39, 79, 106, 107, 116). The identity of these additional proteins will be discussed in Section 3.4, since ultrastructural characteristics alone do not allow one to identify them.

MADBs are not evenly distributed among the different cell regions. In some vascular smooth muscle cells, particularly in smaller-diameter vessels, such as arterioles, the dense bodies are predominantly on the adventitial side of the cell rather than the luminal side, perhaps in response to the difference in stress on the opposite faces of these cells (38, 94), with the stress apparently being compensated for by thin filaments or intermediate filaments. In other tissues Gabella found that although dense-band structures alternated with caveolar areas, resulting in almost equal areas for both plasmalemmal domains in the midportion of the cell, the terminal portions of the cell showed the MADBs occupying nearly 100% of the plasmalemmal area (35–38). This denser concentration of MADBs in the terminal region would make sense if this part of the cell had to bear more stress than other parts of the cell. If so, is the stress due to contractile structures or cytoskeletal structures? Cooke and Fay (17, 19) maintain, based on mainly indirect evidence from physiological studies (see Section 4.5), that intermediate filaments attach an axial cytoskeleton predominantly to the MADBs in the terminal portions of the cell. Thus the increased surface area devoted to MADBs could reflect the attachment of the cytoskeleton.

The importance of the MADBs in transmission of force from the contractile system to the plasmalemma is shown by several experiments. Tissues fixed during contraction show the MADBs in the bottom of invaginated furrows, while caveolar ridges protrude (34, 36, 38, 94). Isolated cells fixed during contraction show protruding blebs with MADBs concentrated at their bases (26–28). This is consistent with thin filaments attached to the MADBs being pulled by their interactions with thick filaments, which are more centrally located. Also, in hypertrophied intestinal muscle, where the increase in diameter of smooth muscle cells should lead to a change in the surface-to-volume relationship from 1.4 in controls to 0.5 in hypertrophied muscle cells, the actual ratio is 0.8 due to the extra surface added by invaginated furrows bearing MADBs. Thin filaments increased far more than did thick filaments, and this was seen as a mechanism for providing additional attachment sites for the increased numbers of thin filaments (40). Haberle et al. (50) showed that the addition of calcium-dependent proteases to smooth muscle tissues skinned with 50% glycerol led to removal of MADBs and, to a variable extent, CDBs. There was a progressive loss of ability to produce force concommitant with the disappearance of MADBs. Tissues treated with protease, but not stimulated to contract, left thick and thin filaments apparently intact and in their normal organization, but tissues fixed during contraction revealed thick and thin filaments detached from the plasma membrane and in central clumps, showing that thick and thin filament interaction had not been inhibited by the protease but that force transmission to the plasmalemma had been eliminated by the removal of MADBs. When leupeptin, an inhibitor of calcium-dependent proteases, was in the dissecting and skinning media, the removal of MADBs and CDBs was completely inhibited and force production was maximal (50). Since MADBs act as the load-bearing attachments to the contractile system, the distribution of MADBs and any changes in structure or orientation during cell contraction should be related to the organization of the contractile system.

2.5. *CDBs (cytoplasmic dense bodies)*

CDBs show many characteristics of the MADBs, but they are distinguished from MADBs by being found free in the cytoplasm. They also have a

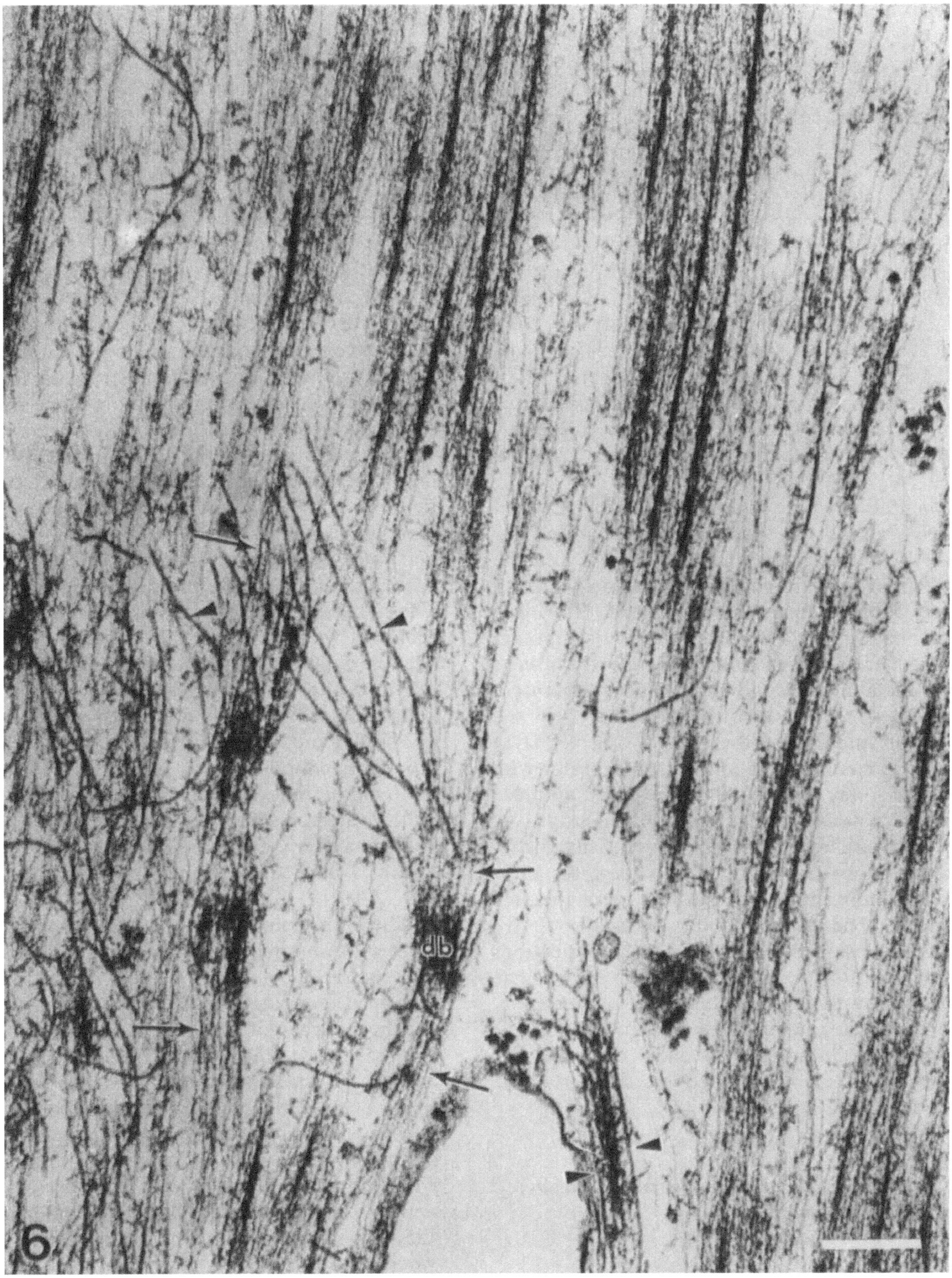

Figure 2-6. Longitudinal section of a saponin-skinned rabbit portal anterior mesenteric vein in which components are more widely separated, revealing relationships among them. Thick filaments are often in loose registration. CDBs (db) and their thin filaments (arrows) tend to line up with thick filaments, while IFs (arrowheads) tend to make looping connections between CDBs. X 70,000. Calibration bar represents 0.2 μm. (Reprinted from Bond and Somlyo, 1982 (11), by permission of the author and Rockefeller University Press.)

different gross morphology, being generally described as fusiform, with the main axis roughly parallel to the cell axis, and having diameters around 100 nm (2,4,5,7,11,17–20,25–28,33–34, 36–40, 50, 53, 62, 79, 90, 99, 100, 106–107, 110,121). In cross sections, filaments having diameters similar to thin filaments have been identified within CDBs (2,11,106,107), sometimes in a latticelike structure whose spacing and arrangement is similar to that of thin filament lattices seen in filament bundles (2,11,106,107). Optical diffraction studies (20) have also given evidence for actin as a CDB component. Intermediate filament profiles are often associated with the lateral surfaces of CDBs, frequently forming a complete ring around them (2,4,11, 18,36–40,73,99,100,106,107,118).

Longitudinal sections are often not very instructive about CDB–filament associations because of the close packing of filaments and the problem of superimposition of filaments in all but the thinnest longitudinal sections. However, Bond and Somlyo (11) used saponin skinning, which revealed associations more clearly in cells where filaments became more widely separated. From these studies, shown in Figure 2-6, and structural studies by others (2,11,106,107,110, 118), it is clear that IFs associate laterally with CDBs, IFs may join neighboring CDBs, and thin filaments associate more or less longitudinally with CDBs. The IFs may be most easily distinguished in longitudinal sections when their paths deviate significantly from the vectors of the thin filaments. The often looping pathways of IFs indicate considerable slack in the connections between CDBs. The clear association of the same CDB with both thin filaments and IFs (see Fig. 2-6) makes the role of CDBs ambiguous. That is, they could be interpreted as either contractile or cytoskeletal structures based on ultrastructural criteria alone.

3. Cytochemical localization of proteins within structural components

3.1. General comments on methods

The most specific cytochemical localizers of proteins are antibodies that have a recognizable marker attached to them. With the limited resolution obtained with light microscopy, several indirect antibody methods with quite large complex markers may be used as long as access to the cell antigen by the antibody and marker(s) is not impaired. However, with the electron microscope, where individual filaments are resolvable, it is desirable to have markers small enough that individual components may be unequivocally labeled. With structures as large as the MADBs and CDBs, this is quite possible; in fact, these were the earliest smooth muscle structures clearly labeled for immunocytochemistry with the electron microscope, using electron-dense proteins such as ferritin and imposil attached to the antibody as a marker (42,43,90). Recently, anti-immunoglobulins attached to colloidal gold particles of 5–10 nm in diameter have become commercially available for indirect antibody labeling, and some have used much smaller colloidal gold particles that they have prepared themselves (51). The great electron density and uniform size and shape of these particles allow them to be seen even in stained sections, making them superior to ferritin. Although individual thick filaments can be labeled (73,99), thin filaments, with diameters of 6–8 nm and frequent dense packing in lattices, are almost impossible to label individually with 5–10 nm particles. Nevertheless, the composition of thin filaments seen in tissue sections may be determined by examining staining of domains where a particular filament type predominates (33,73,99).

There are some rather serious potential problems with immunocytochemistry performed with the transmission electron microscope. Among these are adequate fixation while preserving antigenicity, access of antibody and marker to the antigens, and simultaneous visibility of marker and the component marked. Fixation, preservation of antigenicity, and access problems are interactive, since the best fixation is provided by strong cross-linking such as with glutaraldehyde, while both antigenicity and antibody access to antigens decline as cross-linking is increased (23, 125,129). Access problems are especially aggravated by strong cross-linking in pre-embedding immunocytochemistry, since antibodies must penetrate several micrometers into a tissue block or thick section (23,130). Therefore, postembedding immunocytochemistry is preferred because it minimizes access problems. Cryoultramicrotomy of formalin-fixed, quick-frozen tissues provided an early solution to all the problems except clear visibility of components being labeled (42, 43, 116). Despite the difficulties in obtaining consistent ultrathin sections with cryoultramicrotomes, a few laboratories have provided valuable information on muscle structure using this technique (42, 43, 85, 121). However, in smooth muscles, where the organization is less easily perceived and the location of particular components is much less predictable than with striated muscles, one generally needs heavy-metal staining to identify structural components, and the heavy-metal staining makes it difficult to detect the electron-dense immunocytochemical markers. As a result, immunocytochemistry with cryoultramicrotomy has been useful only for the larger, more visible components of smooth muscles, e.g., MADBs and CDBs (42, 43, 85, 121).

An ideal solution to the problem, which avoids the specialized equipment of ultracryotomy, would be to use a water-soluble embedding medium that avoids the potential loss of antigenicity caused by dehydration with organic solvents, that has sectioning qualities comparable to the epoxy embedding media, and that can be completely removed after sectioning without the danger of chemical denaturation, thereby preserving maximal antigenicity and providing antigen accessibility. Vic Small and his coworkers have perfected embedding with polyvinyl alcohol, a water-soluble plastic that allows embedding directly after fixation, permits ultrathin sectioning on a conventional ultramicrotome, and still allows removal of embedding material by aqueous solutions (33, 73, 98, 99). In addition, Small et al. have utilized negative-staining techniques on the bas-relief surface resulting from embedding medium removal, so that contractile system components are in negative contrast, making it easy to see dense colloidal gold makers on electron-lucent ultrastructural components. For some components, positive staining has also been useful (73). Although the polyvinyl alcohol embedding and sectioning are not as easily performed as with epoxy embedding, the techniques are an order of magnitude easier than cryoultramicrotomy, with far more visible identification of structures. A comparison of antigenicity and visibility of structures with polyvinyl alcohol embedding and with Lowicryl and L.R. White showed polyvinyl alcohol embedding to have distinct advantages (73). The work of Small et al. has allowed the application of immunocytochemical techniques to the composition of the different filaments. Almost as important as the extension by these authors of the resolution of immunocytochemical techniques is their use of serial ultrathin sections at the light microscope level to show the spatial relationships among the localizations of virtually all the important contractile proteins (33, 73, 98, 99). This has, in some cases, provided an entirely new view of their function. Without the work of Small et al., this section would have little new to report, and the chapter as a whole would have much less of the spice of controversy.

3.2. Thick filament proteins

In vertebrate skeletal muscles, the thick filament is composed almost entirely of myosin (57, 58) with additional small amounts of C-protein, H-protein, X-protein (82, 113), and doubtless other minor components yet to be discovered. As shown in Section 2.2, the isolated native thick filament matches rather closely the synthetic thick filaments formed from myosin alone, which lacked a bipolar structure and therefore showed no evidence for a central bare zone structure (20, 21, 54, 91, 97, 100). The localizations of C-protein and perhaps X-protein are related to the staggered overlap of the terminal rod portions of the myosin molecule in the central bare zone of the vertebrate skeletal muscle thick filament (82, 113), a structure apparently missing in the vertebrate smooth muscle thick filament (see Section 2.2). Coupled with the lack of information on smooth muscle proteins equivalent to these minor constituents in skeletal muscles, it is not too surprising that myosin is the only protein that has been unequivocally localized in thick filaments seen in ultrathin sections (73, 99).

A technique that shows the three-dimensional interactions of thick and thin filaments in a longitudinal section should do much to clear up the controversy over thick filament structure. S-1 labeling has been used to show the polarity of thin filaments (discussed in Section 3.3), and this

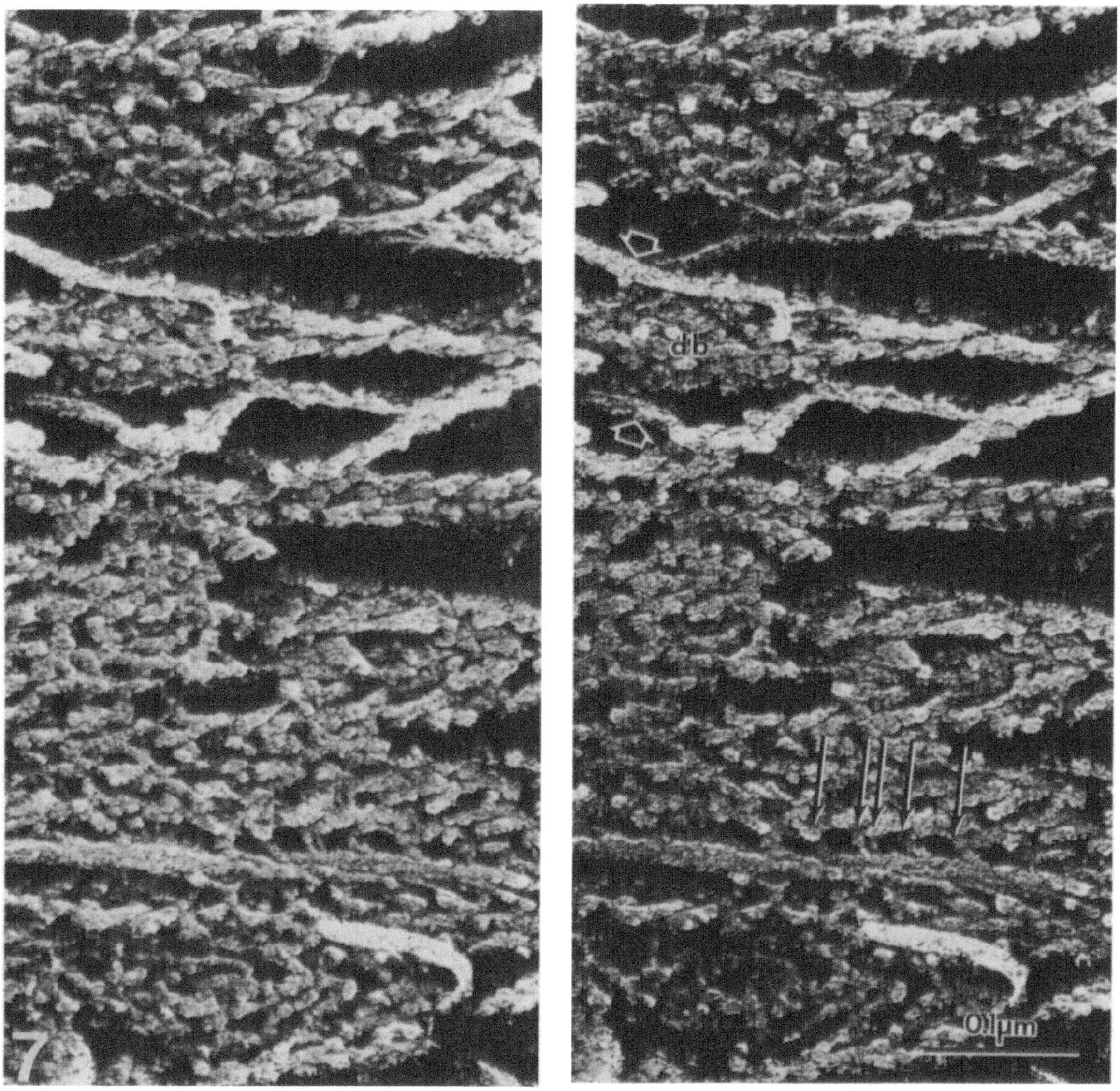

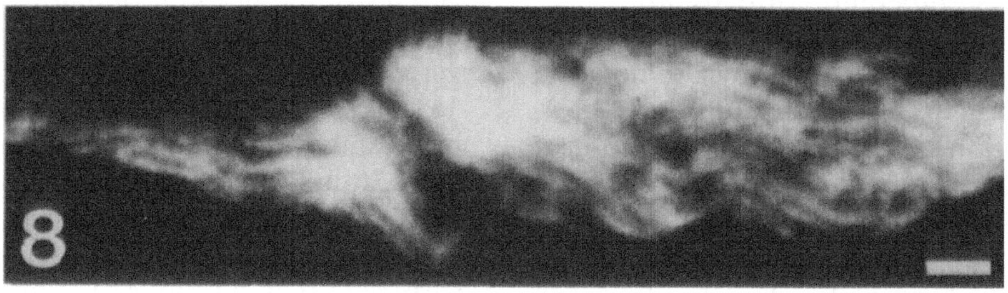

Figure 2-7. Stereo pair ±7° tilt of a portion of saponin-skinned rabbit vas deferens muscle treated with myosin S-1 fragment to label actin and then quick-frozen and deep-etched to reveal surface detail on the filaments. A thick filament has its crossbridges (arrows) attached to adjacent S-1 decorated actin. Intermediate filaments (white arrows) surround a CDB (db) in the upper part of the micrograph. Calibration bar represents 0.2 μm. (Reprinted from Somlyo and Franzini-Armstrong, 1985 (110), by permission of the author and BirkhauserVerlag Ag, Basel/Switzerland.)

Figure 2-8. A broken cell from chicken gizzard stained with fluorescent antimyosin. At the broken end (left), myofibrils show striations. In the intact portion of the cell, many myofibrils take curved paths around the cell. Calibration bar represents 5 μm. (Reprinted from Bagby and Pepe, 1978 (9), by permission of the author and Springer-Verlag.)

technique could conceivably be used to determine the polarity of thick filaments and whether they are bipolar or side-polar by the polarity of thin filaments with which they interact. However, Figure 2-7 shows that this type of experiment does not give unequivocal results. This author interprets the pattern of bridges as being supportive of side-polar thick filaments; Somlyo and Franzini-Armstrong did not (110).

At the light microscope level, antimyosin labeling shows interrupted fibrils with a fairly regular repeating pattern in cultured smooth muscle cells (13, 16, 46, 48, 49); in freshly isolated cells, fibrils show either continuous staining or, in areas where individual fibrils may be clearly seen, some interrupted staining patterns (3, 7, 9) (see Fig. 2-8). Since the interrupted pattern is consistent with that of striated muscle myofibrils, this evidence has been used to build a case for individual fibrils in smooth muscles having a sarcomere organization, even though lack of registration among fibrils in whole cells would obscure the sarcomere organization (3, 4, 7, 9). The interrupted pattern implies a registration of thick filaments that in some instances, such as in Fig. 2-6, has been seen and noted in electron micrographs (2, 11, 106, 107).

3.3. Thin filament proteins

Recently attention has been paid to isolation of native thin filaments and analysis of their constituents (70, 74). Constituents identified thus far are actin, tropomyosin, and caldesmon in molar ratios of 28:4:1, with filamin being an additional, highly variable constituent, while striated muscle thin filaments contain actin, tropomyosin, and a complex of troponins in molar ratios of 7:1:1 (70). The differences between the smooth muscle and striated muscle thin filament constituents have led to a renewed interest in the role(s) of thin filaments in the biochemistry of contraction. In addition, immunocytochemical localizations of all these proteins, showing their spatial relationships to each other, have now been performed both with light and with electron microscopy (33, 73, 99). The results have led to some novel proposals, the implications of which should have a profound effect on future models of organization. This section will review the most documented localizations first, followed by the recent, more controversial localizations.

The earliest ultrastructural means of identifying thin filament components with a chemical tag was the use of myosin, or myosin fragments containing the globular head (e.g., HMM or S-1), which reacted with actin to form arrowhead structures (57, 59). These arrowheads indicated not only the presence of actin, but also that the double helix of actin strands had a polarity, with the barbs of the arrowheads toward the direction of attachment whereas the pointed end was the free end (57, 59). Figure 2-9 and 2-10 show thin filaments attached to MADBs and CDBs respectively, identified by labeling isolated structures or swollen cells with S-1 (11, 118). For both MADBs and CDBs, the arrowheads point away from their respective attachment sites. The thin filaments attached at either end of the CDBs have opposite polarity, as shown by the arrowheads, a situation that is strikingly similar to the reversal of polarity seen at striated muscle Z-lines.

Labeling with S-1 to indicate thin filament bundles of the same polarity should give an indication of the organization of contractile units within the smooth muscle cell. However, in the more usual preparation of tissues, when one has closely packed thin filaments and probable superposition of several layers of thin filaments in a longitudinal section, the polarity of individual thin filaments is not easily determined (107). Also, not all types of electron microscopy reveal the arrowhead structures. This is demonstrated in the work of Somlyo and Franzini-Armstrong (110), where quick-frozen, deep-etched, and rotary shadowed S-1-labeled smooth muscle tissue displays thin filaments as three-dimensional coiled ropes whose polarity cannot be easily determined (Fig. 2-11). Although thin filament polarity is easily seen only when thin filaments are not too densely packed, the presence of actin in thin filaments is easily confirmed by the use of S-1 and is especially useful for distinguishing thin filaments from intermediate filaments in longitudinal sections, as shown in Figure 2-11.

The presence of actin may also be determined by actin antibodies (13, 14, 16, 45, 46, 49, 60, 98, 99) or by phalloidin (49, 131), a toxic substance found in some poisonous mushrooms. The use of actin antibodies was hampered at first by the

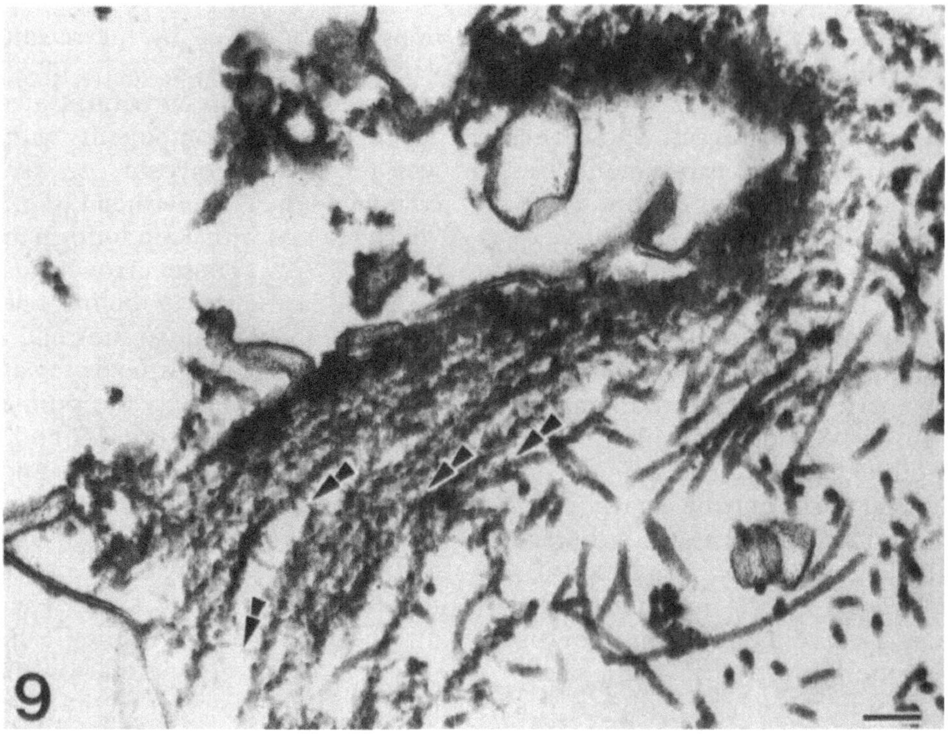

Figure 2-9. Longitudinal sections of an isolated MADB with attached thin filaments. S-1-stained thin filaments reveal an arrowhead pattern (double spearheads) pointing away from the MADB. X 68,000. Calibration bar represents 0.1 μm. (Reprinted from Tsukita, et al., 1982 (118), by permission of the author and Springer-Verlag.)

concept that such a strongly conserved molecule, the structure of which changed little from species to species, could not be used as an antigen to raise antibodies and later by some apparent peculiarities in the immune system response to actin (for reviews, see 46, 49). Both actin antibodies and phalloidin with fluorescent labels show continuously labeled stress fibers in cultured smooth muscle cells viewed with the light microscope (13, 14, 16, 46, 49, 98, 99). Freshly isolated cells labeled with anti-actin show little evidence for fibrillar structure, and the whole cell stains intensely for actin (Bagby, unpublished data). Polyvinyl alcohol sections show only scant evidence for fibrillar organization with anti-actin, since staining of filament-containing areas is continuous, whether viewed with the light or electron microscope (33, 73, 98, 99). The presence of tropomyosin in smooth muscle has been known since the X-ray diffraction studies of Hanson and Lowy (52) showed evidence for organized filament arrays of actin and tropomyosin. Since tropomyosin was found to be localized in striated muscle thin filaments (58), it was always presumed that smooth muscle thin filaments also contained tropomyosin. The work of Small et al. (99) confirmed that both actin and tropomyosin were localized within the smooth muscle thin filament areas, and from their general distribution within these areas, every thin filament seems to contain both these proteins (Fig. 2-12). Prior to the definitive work on constituents of smooth muscle thin filaments (70, 74), most attention was spent on the thick filaments and in particular on the role of myosin light chains, which seemed at first to provide the only calcium-sensitive control for contraction (for reviews, see 1, 22, 61). There had at times been claims of a calcium-sensitive thin filament protein, but the suggestions of a smooth muscle troponin or troponinlike protein had been discounted. However, caldesmon, a highly elongated protein of Mr between 130–135 kDa with little resemblance to skeletal muscle troponin-C, was shown to act with calmodulin to confer calcium sensitivity to the contractile system (33, 70, 74, 105, 123). Its constant although low stoichiometric ratio with actin and tropomyosin (70, 74) indicated caldesmon as a probable thin fila-

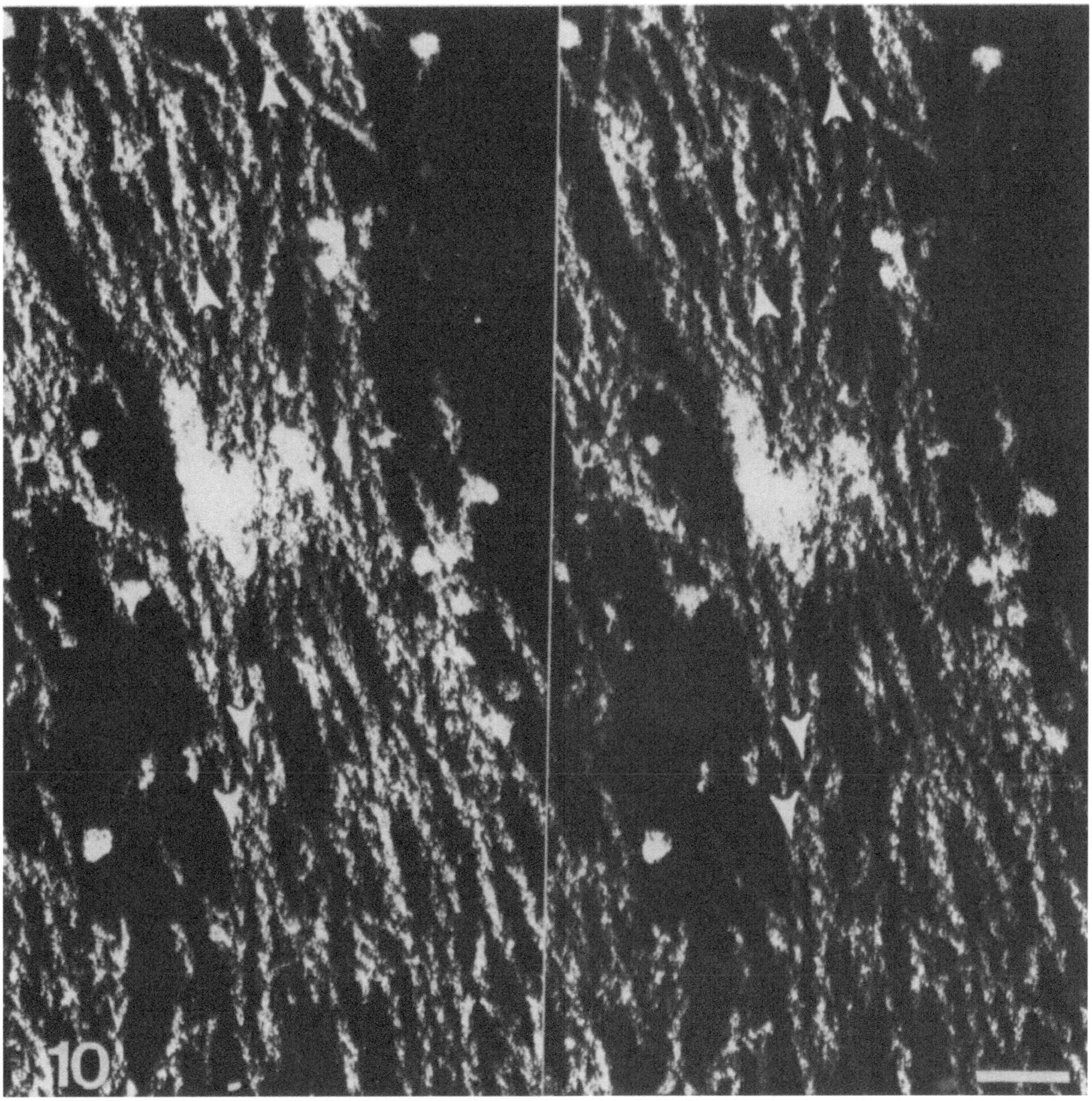

Figure 2-10. Stereo pair of a longitudinally sectioned CDB and accompanying thin filaments stained with S-1. Thin filaments insert at either end, and are shown by the arrowhead pattern (arrowhead markers) to have opposite polarity at either end. Calibration bar represents 0.1 μm. (Reprinted from Bond and Somlyo, 1982 (11), by permission of the author and Rockefeller University Press.)

ment constituent, possibly taking the place of troponins found in striated muscles.

Filamin is another elongated protein with Mr of about 250 kDa that has no established regulatory role in the contractile process, however, it is a potent cross-linker of actin, and it competes with tropomyosin for binding to actin (74, 101, 128, 129). Filamin's high content in smooth muscles, up to 30–40% that of myosin (124), indicates that its function, probably structural and probably associated with thin filaments, is important. In stained isolated guinea pig taenia coli cells it showed a pattern of longitudinal fibrils within the cells (Fig. 2-13) (99). Small and his coworkers, using antibodies to a variety of smooth muscle proteins and the newly developed poly-

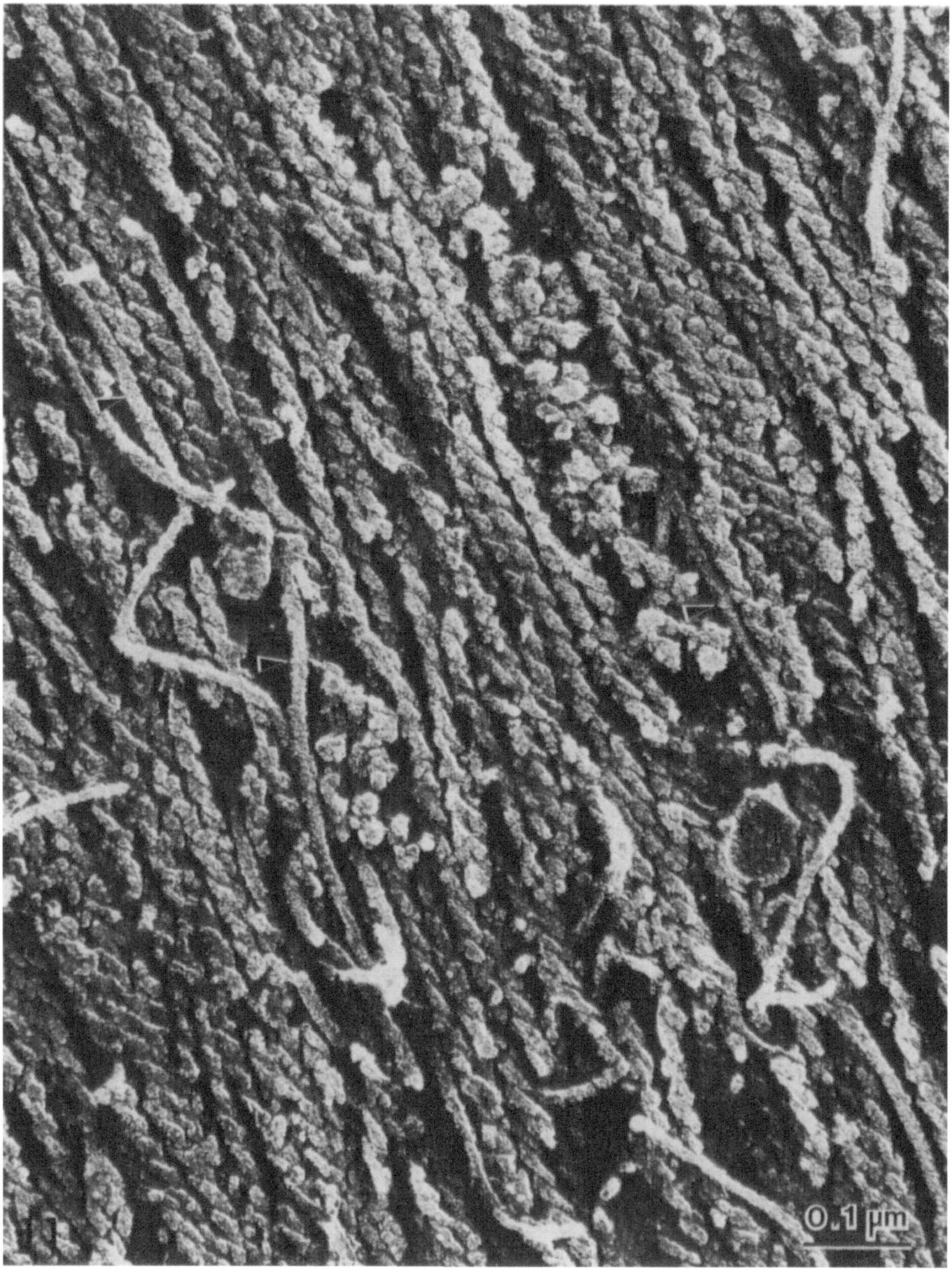
0.1 µm

vinyl alcohol embedding to provide ultrathin sections with superior antigenicity and accessibility to antibodies, did the definitive experiments to localize these proteins to specific filament types (33, 73, 99). Using pseudo-serial sections, they stained tissues with single antibodies first, then used combinations of two antibodies to show spatial relationships between certain proteins. Both anti-actin and antitropomyosin showed uniform distribution among the thin filaments (99), but it was unclear whether actin-binding proteins have uniform distribution among the thin filaments in different areas of the cell. Since the intermediate filament protein desmin was known to be cytoskeletal in function whereas myosin was known to be unequivocally contractile (for reviews, see 4, 101), antibodies to these two proteins were used to mark the two domains within smooth muscle cells, the cytoskeletal and the contractile domains, respectively. Proteins occurring within a particular domain were judged to have the function of that domain. To decide whether a particular protein occupied the cytoskeletal or the contractile domain, one section in a series was double-stained with fluorescent antibodies to the putative protein plus antimyosin or antidesmin and compared to staining of another section in the series by antimyosin or antidesmin alone. If the same pattern was seen in double-staining with antimyosin as with antimyosin alone, the protein was assumed to stain the same domain as antimyosin and to be in the contractile domain. The same argument was applied for single- and double-staining with antidesmin. As confirmation, the antibody that stained in the contractile domain was expected to show complementary staining when used with antidesmin, and an antibody that stained in the cytoskeletal domain was expected to show complementary staining when used with antimyosin. At the electron microscope level, polyvinyl alcohol ultrathin sections on pioloform-coated grids with embedding medium removed were stained with colloidal gold-labeled single antibodies. Double-staining, which was required for marking domains in light microscopy, was unnecessary in electron microscopy since intermediate filament or thick filament profiles marked the cytoskeletal or contractile domains, respectively. Although the size of the gold label made it difficult to localize a particular thin filament protein antibody to an individual thin filament, proximity of the label to thick filaments or to intermediate filaments established whether the putative protein ought to be assigned to the contractile or cytoskeletal domain.

It was shown that filamin was found exclusively among thin filaments in the cytoskeletal domain (Fig. 2-14, 2-15) (73, 99) and in another study (33) that caldesmon was found in the contractile (actomyosin) domain. Therefore, it was hypothesized that there were two types of thin filament, a contractile type composed of actin, tropomyosin, and caldesmon, and a cytoskeletal type composed of actin, tropomyosin, and filamin (33, 73, 99). An independent biochemical study using antibodies to filamin or to caldesmon to isolate and identify thin filaments from chicken gizzard found evidence for two types of thin filaments, one that contained filamin but little caldesmon and another that contained caldesmon but little filamin (70), providing early confirmation of the two-domain hypothesis.

The foregoing evidence for thin filaments occupying both cytoskeletal and contractile domains fits the cultured nonmuscle cell paradigm, since actin in these cells plays just such a dual role (128), but the evidence runs counter to our expectations based on the striated muscle paradigm. As we shall see in the next section, the two-domain hypothesis raises further disturbing questions about our present concepts of CDB and MADB function, which are based on the striated muscle paradigm.

3.4. *Proteins of the MADBs and CDBs*

Since MADBs and CDBs are rather large and can be recognized even in very lightly stained ultrathin

←

Figure 2-11. Longitudinal section of saponin-skinned rabbit portal arterior mesenteric vein incubated with S-1, quickfrozen and deep-etched. Thin filaments reveal a ropelike appearance while the intermediate filaments (arrowheads) are smooth. Calibration bar represents 0.1 µm. (Reprinted from Somlyo and Franzini-Armstrong, 1985 (110), by permission of the author and Birkhauser-Verlag AG, Basel, Switzerland.)

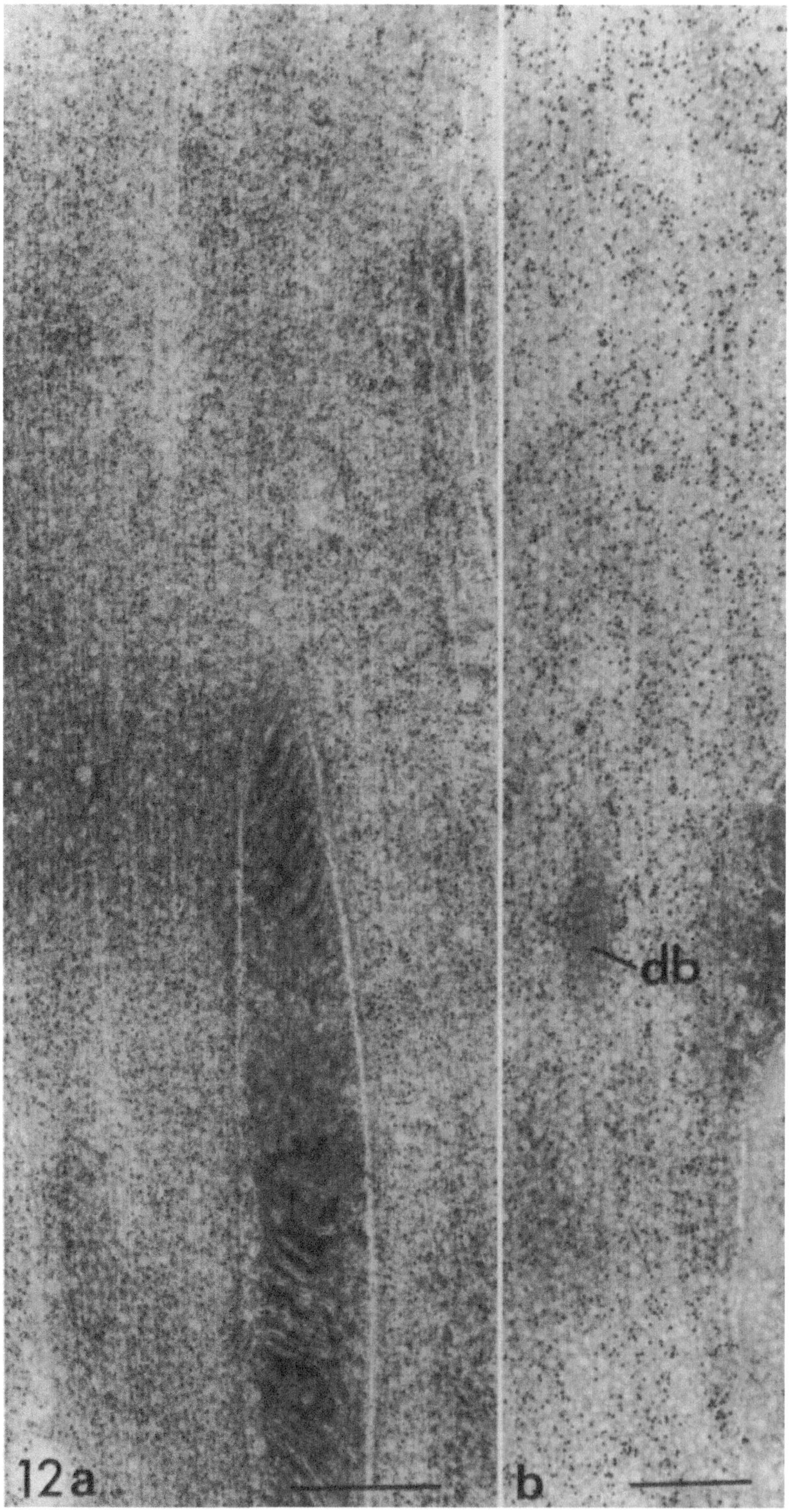

Figure 2-12. Longitudinal section of polyvinyl alcohol embedded guinea pig taenia coli. The water-soluble embedding material was removed and the section was reacted with antibodies to actin (a) or tropomyosin (b), followed by immunogold labeling (5 nm gold for antiactin, 10 nm gold for antitropomyosin) and negative staining of the section to reveal filaments as lighter areas. Both actin and tropomyosin appear to be evenly distributed among all thin filaments. CDBs (db) are not stained by antitropomyosin. Calibration bars represent 0.4 μm. (Reprinted from Small, et al., 1986 (99), by permission of the author and Rockefeller University Press).

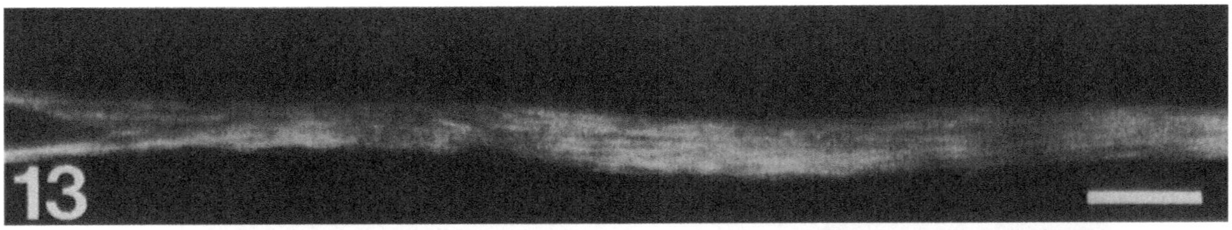

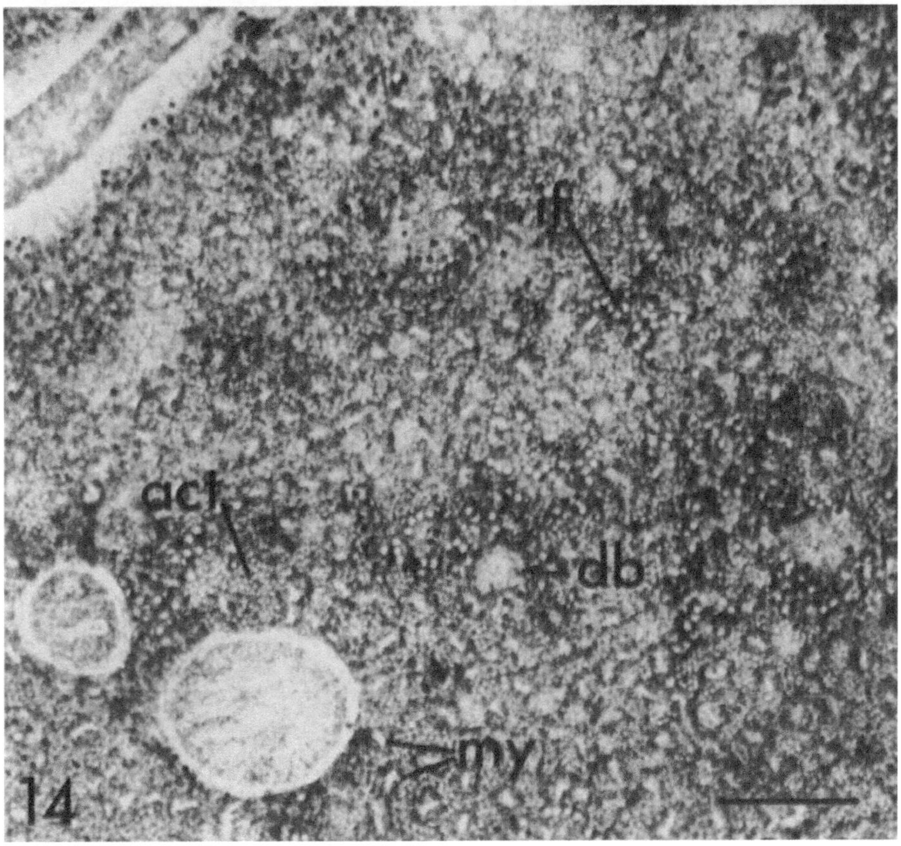

Figure 2-13. Isolated guinea pig taenia coli cells stained with antifilamin. Note fibrillar pattern in the cytoplasm of the cell, presumably due to cytoskeletal thin filament bundles. Calibration bar represents 10 μm. (Reprinted from Small, et al., 1986 (99), by permission of the author and Rockefeller University Press.)

Figure 2-14. Transverse section of polyvinyl alcohol-embedded guinea pig taenia coli, contrasted as in Figure 2-12, but with 10 nm immunogold labeling of antifilamin. Filamin, an actin-binding protein, is localized in the same domain as intermediate filaments (if) and CDBs (db), and it is not found in areas where myosin (my) and actin (act) form close associations. Calibration bar represents 0.2 μm. (Reprinted from Small, et al., 1986 (99), by permission of the author and Rockefeller University Press.)

sections, making electron-dense antibody labels practical, they were the first smooth muscle structures whose composition was studied by immunocytochemistry with the electron microscope (42, 43, 90). Alpha-actinin is an actin-binding protein with Mr of 95–100 kDa that is known to be a major component of Z-discs in striated muscles (58, 67, 71, 76) and of attachment plaques of cultured cells (41, 42), while vinculin is primarily known as an attachment plaque protein (41, 93). These early studies, using two different-sized electro-dense proteins (ferritin and imposil) as antibody labels, found that alpha-actinin was a component of both, whereas vinculin was found only in the MADBs (42, 43, 98). Later studies, mostly with immunogold (20, 71, 85, 121), confirmed these findings (see Figs. 2-16, 2-17). Since both MADBs and CDBs are large enough to be resolved with the light microscope, similar studies were done with serial polyvinyl alcohol sections stained with fluorescent antibodies to vinculin and alpha-actinin, confirming alpha-actinin's presence in both MADBs and CDBs, while only MADBs contained vinculin (98) (see Fig. 2-18).

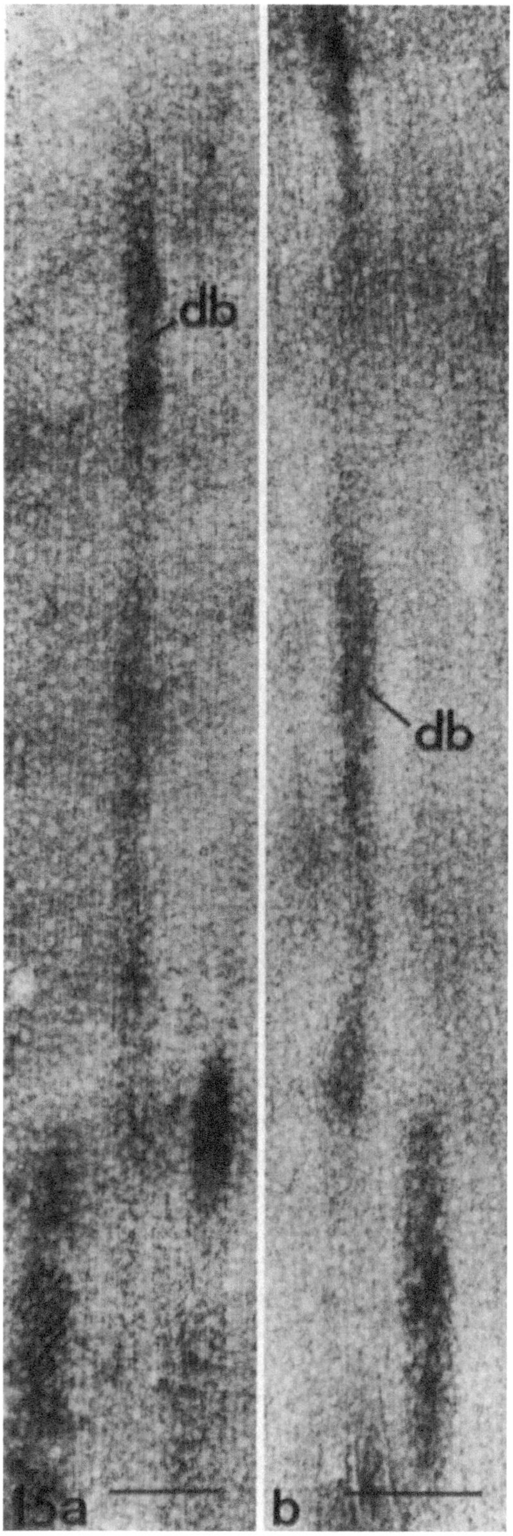

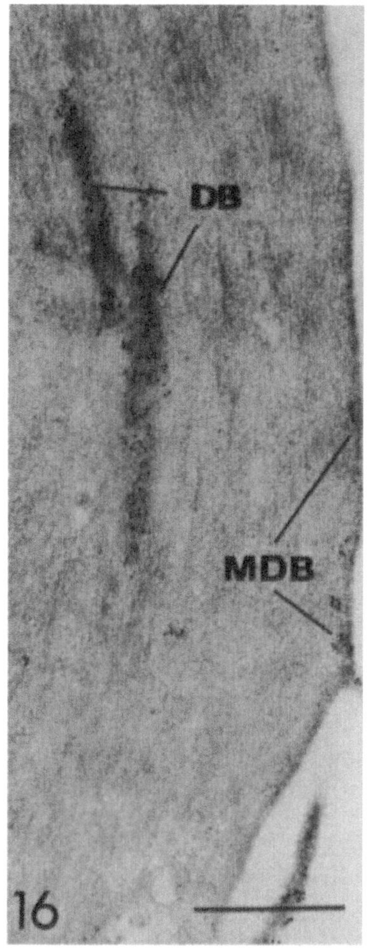

Figure 2-16. Longitudinal section of an isolated *Bufo marinus* stomach muscle cell embedded with Lowicryl and stained with anti-alpha-actinin and contrasted with immunogold. Alpha-actinin is present in both CDBs (DB) and MADBs (MDB). Calibration bar represents 0.5 μm. (Reprinted from Cooke, et al., 1987 (20), by permission of the author and Alan R. Liss, Inc.)

←

Figure 2-15. Longitudinal section of polyvinyl alcohol-embedded guinea pig taenia coli, contrasted as in Figure 2-12, but with 5 nm immunogold labeling of antifilamin (a) and anti-alpha-actinin (b). Anti-alpha-actinin labels CDBs (db) and antifilamin labels thin filaments attached to CDBs but not to other thin filaments. Calibration bar represents 0.4 μm. (Reprinted from Small, et al., 1986 (99), by permission of the author and Rockefeller University Press.)

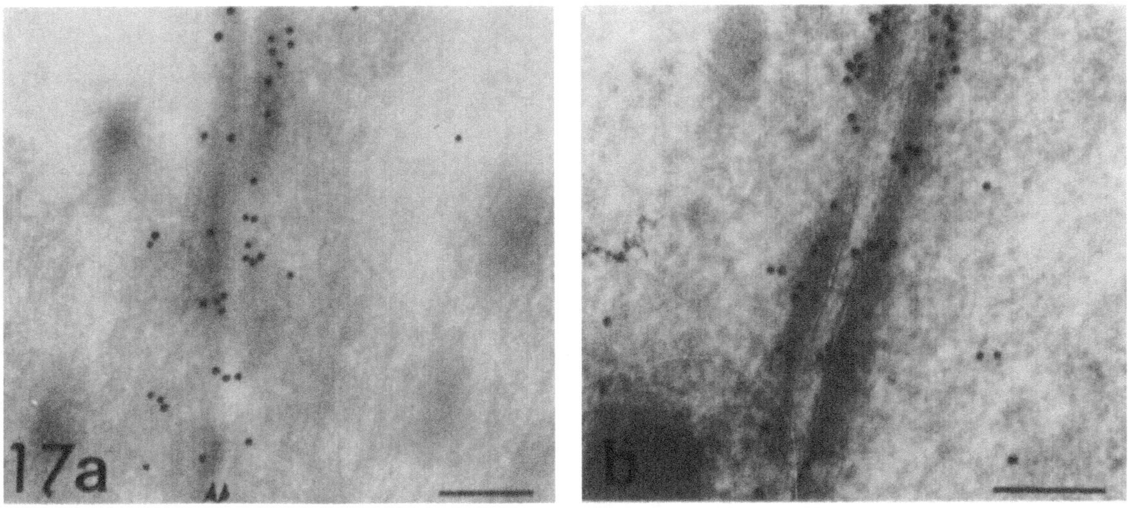

Figure 2-17. Cryoultramicrotome sections stained with antitalin (a) and antivinculin (b), immunogold labeling. Both talin and vinculin are found in MADBs but not in CDBs. Calibration bars represent 0.2 μm. (Reprinted from Volberg, et al., 1987 (121), by permission of the author and Springer-Verlag.)

The use of isolated cells for fluorescent antibody staining of these structures has led to very useful data for cell-organization studies. The MADBs have been seen as longitudinal strips or patches using anti-alpha-actinin with isolated chicken gizzard cells (3) or toad stomach cells (28), while with isolated guinea pig cells anti-alpha-actinin staining reveals MADBs as longitudinal strips running nearly the length of the cell (98), and antivinculin staining shows even more clearly defined longitudinal continuous strips (98) as shown in Figure 2-19. The apparently longitudinal orientation of MADBs, which are accepted as attachment sites for thin filaments and intermediate filaments (see Section 2.4), seems to contradict earlier cell models based on *helical* membrane attachment sites (6, 30, 96, 100), which were proposed to explain an apparently helical orientation of myofilaments (31, 95, 96). However, Gabella has stated that these longitudinal dense-band structures tend to become helical during contraction (38).

There are a variety of other proteins that have been found associated with the attachment plaques of cultured smooth muscle cells, including talin (12, 121) (see Fig. 2-17), fibronectin (apparently only on the exterior of the plasmalemma) (65), Sgp 130, a sialoglycoprotein (85), and metavinculin (41, 92). The structural relationships of these proteins to each other is unclear; some may provide attachment to actin, some may anchor the MADB to the plasmalemma, and still others appear to interact with the extracellular matrix (41). Both talin and alpha-actinin are found closer to the actin bundles than vinculin and may act as links between thin filament bundles and MADBs (42, 43, 121). Despite the rather detailed information we have about the chemical composition of MADBs, it is not clear which proteins within them specifically bind to intermediate filaments. If we had this information, it would be easier to use immunocytochemical techniques to discover whether MADBs in different regions of the cell have different affinities for intermediate filaments. Based on the tendency for IFs and CDBs to cluster in the axis of the cell when the tissue is stretched (7, 17, 19), it has been proposed that intermediate filaments attach primarily to MADBs in the terminal portions of the cells but not to MADBs in the middle portions (4, 17, 19). Unfortunately, immunocytochemical methods have not been directed toward testing for the implied differences in MADB composition.

The composition of CDBs has not been studied in great detail. Alpha-actinin has been definitely localized in CDBs by a number of investigators (20, 42, 43, 90, 121), and vinculin is definitely *not* a component of CDBs (42, 43, 98, 121); but other than actin, whose presence in CDB cores was proposed based on ultrastructural characteristics

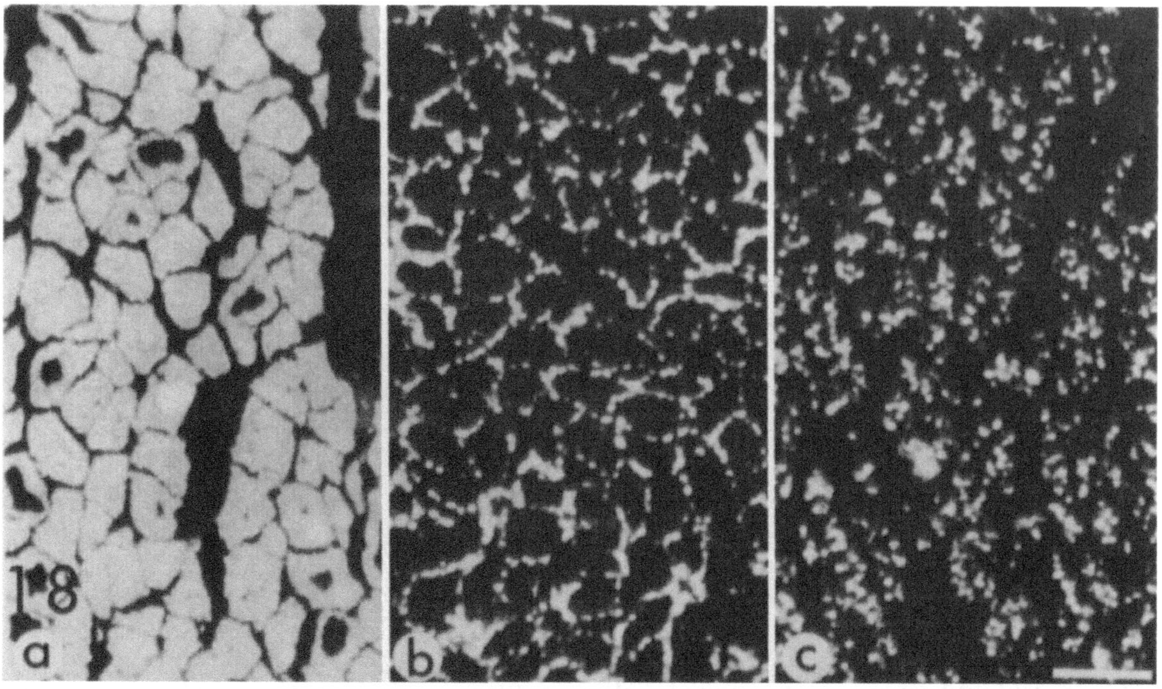

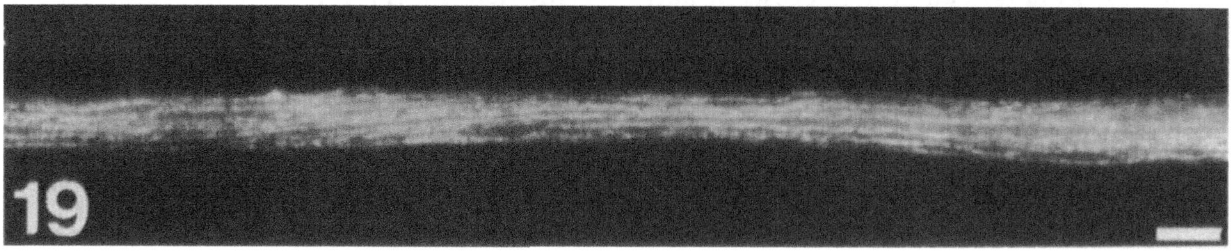

Figure 2-18. Serial ultrathin transverse sections of polyvinyl alcohol-embedded guinea pig taenia coli stained with fluorescent antibodies to actin (a), vinculin (b), and alpha-actinin (c), showing the uniform cytoplasmic distribution of actin, the peripheral punctate localization of vinculin (presumably in MADBs), and the punctate localization of alpha-actinin in both cytoplasm (presumably in CDBs) and periphery (presumably in MADBs). Calibration bar represents 5 μm. (Reprinted from Small, 1985 (98), with permission of the author and IRL Press, Ltd.)

Figure 2-19. Isolated guinea pig taenia coli cell stained with fluorescent anti-vinculin, showing its localization on longitudinal structures on the plasma membrane, which are presumably MADBs. Calibration bar represents 5 μm. (Reprinted from Small, 1985 (98), with permission of the author and IRL Press, Ltd.)

(see Section 2.5), and whose probable presence in CDBs was noted with anti-actin staining (99), we are ignorant of additional components of CDBs.

Based on the opposite polarity of thin filaments attached at either end, as revealed by S-1 labeling, giving an appearance consistent with CDBs being Z-line equivalents (see Section 3.3), one would classify CDBs as myofibrillar/contractile. However, based on experiments described but not shown, Small et al. (99) placed cytoplasmic anti-alpha-actinin-stained structures (presumably CDBs) in the cytoskeletal domain due to their coincident localization with filamin and desmin. In Figure 2-15, one can see what appears to be filamin-containing thin filaments emanating from a dense body, which presumably would contain alpha-actinin. Lehman et al. (70) have circumstantial biochemical evidence that supports Small's view. The antibody precipitation that was used to separate the two types of thin filaments (Section 3.3) also precipitates any associated cytoskeletal proteins, and the filamin-containing thin filaments appeared to be associated with alpha-actinin and desmin, while the caldesmon-containing thin filaments were not (70). In cultured chicken gizzard smooth muscle cells stained with rhodamine-labeled antimyosin and fluorescein-labeled anti-alpha-actinin, "fibrils" stained with one antibody were usually unstained by the other, indicating two classes of fibril, one contractile, one cytoskeletal (Bagby and Frierson, unpublished data).

4. Organization of contractile/cytoskeletal components

4.1. Puzzles and paradoxes

Sections 2 and 3 established the ultrastructure and the biochemical composition of individual components in vertebrate smooth muscles, using biochemical criteria to determine, where possible, whether a component was part of the contractile system or of the cytoskeletal system. In the past, various models were proposed to describe how the contractile components and/or cytoskeletal components were organized (for reviews of these models, see 4, 5). The models were proposed as a means of reconciling data that seemed to be inconsistent with the organization present in cross-striated muscle, but they still contained assumptions of striated muscle mechanisms where data were insufficient to suggest otherwise. It is useful at this point to examine which smooth muscle data are the most troublesome to reconcile with the striated muscle paradigm and thereby lead to apparent paradoxes. It is also helpful to examine smooth muscle data that seem inconsistent with other smooth muscle data. We can think of all the data gathered from smooth muscles as being part of a puzzle. All data gathered from smooth muscle, assuming the data are valid, will eventually fit together to make a consistent model for smooth muscle, just as all the pieces of a puzzle will yield a picture when all the pieces are fitted together. However, we do not have all the pieces to the smooth muscle puzzle, so we try to fit the known pieces together to make *some* picture. Completing puzzles is much quicker if we have the picture on the puzzle box. We use various paradigms as our picture on the puzzle box, and we try to make the pieces join together to make the data fit the paradigm. Occasionally, we have pieces that fit a neighboring puzzle piece, but a picture begins to form that does not match the paradigm we are using, so we call this situation a paradox. The following subsections present some puzzles and paradoxes that have been around for some time. Suggestions of possible solutions are made at the end of each subsection. A concluding summary section (Section 5) includes suggestions for future research to gather some important missing data.

4.2. Are there extra thin filaments?

In vertebrate skeletal muscles, each thin filament interacts with three thick filaments, and each thick filament has six thin filaments surrounding it — one thin filament for each of six bridges arranged in a helix around the thick filament, resulting in a hexagonal lattice and leading to a thin-filament: thick-filament ratio of 2:1 in the single-overlap region of the A-band (58). In extremely shortened striated muscles, where there is double-overlap of thin filaments, the ratio would be 4:1. The thin: thick filament ratios in vertebrate smooth muscles range from 12:1 to 30:1 in the literature (for reviews, see 4, 106), depending upon the tissue examined and conditions of fixation, etc., but none of them shows ratios as low as in vertebrate striated muscles. This discrepancy occurs partly because the ratio from skeletal muscles is taken only from the overlap regions in the A-Band, while ratios from smooth muscles are taken from cross sections that would randomly sample all bands of sarcomeres, should some type of sarcomere exist. An attempt was made in our laboratory to compensate for this discrepancy by designating areas of thick filament concentration as *A-Band areas*. Even these areas have ratios of 7:1 and 9:1 in guinea pig taenia coli at 1.5 L_o and 0.5 L_o, respectively, and of 14:1 in *Bufo marinus* circular stomach muscle at both 1.2 L_o and 0.6 L_o (Bagby and Kreyling, unpublished data). Both the much higher thin:thick filament ratio and the relative constancy of the ratio, over a length change that would have doubled the ratio in the vertebrate skeletal muscle, present a paradox if the vertebrate striated muscle paradigm is applied.

Related to this data is the finding that, while the expected increase in segregation of thin filaments into thick-filament-lacking areas occurs with stretch (7, 19, 53), and while thick filaments have a tendency to be found in loosely registered

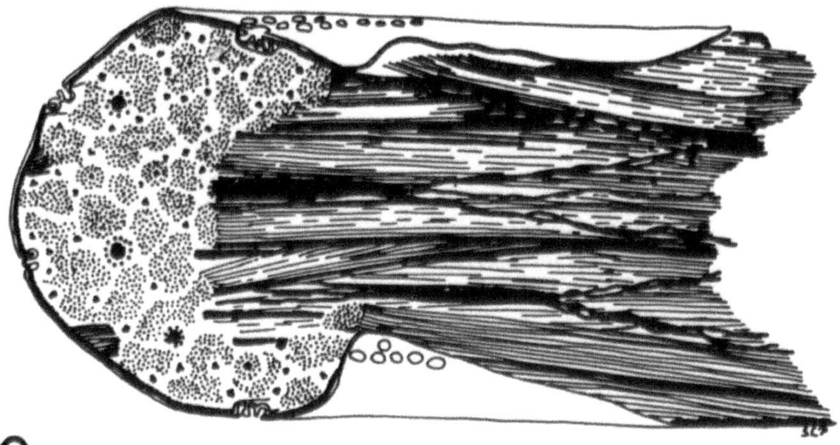

20

Figure 2-20. 3-D illustration of the relationships between thick and thin filaments. Thin filaments in bundles form networks. Thick filaments are mostly parenchymal to thin filament bundles, but occasionally they interdigitate with some bundles to form rosette structures. Intermediate filaments and CDBs form a cytoskeletal network that may not interact with the contractile components. (Reprinted from Cooke, 1982 (18), by permission of the author and Plenum Publishing Co.)

bundles of 3–5 thick filaments (2, 11), as would be expected from a sarcomere organization like that of vertebrate skeletal muscle, there were rarely areas where there was segregation of thick filaments into thin-filament-lacking areas (7). This pattern was also present in micrographs in some publications comparing stretched and shortened smooth muscles (19, 53) where the authors did not specifically describe this type of filament distribution.

The filament ratio data and the data about filament distribution with stretch have sometimes been explained by speculations that thin filaments may be much longer than thick filaments (4, 5, 49, 77). In a muscle showing a 10:1 thin:thick filament ratio from cross sections, and whose thick filaments are 2.2 μm long (2), if the thin filaments are 1.5 μm long (maintaining the length of thin filaments as 67% of the length of thick filaments, as in vertebrate skeletal muscle), there would be an actual 15:1 ratio, but if thin filaments were 11 μm long, the actual ratio would be 2:1 (77). The thin:thick filament ratio measured from random cross sections would be high, because the same thin filament would be repeatedly sampled at more sectioning levels than the thick filament, even though the actual ratios of thin:thick filaments could be low. Unfortunately, there are great difficulties in making accurate measurements of thin filament lengths in smooth muscle sections, and measurements from isolated thin filaments, which may show relatively short thin filaments (74), are suspect because one cannot be sure filaments are isolated intact.

Another explanation is that there are some thin filaments that do not interact with thick filaments. Cooke (18) devised a model based on serial section reconstruction where thin filament bundles split and converged in a network, and thick filaments were peripheral to these bundles, apparently able to interact with only the peripheral thin filaments in these bundles (Fig. 2-20). The non-myosin-interacting thin filament is essentially the same as the cytoskeletal thin filament proposed by Small et al. (33, 99). In this solution to the paradox, the higher thin:thick filament ratio is due to counting *both* contractile domain and cytoskeletal domain thin filaments. If the two-domain hypothesis is correct, the ratio between *contractile* domain thin filaments and thick filaments might be low enough to tempt one to apply the vertebrate striated paradigm to the contractile domain of vertebrate smooth muscle cells.

4.3. *Do fibrils exist?*

Fibrillar organization (organization of filaments into bundles) in vertebrate smooth muscle cells has been inferred from studies of isolated cells viewed with polarized light (4–7, 95, 96, 100) or with 200 KV TEM (5), and especially with isolated cells stained with antimyosin (3–7), anti-alpha-actinin (3–5, 7, 20, 28, 98), and antifilamin (99). Staining of tissue sections with fluorescent anti-myosin, antifilamin, antidesmin, and anti-caldesmon (33, 99) has shown some evidence for fibrillar organization also, as have ultrathin sections stained with gold-labeled antibodies to these same proteins (33, 73, 99).

On the other hand, ultrathin sections stained with antibodies to actin or tropomyosin revealed little evidence for organization of filaments into bundles, whether the sections were viewed with light or electron microscopy (33, 73, 99) (see Fig. 2-12). Also, normal tissues fixed and processed for conventional TEM rarely reveal any fibrillar organization (for a review of data on fibrillar structure, see 4, 5). However, chemically skinned smooth muscle tissues show frequent separation of components into fibrillar bundles (11, 20, 62), and skinned cells treated to produce rigor show especially clear division into bundles (62, 97, 100). Hypertrophic smooth muscle cells also tend to show more obvious bundles than normal cells, having increased intermediate filaments running between the bundles (40).

Why are fibrils apparent in some cases, but not in others? There are probably several reasons. Even if there are functional bundles of filaments that act independently of other bundles, there is usually nothing marking the boundaries of bundles comparable to the fenestrated collars of SR in most striated muscles since SR is sparser in smooth muscles (108). In ascidian non-striated muscles there are abundant IFs between bundles, making it easier to see bundles even though SR is sparse in these muscles also (114, 115). Since this arrangement is sometimes apparent in hypertrophied but not in normal vertebrate smooth muscles (40), it may be that cytoskeletal thin filaments, along with IFs, mark the divisions between fibrils, but most techniques do not distinguish between cytoskeletal and contractile thin filaments, and the IFs are normally too sparse to be good markers. However, antibodies that preferentially stain the *contractile* domain, such as antimyosin and caldesmon, and that leave the cytoskeletal domain unstained, would enhance fibrillar appearance, as is shown by several investigators (3, 6, 9, 33, 99) (see Fig. 2-8). Likewise, staining cytoskeletal components specifically, as with anti-alpha actinin, antifilamin, and antidesmin, should stain material between contractile fibrils, leading to a fibrillar appearance also, which would explain the fibrils observed with these stains (3, 28, 33, 98, 99) (see Fig. 2-13). Antibodies to proteins belonging to *both* domains, such as actin and tropomyosin, would *not* be expected to reveal fibrillar structure, and they generally do not (33, 99). Since polarized light enhances the A-Band visibility in striated muscles due to the presence of parallel thick filaments (56), in smooth muscles this technique should also enhance contractile domain visibility while suppressing cytoskeletal domain visibility. It is not too surprising that polarized light studies of isolated smooth muscle cells have revealed fibrillar structure (6, 95). The picture that emerges is one in which there are interspersed fibrils, some contractile, some cytoskeletal, whose boundaries are not apparent in conventional TEM because *both* contain thin filaments.

Why does skinned muscle (20, 62) and especially skinned muscle in the *rigor* state (62, 97, 100) lead to bundles being more spparent? The skinning process can lead to preferential extraction of certain components (50, 63). In their experiments with skinned smooth muscle tissues, Kossman et al. (63) showed that filamin was the most readily lost thin filament protein. This result, coupled with the preferential loss of MADBs and CDBs that was shown to take place with skinned tissues if calcium dependent proteases were not inhibited with leupeptin (50), could lead to preferential loss of the cytoskeletal domain components. It may also be that in the case of skinned rigor muscles, where thick filaments are firmly bound to thin filaments of the contractile domain, cytoskeletal thin filaments are preferentially removed, leading to more obvious bundles being seen in these tissues (62, 97, 100).

4.4. *Do myofibrils have sarcomere structure?*

In the previous subsection, reasonably convincing evidence was presented for the existence of fibrils in the contractile domain as well as for the probable existence of cytoskeletal fibrils. The contractile fibrils (myofibrils) must contain, as a bare minimum, myosin, actin, and probably tropomyosin for there to be a contractile mechanism similar to that of striated muscles (58). For a sarcomere organization comparable to that of striated muscles, alpha-actinin should also be present (7, 67, 71), and there should be a regular repetition of bands of thick filaments and thin filaments, presumably with Z-disc or Z-substance for attachment of thin filaments. Throughout the animal kingdom, cross-striated or obliquely striated muscles all have some type of sarcomere with these bare minimum requirements (58, 69, 86). With this in mind, many investigators, including this author, used fluorescent antibodies to look for fibrils with interrupted staining patterns with the assumption that some sort of sarcomere might exist in vertebrate smooth muscles also. Immunofluorescent staining of cultured smooth muscle cells or even freshly isolated smooth muscle cells have shown interrupted (striated) patterns of staining in fibrils using antimyosin (7, 9, 13, 16, 46, 48), anti-alpha-actinin (3, 28), and even tropomyosin (15). But anti-actin staining has almost universally led to continuously staining fibrils (13, 14, 16, 46, 47, 49), making it difficult to postulate a sarcomere structure like that of skeletal muscles (see Bagby (3) and Bagby and Corey-Kreyling (7) for more thorough reviews of evidence for and against sarcomere structure). The existence of cytoskeletal thin filaments (33, 70, 73, 99), which need not be segregated into bands to perform their cytoskeletal function, could explain the continuous staining seen with anti-actin since continuously staining cytoskeletal fibrils would tend to mask any discontinuous staining in contiguous contractile fibrils. There has been some supporting evidence from TEM for a sarcomere or at least a minisarcomere organization being present. Somlyo and coworkers have found that thick filaments tend to be found in groups of three to five in reasonable registration (2, 11) (see Fig. 2-7), and thin filaments decorated with S-1 fragment show that thin filaments at one pole of a CDB have opposite polarity to those at the opposite pole (11, 118) (see Fig. 2-10), consistent with CDBs being Z-line-equivalent structures in vertebrate smooth muscles (11, 118).

We have seen that proteins belonging to the contractile domain, according to the two-domain hypothesis (33, 99), are myosin, actin, tropomyosin, and caldesmon (see Section 3.3). If we assign caldesmon a function similar to that of the striated muscle troponins, the composition of the vertebrate smooth muscle myofibril is comparable to that of striated muscle myofibrils, with one important exception: alpha-actinin. Prior to the localization experiments by Smalls' group (33, 73, 99), alpha-actinin was usually assumed to be part of the contractile system, since it is a major component of Z-lines in striated muscles (67, 71, 75), and it was known to provide for attachment of thin filaments in the sarcomeres (57, 58). Indeed, without the Z-discs (and alpha-actinin) there could be no sarcomere structure, since the striated muscle contractile mechanism depends upon thin filaments at each end of the sarcomere having opposite polarity for them to be able to form bridges with the near ends of the bipolar thick filaments, and the attachment of thin filaments to the opposite faces of the Z-discs provides the mechanism for the change in polarity of thin filaments (for a review of sarcomere structure, see 58). The Z-discs, along with the M-zline, also provided for registration of I-bands and A-Bands, respectively, leading to the high degree of order in most striated muscles. Unless some sort of Z-line equivalent exists in vertebrate smooth muscle myofibrils, it is difficult to see how there would be enough registration of filaments for a sarcomeric organization. Although the evidence for two types of thin filaments (33, 70, 73, 99) has helped to resolve some problems (see Sections 4.2, 4.3), at first sight, the proposal for alpha-actinin (and therefore CDBs) being strictly in the cytoskeletal domain seems to cause more conflict than resolution.

Let us consider myofibril organizations consistent with all CDBs being in the cytoskeletal domain: that is, CDBs are not found *within* myofibrils. CDBs may still be *terminal* attachment points for myofibrils even if they are not present *within* the myofibril. One possibility is that myofibrils are only one sarcomere long, with the ends of the contractile domain thin filaments attached to either CDBs or MADBs. This type of organization is compatible with some experiments on CDB distribution (3, 7, 19) (see Section 4.5), but it seems in conflict with most of the immunofluorescent staining, which shows *repetitive* banding patterns, indicating several sarcomeres in a myofibril. Another possibility is that there is a fairly regular repetition of thick filament bundles (bands?) within a bundle of contractile thin filaments, many of which have no attachments to CDBs, but some of which could attach to CDBs at one end of the myofibril. Small seems to favor the latter possibility rather than the one-sarcomere model, since he speaks of the contractile domain as an "actomyosin" domain (99), and an earlier model for myofibrils shows rather randomly organized fibrils of thick and thin filaments with no internal CDBs (96, 100). However, the evidence from S-1 staining and from numerous structural studies shows thin filaments attached to *both* ends of CDBs, implying that CDBs are *internal* structures in a fibril rather than merely terminal attachment points (for reviews of CDB structure and function, see 4, 5, 106, 107). Also, immunofluorescent staining with anti-alpha-actinin reveals interrupted fibrils or strings (3, 20, 28), which are shown especially clearly in the computer-aided reconstructions by Fay et al. (20, 28). If CDBs are excluded from the contractile domain, these fibrils with repeating patterns of alpha-actinin staining must be *cytoskeletal* fibrils. This would lead to an interesting paradox, since S-1 staining reveals myosin-interacting sites on actin filaments attached to CDBs, implying that the cytoskeletal thin filaments attached to CDBs also have the ability to interact specifically with myosin.

Since the immunocytochemical evidence for alpha-actinin being strictly cytoskeletal (see Section 3.4) is not presented as convincingly as the evidence for the two types of thin filaments (33, 73, 99), and since the biochemical evidence for alpha-actinin being cytoskeletal was its close association with filamin-containing thin filaments during extraction procedures (70), the assignment of alpha-actinin exclusively to the cytoskeletal domain seems to be unjustified at the present time. Therefore, the possibility of a sarcomere or minisarcomere structure that includes alpha-actinin should still be considered.

4.5. What are the terminal attachment points for contractile and cytoskeletal units?

Most of the models for smooth muscle cells differ from each other in one important aspect, namely, where the contractile and cytoskeletal units have their terminal attachments. It has been obvious since the studies of Pease and Molinari in 1960 (81) that some thin filaments attach to MADBs (for reviews, see 3, 4, 36, 38, 106, 107), and it was shown by S-1 labeling (107, 118) that the polarity of attached thin filaments indicates that the MADBs are analagous to the terminal Z-lines at the ends of skeletal muscle fibers (117). It has also been shown that in many cases MADBs appose MADBs in adjacent cells with either specialized junctions, elastic fibers, or other extracellular filaments concentrated on the outer plasma membranes of MADB areas, providing for the transmission of force from cell to cell throughout the smooth muscle tissue (36, 38, 39, 121). Therefore, we may say with certainty that the contractile units have at least one terminal attachment to MADBs. To produce shortening, each contractile unit should have an *origin* and an *insertion*, just as a skeletal muscle does. The term *origin* is usually given to the attachment that moves least during muscle shortening, but since we don not have much certainty as to where both ends attach, we will call the ends attached to the plasma membrane the origins.

But where are the insertions? Early work viewed the CDBs as free-floating (for a review of early concepts, see 78). This concept rendered the CDBs as acceptable Z-line equivalents but not as terminal Z-lines. Therefore, it is not too surprising that most early models depicted contractile units (or myofilament bundles) being attached at *both* ends to the plasma membrane (for a critical review of the features of these models, see 4). However, in 1972 Cooke and Fay (19) introduced a model of a cytoskeleton composed of CDBs and IFs, based on a combination of physiological and structural evidence. They were the first to show the importance of the length–tension relationship, the only objective means of determining relative muscle cell length (44, 77), as determining the distribution of contractile and cytoskeletal components. They showed that CDBs and IFs were distributed axially in highly stretched muscles, and more randomly in shortened muscles (17, 19). To account for the changed distribution of CDBs with stretch, they proposed a model in which IFs linked CDBs in a cytoskeletal network that attached to the plasma membrane by means of IFs to MADBs, primarily in the terminal regions of the cell. This is in marked contrast to both vertebrate striated muscles organization and a recently proposed model for ascidian "smooth" muscle (115) where thin filaments attach to terminal regions and IFs attach to lateral plasmalemma, but Cooke (17) showed ultrastructural evidence for the sparse attachment of IFs to lateral plasmalemma in guinea pig taenia coli. Although Cooke and Fay (9) proposed that contractile units attached only to MADBs and did not interact with this cytoskeleton, they did establish CDBs as being part of a cytoskeleton and, therefore, as potential insertions for contractile units.

Our laboratory repeated the Cooke and Fay experiments, not because we did not accept their conclusions, but because we wanted to extend their study by thoroughly describing the changes in distribution of thick and thin filaments. However, contrary to their results, we found that CDB distribution depended upon the contractile state of the muscle in addition to its length, CDBs being less axially concentrated if stretched muscles were actively contracting (7), as if contractile fibrils were attached to MADBs on one end and to CDBs on the other end (for the model developed from these resuslts, see 4), as shown in the model in Figure 2-21. This model is reproduced here not because it is perfect or proven to be correct in every aspect, but because it is consistent with most of foregoing data, including, surprisingly enough, the recent data supporting the two-domain hypothesis (33, 70, 73, 99). With regard to the two-domain hypothesis, the model provides a way that CDBs can be considered cytoskeletal and yet attach to contractile thin filaments if these attachments are the *terminal* insertions of contractile units. Recent results from Cooke's group (20) on CDB movements in isolated cells during contraction tend to corroborate the theory that contractile units either incorporate CDBs or are terminally attached to them. The model also explains the peripheral-to-central layering seen by both Cooke's group (19) and Bagby's (7) in cross sections of highly stretched, relaxed guinea pig taenia coli, where thin filaments are most peripheral, followed by a broad layer of thick and thin filaments, with thin filaments, CDBs, and IFs forming the axial core (7, 19). However, the model is not strictly applicable to smooth muscles having sparse IFs. Both Cooke (20) and this author (Bagby, unpublished data) have noted the apparent lack of IFs in *Bufo* marinus (toad) circular stomach muscle, which would seem to make a cytoskeletal network impossible. However, highly stretched, relaxed *Bufo* stomach muscle shows an axial core of CDBs and lattice bundles of thin filaments (7) as shown in Figure 2-22. According to the two-domain hypothesis (99), the thin filaments containing filamin are the predominant ones that interact with CDBs. It is possible that *cytoskeletal* thin filaments attached to CDBs form this core, whereas *contractile* thin filaments are found peripherally in the contractile units. To have the axial concentration of CDBs occur in highly stretched relaxed muscles that have little or no IFs, these cytoskeletal thin filament bundles would have to have their primary terminal attachments to MADBs in the terminal regions of the cell. Thus, the basic cytoskeletal arrangement could be operative even in cells that lack IFs or have too little IF to provide much mechanical stability to CDBs. In cells that have *both* IFs and cytoskeletal thin filaments attached to CDBs, both IFs and cytoskeletal thin filaments must be mechanically linked to terminal MADBs, rather than midcell MADBs, to account for CDBs becoming axial during passive stretch.

Using mechanical stresses to perturb cells so that the attachment points of cytoskeletal and contractile components can be deduced from CDB distributions is a tricky business at best. It may be that differences in the agonist used for contraction (Bagby and Corey-Kreyling (7) used acetylcholine; Cooke and Fay (19) used K+), the time taken to perform the length–tension study, or the time the muscle remains at a particular length prior to fixation have effects on CDB distribution. With regard to the time factor, Rasmussen et al. (84) have summarized evidence that phosphorylation of cytoskeletal elements occurs much later than phosphorylation of myosin light chains, and they have proposed that the *sustained* contraction that occurs while myosin light chains are not phosphorylated may be due to the events in the cytoskeletal domain. They propose that the cytoskeletal events, triggered by slow phorphorylation of cytoskeletal components, are responsible for the tension usually ascribed to a latch-bridge (1) between myosin and

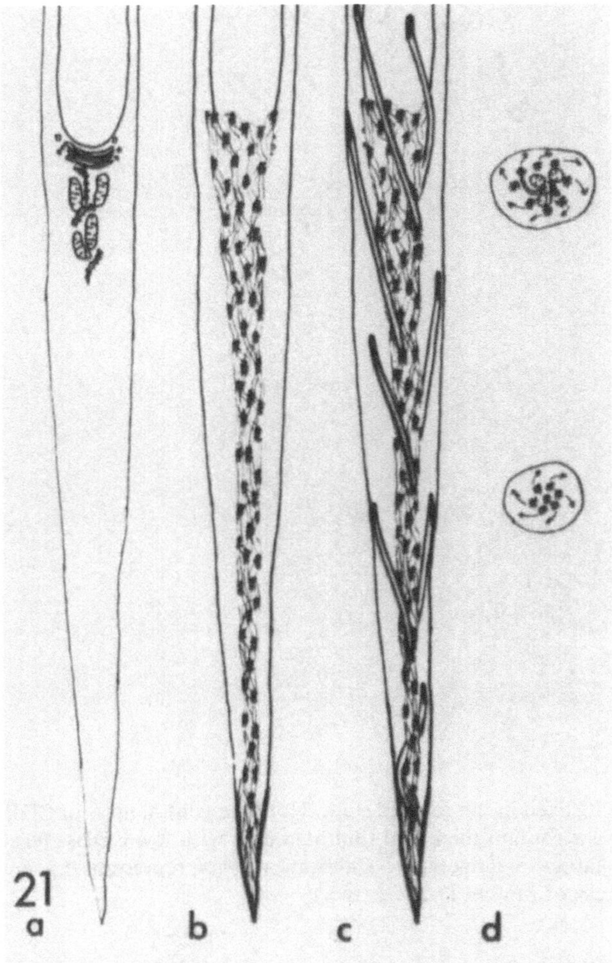

Figure 2-21. A model of the vertebrate smooth muscle cell in which cytoskeletal and contractile components interact. The model's construction progresses from the innermost components (a) to the outermost (b, c). (a) The innermost cell components are the nucleus and membranous organelles concentrated at either end of the nucleus. (b) A cytoskeleton of CDBs and IFs surrounds the innermost components and is located axially in distal regions of the stretched relaxed cell due to primary attachments to the terminal areas, presumably to MADBs. (c) A few myofibrils are shown. These are attached at one end to MADBs and follow helical paths until they attach at their other end to a CDB in the cytoskeleton. (d) Transverse sections of the model at two levels showing the helical paths CDBs should take toward the periphery when myofibrils contract. (Reprinted from Bagby, 1983 (4), by permission of the author and CRC Press, Inc.)

actin-containing filaments. It is clear that the possibility of an "active" cytoskeleton will necessitate additional controls in future length–tension/ultrastructure studies.

The picture that emerges from considering both length–tension/ultrastructural studies and immunocytochemical localizations is that of a cytoskeleton of IFs, filamin-containing thin filaments, and CDBs attached to the MADBs in terminal portions of the cell while the contractile units of thick filaments and caldesmon-containing thin filaments attach by at least one end to MADBs in any region of the cell, and that at least some of the contractile units attach by one end to CDBs in the axial cytoskeleton.

4.6. *What is the path of contractile units?*

The preceding subsection dealt with attachment points for contractile units. To determine the paths of contractile units, it would seem to be a matter of connecting the two points by a straight line, but it is not as simple as that. From the very earliest studies of isolated smooth muscle cells, it was apparent that the orientation of the contractile material, as viewed with polarized light, changed during shortening such that some helical organization provided the most reasonable explanation for the patterns seen (30, 31, 95, 96, 100). Some disagreed with this type of order (27) or attributed it either to surrounding active cells causing passive cells to buckle or to connective tissue attached to cell membranes influencing the cell shape in shortened tissues (34, 36). Early models by Bagby and coworkers (6, 30) and by Small's group (96, 100) based the helical appearance on straight myofilament bundles or on contractile units running from one MADB to another MADB across the cell, with the helical appearance being due to MADB attachment sites having a helical path around the inner surface of the plasmalemma. However, the finding that antivinculin, which stains MADBs, shows longitudinal rows on the plasmalemma (98) (see Fig. 2-19) argues against the helical appearance being due to helical attachment sites. Cells stained with antimyosin (Fig. 2-8) often show myofibrils that follow curved paths (6, 9) and curved fibrils are also seen in living cells viewed with polarized light (6, 7), but curved paths of myofibrils are not consistent with the striated muscle paradigm where myofibrils remain straight as they shorten. Could helical patterns be an artifact unrelated to contractile function? The recent independent work of Warshaw et al. (126) used marker beads attahced

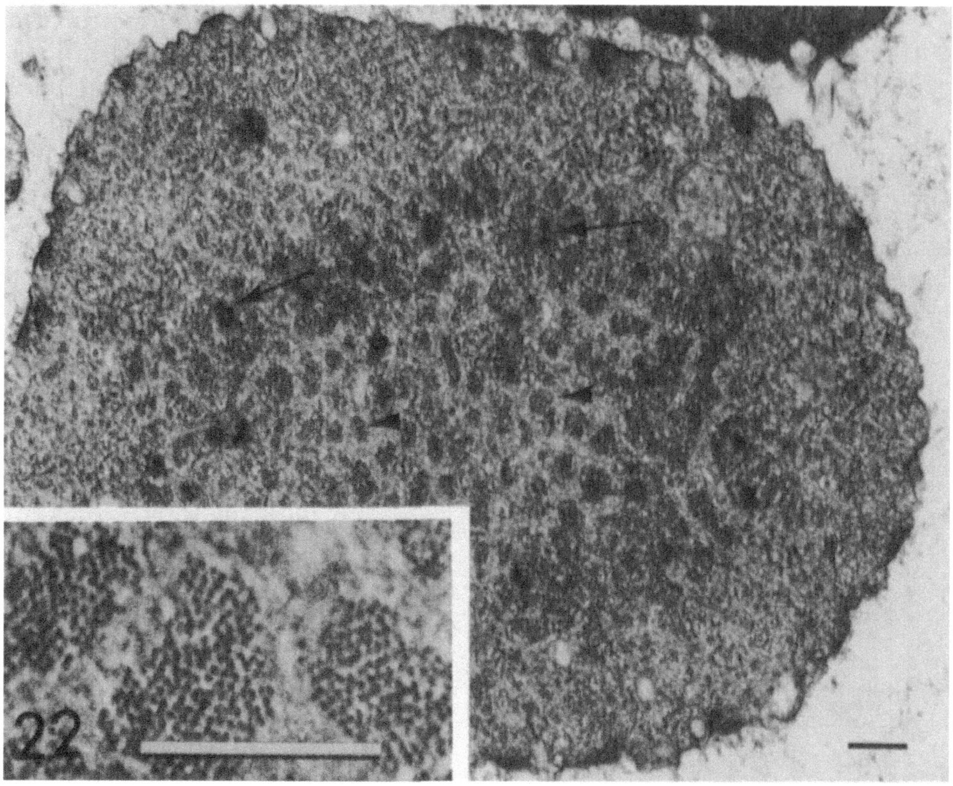

Figure 2-22. Transverse section of *Bufo marinus* stomach muscle at 1.6 L_o fixed in the relaxed state. Note the central mass of CDBs (arrows) and thin filament bundles (arrowheads) while peripheral regions contain thick and thin filaments with few CDBs. Inset: higher magnification of central thin filament bundles showing the lattice arrangement. Calibration bars represent 0.2 μm. (Reprinted from Bagby and Corey-Kreyling, 1984 (7), p. 66, by courtesy of Marcel Dekker, Inc.)

to the plasmalemma of isolated smooth muscle cells to show that these beads traced a helical path during cell shortening. They concluded that the torsion of the cell membrane was probably due to attached contractile units that must be in some helical arrangement.

The model in Figure 2-21 could explain the helical movement of the cell surface (126) and/or peripheral movements of CDBs toward the periphery during contraction (7) being due to the myofibrils, which are attached to MADBs (which need not be helically aligned), and which take a slightly helical path around the periphery of the cell, spiraling toward the axial cytoskeleton and attaching to it terminally by means of thin filaments inserted into CDBs (4). To be consistent with the length–tension/ultrastructure studies (7, 17, 19) and the proposed assignment of all CDBs to the cytoskeletal domain (70, 99), the peripheral myofibrils would *not* contain CDBs that divided sarcomeres, but they might still have reasonably regular repeating bands of thick filaments interspersed with contractile-domain thin filaments, as proposed by Small (96, 100). Since thick filaments are apparently not bipolar (see Section 2.2), the requirements for a Z-line equivalent that changes the polarity of attached thin filaments might not be necessary. (One of the functions of the Z-disc in striated muscles is to provide for a change of thin filament polarity to match the opposite polarities found on each end of bipolar filaments in adjacent sarcomeres (57, 58) between bands of thick filaments.) The periodic strings of stained material seen with anti-alpha-actinin staining (3, 20, 28) could thus be interpreted as interrupted linear MADBs when seen in the periphery or as cytoskeletal fibrils with periodic CDBs when seen in the more axial regons.

This subsection has been more speculative than the preceding ones, but it is believed that the speculations will be useful in directing future ultrastructure research.

5. Summary and suggestions for future work

We have seen, convincingly it is hoped, that the organization of the vertebrate smooth muscle cell contractile system is quite different from that suggested by the vertebrate skeletal muscle paradigm, and also that it does not conform to any *one* paradigm based on another contractile system. However, the probable organization of vertebrate smooth muscle cells is brought into sharper focus by comparison to other contractile systems. The most useful data for determining organization were those obtained from experiments that combined measures of contractile function with structural observations, and those obtained from immunocytochemical localizations. These types of data tended to point toward the same organization, an organization that is markedly different from that formerly proposed from ultrastructural observations alone.

The following is a summary of conclusions from the data reviewed:

1. Thick filaments are composed of myosin (73, 99) and appear to be side-polar (face-polar) (20, 21, 54, 91, 97, 100) rather than bipolar.
2. All thin filaments appear to contain actin and tropomyosin (33, 70, 74, 90), but they can be divided into two types, one of which contains filamin and occupies the cytoskeletal domain (70, 73, 99), and another that contains caldesmon and occupies the contractile domain (33, 70). All thin filaments appear to be decorated by S-1 staining (11, 110, 118).
3. MADBs (membrane-associated dense bodies) are usually arranged in longitudinal bands on the inner surface of the plasmalemma (2, 4, 18, 34, 36–39, 98, 106, 107). They contain alpha-actinin (3, 20, 28, 42, 43, 71, 98, 121), vinculin (42, 43, 85, 98, 121), and talin (121) on the cytoplasmic side, with metavinculin as a possible intramembrane component (92), and they appear to be associated with fibronectin (65) and sialoglycoproteins (85) and other extracellular proteins on the extracellular surface. Both thin filaments and IFs (intermediate filaments) attach to them (for reviews, see 4, 5, 36, 38, 106, 107). S-1 decoration leads to arrowheads pointing away from the MADBs (107, 118), consistent with their being equivalent to terminal Z-lines of skeletal muscle myofibrils.
4. CDBs (cytoplasmic dense bodies) are found throughout the cytoplasm and contain alpha-actinin (3, 20, 28, 42, 43, 71, 90, 99) but not vinculin (42, 43, 121) or talin (121). Thin filaments appear to be a part of the fibrous material of CDBs (11, 106, 107), and they project from either pole (11, 106, 107, 118). Thin filaments decorated with S-1 are shown to have opposite polarities at opposite poles of CDBs (11, 118), with arrowheads pointing away from their attachment (11, 118), consistent with CDBs acting as Z-line equivalents.
5. Although the preceding conclusion is consistent with CDBs acting as Z-lines within myofibrils, some rather sparse immunochemical and biochemical evidence (70, 99) suggests that *all* CDBs are in the cytoskeletal domain. Length–tension/ultrastructural evidence, which shows an axial cytoskeletal domain and a peripheral contractile domain in highly stretched cells (7, 19), shows CDBs predominantly in the cytoskeletal domain also.
6. An earlier model for organization (4) is shown to be consistent with the recent immunocytochemical data (33, 73, 99) as well as with most length–tension/ultrastructural data (7, 19), except that the axial cytoskeleton in the model should contain cytoskeletal thin filaments as well as IFs and CDBs. It also is consistent with recent experiments (126) suggesting a helical organization.

The conclusions reached from the data reviewed are not likely to meet with universal approval, since they are probably not what many investigators had expected. Also, there are some points on which there is an apparent conflict, in which case one set of data has been relied on instead of another, based on how well the data fits to form a consistent model. It may have been premature to guess how the smooth muscle puzzle is put together, but proposing solutions often gives impetus for new studies to prove or disprove a model.

The following are suggestions for future work to help resolve some present conflicts or uncertainties:

1. Experiments that combine length–tension measurements with immunocytochemical localization of muscle proteins. Thus, one would expect axial localization of filamin and desmin

(or vimentin) with stretched, relaxed tissues, but not in shortened tissues.
2. Three-dimensional reconstructions of different portions of smooth muscle cells fixed at known lengths and states of contraction, using serial semi-thin transverse sections viewed with high-voltage TEM to measure, for example, thin filament length.
3. Three-dimensional reconstructions of smooth muscle tissues prepared and sectioned as above but with immunocytochemical staining for viewing with either light or electron microscopy.
4. Use of antibodies to alpha, beta, and gamma isomers of actin (24, 55, 66, 87, 120) to determine whether the cytoskeletal domain contains one type of actin while the contractile domain contains another. Similar experiments with isomers of tropomyosin (24).
5. Careful documentation of the relative cell lengths, contractile conditions, and localities that correspond to the occurrence of lattice, row, or rosette grouping of thin filaments.
6. Determination of whether certain thin filament groupings (e.g., the lattice) are peculiar to only one domain by using antifilamin and anticaldesmon to mark cytoskeletal and contractile thin filaments, respectively.
7. Studies of skinned smooth muscles stained with both S-1 and antifilamin or anticaldesmon to determine whether CDBs having opposite polarity thin filaments at either end (putative Z-line equivalents) are attached to cytoskeletal thin filaments or contractile thin filaments or both.

The last five years have provided some very useful data due to immunocytochemical techniques being applied to both semithin and ultrathin sections. If these techniques are applied in combination with careful attention to the relative length and contractile state, and 3-D reconstruction techniques are applied where needed, the next five years should provide all the data needed to provide a generally accepted model of the contractile system of vertebrate smooth muscle cells. It has been exciting to play even a small role in the development of present models, and we look forward with anticipation to what the future will bring. It is to be hoped that the following complete quotation, the first part of which was used to begin this chapter, will apply then.

"For now we see through a glass, darkly; but then face to face: now I know in part; but then shall I know (fully) even as also I am known." (80)

6. Conclusions

Recent ultrastructural and immunocytochemical data suggest that former concepts of myofilament organization and interaction in vertebrate smooth muscle cells must be revised. Based on the data reviewed, it is suggested that myosin-containing thick filaments are side-polar (face-polar) rather than bipolar, and that there are two types of thin filament: contractile thin filaments composed of actin, tropomyosin, and caldesmon; and cytoskeletal thin filaments composed of actin, tropomyosin, and filamin. The proposal for two domains (contractile and cytoskeletal) in smooth muscle, with different types of thin filaments in each domain, is helpful in explaining many puzzling aspects of cell organization, especially the high thin:thick filament ratio. Although CDBs (cytoplasmic dense bodies) and MADBs (membrane-associated dense bodies) are attachment sites for both thin filaments and the cytoskeletal IFs (intermediate filaments), they have quite different compositions; both CDBs and MADBs contain alpha-actinin, but MADBs contain vinculin, talin, and other proteins not found in CDBs. While MADBs are accepted as the terminal attachment sites for both the contractile system and the cytoskeleton, there is conflicting evidence as to whether CDBs act as Z-lines in the contractile domain or as focal points of a cytoskeletal matrix. Based on the immunocytochemical data and length–tension/ultrastructural data, both of which suggest segregation into cytoskeletal and contractile domains, a model is presented in which contractile fibrils composed of loosely registered thick filaments and contractile-domain thin filaments originate from MADBs and take a gentle helical course around an axial cytoskeleton of CDBs, IFs, and cytoskeletal thin filaments before inserting on CDBs. Future experiments to test the model are also proposed.

Acknowledgments

I should like to thank Prof. Pietro Motta for inviting me to write this chapter. I especially thank those who graciously supplied illustrations and all those whose investigations provided the data base for writing this chapter. Funding for the author's work reviewed in this chapter was provided by the National institutes of Health and the American Heart Association, Tennessee Affiliate. I am very grateful to Mrs. Debbie Pendleton, without whose patient work on the word processor the many corrections to the manuscript would have been impossible. My wife and family have been deprived of my attention during the writing and I thank them for their continued patience. Finally, I thank God the Father, the Son (Jesus Christ), and the Holy Spirit for being an everpresent refuge in difficult times and as the ultimate source of inspiration for my work and writing.

References

1. Aksoy MO, Murphy RA: Regulation of the dynamic properties of smooth muscle: Ca^{++}-stimulated cross-bridge phosphorylation. In: Biochemistry of Smooth Muscle, Vol I. NL Stephens (ed), Baca Raton, FL: CRC Press, p 141–166, 1983.
2. Ashton, FT, Somlyo, AV, Somlyo AP: The contractile apparatus of vascular smooth muscle: intermediate high voltage stereo electron microscopy. *J Mol Biol* 98: 17–29, 1975.
3. Bagby RM: Double-immunofluorescent staining of isolated smooth muscle cells. I. Preparation of anti-chicken gizzard alpha-actinin and its use with anti-chicken gizzard myosin for co-localization of alpha-actinin and myosin in chicken gizzard cells. *Histochemistry* 69: 113–130, 1980.
4. Bagby RM: Organization of contractile elements. In: The Biochemistry of Smooth Muscle, Vol I. NL Stephens (ed), Boca Raton, FL: CRC Press, p 1–84, 1983.
5. Bagby RM: Toward a comprehensive 3-D model of the contractile system of vertebrate smooth muscle cells. *Int Rev Cytol* 105: 67–128, 1986.
6. Bagby RM, Abercrombie RK: Observations on the three-dimensional organization of myofibrils in vertebrate smooth muscle. In: Motility in Cell Function. FA Pepe (ed), New York: Academic Press, p 427–431, 1979.
7. Bagby RM, Corey-Kreyling MD: Structural aspects of the contractile machinery of smoot muscle: Is the organization of smooth muscle compatible with a sliding-filament mechanism: In: Smooth Muscle Contraction. NL Stephens (ed), New York: Marcel Dekker, p 47–74, 1984.
8. Bagby RM, Fisher BA: Effects of DMSO, pH, stretch and calcium ion on the thick filaments in an amphibian smooth muscle. *Eur J Cell Biol* 19: 196–200, 1979.
9. Bagby RM, Pepe FA: Striated myofibrils in anti-myosin-stained isolated chicken gizzard smooth muscle cells. *Histochemistry* 58: 219–235, 1978.
10. Bagby RM, Young A, Dotson R, Fisher BA, McKinnon K: Contraction of single smooth muscle cells from *Bufo marinus* stomach. *Nature (Lond)*, 234: 351–352, 1978.
11. Bond M, Somlyo AV: Dense bodies and actin polarity in vertebrate smooth muscle. *J Cell Biol* 95: 403–413, 1982.
12. Burridge K, Connell L: Talin: a cytoskeletal component concentrated in adhesion plaques and other sites of actin-membrane interaction. *Cell Motil*, 3: 405–417, 1983.
13. Chamley JH, Campbell GR, McConnell JD, Gröschel-Steward U: Comparison of vascular smooth muscle cells from adult human, monkey, and rabbit in primary culture and in subculture. *Cell Tissue Res* 177: 503–522, 1977.
14. Chamley JH, Gröschel-Steward U, Campbell GR, Burnstock G: Distinction between smooth muscle, fibroblasts and endothelial cells in culture by the use of fluoresceinated antibodies against smooth muscle actin. *Cell Tissue Res* 177: 445–457, 1977.
15. Chamley-Campbell J, Campbell GR, Gröschel-Stewart U, Burnstock G: FITC-labeled antibody staining of tropomyosin-containing fibrils in smooth, cardiac, and skeletal muscle cells, prefusion myoblasts, fibroblasts, endothelial cells and 3T3 cells in culture. *Cell Tissue Res* 183: 153–166, 1977.
16. Chamley-Campbell J, Campbell GR, Ross R: The smooth muscle cell in culture. *Physiol Rev* 59: 1–61, 1979.
17. Cooke PH: A filamentous cytoskeleton in vertebrate smooth muscle fibers. *J Cell Biol* 68: 539–556, 1976.
18. Cooke PH: Organization of contractile fibers in smooth muscle. In: Cell and Muscle Motility, Vol 3. RM Dowben, JW Shay (eds), New York: Plenum Press, p 57–77, 1983.
19. Cooke PH, Fay FS: Correlation between fiber length, ultrastructure, and the length–tension relationship of mammalian smooth muscle. *J Cell Biol* 52: 105–116, 1972.
20. Cooke PH, Kargacin G, Craig R, Fogarty K, Fay FS: Molecular structure and organization of filaments in single, skinned smooth muscle cells. In: Regulation and Contraction of Smooth Muscle. New York: Alan R. Liss, Inc., p 1–25, 1987.
21. Craig R, Megerman J: Assembly of smooth muscle myosin into side polar filaments. *J Cell Biol* 75: 990–996, 1977.
22. Driska SP: Mechanical properties, contractile proteins, and regulation of contraction of vascular smooth muscle. In: Physiology and Pathophysiology of the Heart. N Sperelakis (ed), Boston: Martinus-Nijhoff Publishing,

p 757–779, 1984.

23. Eldred WD, Zucker C, Karten HJ, Yazulla S: Comparison of fixation and penetration enhancement techniques for use in ultrastructural immunocytochemistry. *J. Histochem. Cytochem.* 31: 285–292, 1983.
24. Fatigati V, Murphy, RA: Actin and tropomyosin variants in smooth muscles. *J Biol Chem* 259: 14383–14388, 1984.
25. Fay FS, Cooke PH: Reversible disaggregation of myofilaments in vertebrate smooth muscle. *J. Cell Biol* 56: 399–411, 1973.
26. Fay FS, Cooke PH, Canaday PG: Contractile properties of isolated smooth muscle cells. In: Physiology of Smooth Muscle. E Bulbring, MF Shuba (eds), New York: Raven Press, 249–264, 1976.
27. Fay FS, Delise CM: Contraction of isolated smooth muscle cells — structural changes. *Proc Natl Acad Sci USA* 70: 641–645, 1973.
28. Fay FS, Fujiwara K, Rees DD, Fogarty KE: Distribution of alpha-actinin in single isolated smooth muscle cells. *J Cell Biol* 96: 783–795, 1983.
29. Feramisco JR, Blose SH: Distribution of fluorescently labeled alpha-actinin in living and fixed fibroblasts. *J Cell Biol* 86: 608–615, 1980.
30. Fisher BA: A model for vertebrate smooth muscle contraction derived from studies of circular stomach muscle from the tropical toad *Bufo marinus*. Ph.D. dissertation, University of Tennessee, Knoxville, 1974.
31. Fisher BA, Bagby RM: Reorientation of myofilaments during contraction of a vertebrate smooth muscle. *Am J Physiol* 232: C5–C14, 1977.
32. Fujiwara K, Pollard TD: Simultaneous localization of myosin and tublin in human tissue culture cells by double antibody staining. *J Cell Biol* 77: 182–195, 1978.
33. Fürst DO, Cross RA, DeMey J, Small JV: Caldesmon is an elongated, flexible molecule localized in the actomyosin domains of smooth muscle. *EMBO J* 5: 251–257, 1986.
34. Gabella G: Quantitative morphological study of smooth muscle cells of the guinea pig taenia coli. Structural changes in smooth muscle cells during isotonic contraction. *Cell Tissue Res* 170: 161–201, 1976.
35. Gabella G: Arrangement of smooth muscle cells and intramuscular septa in the taenia coli. *Cell Tissue Res* 184: 195–212, 1977.
36. Gabella G: Smooth muscle cell junctions and structural aspects of contraction. *Br Med Bull* 35: 213–218, 1979.
37. Gabella G: An introduction to the structural variety of smooth muscles. In: Vascular Neuroeffector Mechansims. J Bevan et al. (eds), New York: Raven Press, p 13–35, 1983.
38. Gabella G: Structural apparatus for force transmission in smooth muscles. *Physiol Rev* 64: 455–477, 1984.
39. Gabella G: Chicken gizzard: The muscle, the tendon and their attachment. *Anat Embryol* 171: 151–162, 1985.
40. Gabella G: Muscle hypertrophy in the partially obstructed intestine. In: Hypertrophic Response in Smooth Muscle. CL Seidel, NW Weisbrodt (eds), Boca Raton, FL: CRC Press, Inc., p 45–76, 1987.
41. Geiger B: Microfilament-membrane interaction. *Trends Biochem Sci* 10: 456–460, 1985.
42. Geiger B, Dutton AH, Tokuyasu KT, Singer SJ: Immunoelectron microscope studies of membrane–microfilament interactions: distributions of alpha-actinin, tropomyosin, and vinculin in intestinal epithelial brush border and chicken gizzard smooth muscle cells. *J Cell Biol* 91: 614–628, 1982.
43. Geiger B, Tokuyasu KT, Dutton A, Singer SJ: Vinculin, an intracellular protein localized at specialized sites where microfilament bundles terminate at cell membranes. *Proc Natl Acad Sci USA* 77: 4127–4131, 1980.
44. Gordon AM, Huxley AF, Julian F: The variation in isometric tension with sarcomere length in vertebrate muscle fibers. *J Physiol (Lond)* 184: 170–192, 1966.
45. Gordon WE: Immunofluorescent and ultrastructural studies of "sarcomeric" units in stress fibers of cultured non-muscle cells. *Exp Cell Res* 117: 253–260, 1978.
46. Gröschel-Stewart U: Immunocytochemistry of cytoplasmic contractile proteins. *Int Rev Cytol* 65: 193–254, 1980.
47. Gröschel-Stewart U, Ceurremanns S, Lehr I, Mahlmeister C: Production of specific antibodies to contractile proteins and their use in immunofluorescence microscopy. II. Species specific and species nonspecific antibodies to smooth and striated chicken muscle actin. *Histochemistry* 50: 271–279, 1977.
48. Gröschel-Steward U, Chamley JH, Campbell GR, Burnstock G: Comparison of the reaction of cultured smooth and cardiac muscle cells and fibroblasts to specific antibodies to myosin. *Histochemistry* 43: 215–224, 1975.
49. Gröschel-Stewart U, Drenckhahn D: Muscular and cytoplasmic contractile proteins. *Collagen Rel Res* 2: 381–463, 1982.
50. Haberle JR, Coolican SA, Evan A, Hathaway DR: The effects of a calcium dependent protease on the ultrastructure and contractile mechanics of skinned uterine smooth muscle. *J Muscle Res Cell Motil* 6: 347–366, 1985.
51. Hainfeld JF: A small gold-conjugated antibody label: improved resolution for electron microscopy. *Science* 236: 450–453, 1987.
52. Hanson J, Lowy J: The structure of F-actin and of actin filaments isolated from muscle. *J Mol Biol* 6: 46–60, 1963.
53. Heumann HG: Smooth muscle: contraction hypothesis based on the arrangement of actin and myosin filaments in different states of contraction. *Philos Trans R Soc Lond B* 265: 213–217, 1973.
54. Hinssen H, D'Haese J, Small JV, Sobieszek A: Mode of filament assembly of myosins from muscle and non-muscle cells. *J Ultrastruct Res* 64: 282–302, 1978.
55. Hirai S, Hirabayashi T: Developmental change of protein constituents in chicken gizzards. *Dev Biol* 97: 483–493, 1983.
56. Huxley AF: Muscle structure and theories of contraction. *Prog Biophys Biophys Chem* 7:255–318, 1957.
57. Huxley HE: Electron microscope studies on the structure of natural and synthetic protein filaments from striated muscle. *J Mol Biol* 7: 281–308, 1963.
58. Huxley HE: Molecular basis of contraction in cross-striated muscles. In: The Structure and Function of

Muscle, Vol I. GH Bourne (ed), New York: Academic Press, p 301–387, 1972.
59. Ishikawa H, Bischoff R, Holtzer H: Formation of arrowhead complexes with heavy meromyosin in a variety of cell types. *J Cell Biol* 43: 312–328, 1969.
60. Jockush BM, Huckriede A, Wiegand C, Fuchtbauer A: Structural proteins involved in cellular motility as studied by microinjection. *Exp Biol Med* 10: 69–80, 1985.
61. Kamm KE, Stull JT: The function of myosin and myosin light chain kinase phosphorylation in smooth muscle. *Annu Rev Pharmacol Toxicol* 25: 593–620, 1985.
62. Kargacin GJ, Fay FS: Physiological and structural properties of saponin-skinned single smooth muscle cells. *J Gen Physiol* 90: 49–73, 1987.
63. Kossmann T, Furst D, Small JV: Structural and biochemical analysis of skinned smooth muscle preparations. *J Muscle Res Cell Motil* 8: 135–144, 1987.
64. Kreis TE, Birchmeier W: Stress fiber sarcomeres of fibroblasts are contractile. *Cell* 22: 555–561, 1980.
65. Kurisu K, Ohsaki Y, Nagata K, Kukita T, Yoshikawa H, Inai T: Immunoelectron microscopic localization of fibronectin in the smooth muscle layer of mouse intestine. *J Histochem Cytochem* 35: 411–417, 1987.
66. Kuroda M: Change of actin isomers during differentiation of smooth muscle. *Biochim Biophys Acta* 843: 208–213, 1985.
67. Lane BP, Elias J, Drummond E: Immunoelectronmicroscopic localization of alpha-actinin in skeletal muscle cells. *J Histochem Cytochem* 25: 69–72, 1977.
68. Langanger G, Moermans M, Daneels G, Sobieszek A, Debrabander M, DeMey J: The molecular organization of myosin in stress fibers of cultured cells. *J Cell Biol* 102: 200–209, 1986.
69. Lanzavecchia G, Arcidiocono G: Contraction mechanism of helical muscles. *J Submicrosc Cytol* 13: 253–266, 1981.
70. Lehman W, Sheldon A, Madonia W: Diversity in smooth muscle thin filament composition. *Biochim Biophys Acta* 914: 35–39, 1987.
71. Lemanski LF, Paulson DJ, Hill CS, Davis LA, Riles LC, Lim S: Immunoelectron microscopic localization of alpha-actinin on Lowicryl-embedded thin-sectioned tissues. *J Histochem Cytochem* 33: 515–522, 1985.
72. Lowy J, Small JV: the organization of myosin and actin in vertebrate smooth muscle. *Nature (Lond)* 227: 46–51, 1970.
73. Malecki M, Small JV: Immunocytochemistry of contractile and cytoskeletal proteins in smooth muscle: Lowicryl, LR White, and polyvinylalcohol compared. *Protoplasma* 139: 160–169, 1987.
74. Marston SB, Smith CWJ: The thin filaments of smooth muscles. *J Muscle Res Cell Motil* 6: 669–708, 1985.
75. Masaki T: Immunochemical comparison of myosins from chicken cardiac, fast white, slow red, and smooth muscle. *J Biochem* 76: 441–449, 1974.
76. Masaki T, Endo S, Ebashi S: Localization of 6s component of alpha-actinin at Z band. *J Biochem* 62: 630–632, 1967.
77. Murphy RA: Mechanics of vascular smooth muscle. In: Handbook of Physiology. Section 2 The Cardiovascular System. Vol II. Vascular Smooth Muscle. DF Bohr, AP, Somlo, HV Sparks, (eds), Bethesda, MD: American Physiological Society, p 325–351, 1980.
78. Needham DM: Machina Carnis. The Biochemistry of Muscular Contraction in its Historical Development. Cambridge: Cambridge University Press, 1971.
79. Oki M, Tanaka O, Domoto T, Gonda T: Contractile units in mammalian visceral smooth muscle cells. *Shimane J Med Sci* 4: 9–22, 1980.
80. Paul of Tarsus: First epistle to the Corinthians, Ch. 13, v. 12. In: *The Holy Bible*. King James Version, ca A.D. 51.
81. Pease DC, Molinari S: Electron microscopy of muscular arteries; pial vessels of the cat and monkey. *J Ultrastruct Res* 3: 447–468, 1960.
82. Pepe FA, Drucker B: The myosin filament III. C-protein. *J Mol Biol* 99: 609–617, 1975.
83. Prosser CL: Evolution and diversity of nonstriated muscles in vascular smooth muscle. In: Handbook of Physiology, Section 2 The Cardiovascular System, Vol II. Vascular Smooth Muscle. DF Bohr, AP Somlyo, HV Sparks (eds), Bethesda, MD: American Physiological Society, p 635–670, 1980.
84. Rasmussen H, Takua Y, Park S: Protein kinase C in the regulation of smooth muscle contraction. *FASEB J* 1: 177–185, 1987.
85. Rogalski AA: A plasma membrane integral sialoglycoprotein (Sgp 130) molecularly distinguishes nonjunctional dense plaque sites of microfilament attachment. *J Cell Biol* 105: 819–831, 1987.
86. Rosenbluth J: Obliquely striated muscle. In: The Structure and Function of Muscle, Vol I. GH Bourne (ed), New York: Academic Press, p 389–420, 1972.
87. Rubenstein PA: Differential behavior of gizzard isoactions. *Arch Biochem Biophys* 210: 598–608, 1981.
88. Sanger JM, Mittal B, Pochapin M, Sanger JW: Observations of microfilament bundles in living cells microinjected with fluorescently labelled contractile proteins. *J Cell Sci* Suppl 5: 17–44, 1986.
89. Sanger JW, Mittal B, Sanger JM: Interaction of fluorescently labeled contractile proteins with the cytoskeleton in cell models. *J Cell Biol* 99: 918–928, 1984.
90. Schollmeyer JE, Furcht LT, Goll DE, Robson RM, Stromer MH: Localization of contractile proteins in smooth muscle cells and in normal and transformed fibroblasts. In: Cell Motility, Cold Spring Harbor Conference on Cell Proliferation, Vol 3, Book A. RD Goldman, TD Pollard, JL Rosenbaum (eds), Cold Spring Harbor, NY: Cold Spring Harbor Laboratory, p 361–387, 1976.
91. Shoenberg CF, Stewart M: Filament formation in smooth muscle homogenates. *J Muscle Res Cell Motil* 1: 117–126, 1980.
92. Siciliano JD, Craig SW: Meta-vinculin — a vinculin-related protein with solubility of a membrane system. *Nature (Lond)* 300: 533–534, 1982.
93. Singer II: Association of fibronectin and vinculin with focal contacts and stress fibers in stationary hamster fibroblasts. *J Cell Biol* 92: 398–408, 1982.
94. Sleek GE, Duling BR: Coordination of mural elements

and myofilaments during arteriolar constriction. *Circ Res* 59: 620–627, 1986.
95. Small JV: Contractile units in vertebrate smooth muscle cells. *Nature (Lond)* 249: 324–327, 1974.
96. Small JV: Studies on isolated smooth muscle cells: the contractile apparatus. *J Cell Sci* 24: 327–349, 1977.
97. Small JV: The contractile apparatus of the smooth muscle cell: structure and composition. In: The Biochemistry of Smooth Muscle. NL Stephens (ed), Baltimore, MD: University Park Press, p 379–411, 1977.
98. Small JV: Geometry of actin-membrane attachments in the smooth muscle cell: the localisations of vinculin and alpha-actinin. *EMBO J* 4: 45–49, 1985.
99. Small JV, Fürst DO, DeMey J: Localization of filamin in smooth muscle. *J Cell Biol* 102: 210–220, 1986.
100. Small JV, Sobieszek A: The contractile apparatus of smooth muscle. *Int Rev Cytol* 64: 241–306, 1980.
101. Small JV, Sobieszek A: Contractile and structural proteins of Smooth Muscle. In: Biochemistry of Smooth Muscle, Vol I. NL Stephens (ed), Boca Raton, FL: CRC Press, p 85–140, 1983.
102. Small JV, Squire JM: Structural basis of contraction in vertebrate smooth muscle. *J Mol Biol* 67: 117–149, 1972.
103. Smith RC, Cande WZ, Craig R, Tooth PJ, Scholey JM, Kendrick-Jones J: Regulation of myosin-filament assembly by light-chain phosphorylation. *Philos Trans R Soc Lond B* 302: 73–82, 1983.
104. Sobieszek A: The fine structure of the contractile apparatus of the anterior byssus retractor muscle of *Mytilus edulis*. *J Ultrastruct Res* 43: 313–343, 1973.
105. Sobue K, Muramoto Y, Fujita M, Kakiuchi S: Purification of a calmodulin binding protein from chicken gizzard that interacts with F-actin. *Proc Nat Acad Sci USA* 78: 5652–5655, 1981.
106. Somlyo AV: Ultrastructure of vascular smooth muscle. In: Handbook of Physiology, Section 2 The Cardiovascular System, Vol II. Vascular Smooth Muscle. DF Bohr, AP Somlyo, HV Sparks (eds), Bethesda, MD: American Physiological Society, p 33–67, 1980.
107. Somlyo AV, Ashton FT, Lemanski LF, Vallieres J, Somlyo AP: Filament organization and dense bodies in vertebrate smooth muscle. In: The Biochemistry of Smooth Muscle. NL Stephens (ed), Baltimore, MD: University Park Press, p 445–471, 1977.
108. Somlyo AV, Ashton FT, Lemanski LF, Vallieres J, Somlyo AP: Excitation–contraction coupling and the ultrastructure of smooth muscle. *Circ Res* 57: 497–507, 1985.
109. Somlyo AP, Devine CE, Somlyo AV, Rice RV: Filament organization in vertebrate smooth muscle. *Philos Trans R Soc Lond B* 265: 223–229, 1973.
110. Somlyo AV, Franzini-Armstrong C: New views of smooth muscle structure using freezing, deep-etching and rotary shadowing. *Experientia* 41: 841–856, 1985.
111. Somlyo AV, Goldman YE, Fujimori T, Bond M, Trentham DR, Somlyo AP: Cross-bridge kinetics, cooperativity, and negatively strained cross-bridges in vertebrate smooth muscle. A laser-flash photolysis study. *J Gen Physiol* 91: 165–192, 1988.
112. Somlyo AP, Somlyo AV, Devine CE, Rice RV: Aggregation of thick filaments into ribbons in mammalian smooth muscle. *Nature New Biol (Lond)* 231: 243–246, 1971.
113. Starr R, Almond R, Offer G: Location of C-protein, H-protein and X-protein in rabbit skeletal muscle fibre types. *J Muscle Res Cell Motil* 6: 227–256, 1985.
114. Terakado K: Fine structure of ascidian smooth muscle. *Zool Sci* 4: 751–762, 1987.
115. Terakado K: The pattern of organization of intermediate filaments and their asymmetrical association with dense bodies in smooth muscle of an ascidian *Halocynthia roretzi*. *Cell Tissue Res* 252: 23–32, 1988.
116. Tokuyasu KT: Application of cryoultramicrotomy to immunocytochemistry. *J Microsc* 143: 139–149, 1986.
117. Trotter JA, Eberhard S, Samora A: Structual domains of the muscle-tendon junction. 1. The internal lamina and the connecting domain. *Anat Rec* 207: 573–591, 1983.
118. Tsukita S, Tsukita S, Ishikawa H: Association of actin and 10 nm filaments with the dense body in smooth muscle cells of the chicken gizzard. *Cell Tissue Res* 229: 233–242, 1983.
119. Uehara Y, Campbell GR, Burnstock G: Cytoplasmic filaments in developing and adult vertebrate smooth muscle. *J Cell Biol* 50: 484–497, 1971.
120. Vandekerckhove J, Weber K: Chordate muscle actins differ distinctly from invertebrate muscle actins. The evolution of the different vertebrate muscle actins. *J Mol Biol* 179: 391–413, 1984.
121. Volberg T, Sabanay H, Geiger B: Spatial and temporal relationships between vinculin and talin in the developing chicken gizzard smooth muscle. *Differentiation* 32: 34–43, 1986.
122. Walmsley JG, Murphy RA: Force–length dependence of arterial lamellar, smooth muscle, and myofilament orientations. *Am J Physiol* 253: H1141–H1147, 1987.
123. Walsh MP: Caldesmon, a major actin- and calmodulin-binding protein of smooth muscle. In: Regulation and Contraction of Smooth Muscle. New York: Alan R. Liss, Inc., p 119–141, 1987.
124. Wang K, Ash J, Singer SJ: Filamin, a new high-molecular-weight protein found in smooth muscle and non-muscle cells. *Proc Nat Acad Sci USA* 72: 4483–4486, 1975.
125. Wang K, Feramisco JR, Ash JF: Fluorescent localization of contractile proteins in tissue culture cells. In: Methods in Enzymology, Vol 85, Part B, The Contractile Apparatus and the Cytoskeleton. DW Frederiksen, LW Cunningham (eds), p 514–562, 1982.
126. Warshaw DM, McBride WJ, Work SS: Corkscrew-like shortening in single smooth muscle cells. *Science* 236: 1457–1459, 1987.
127. Weber K, Gröschel-Stewart U: Antibody to myosin: the specific visualization of myosin-containing filaments in nonmuscle cells. *Proc Natl Acad Sci USA* 71: 4561–4564, 1974.
128. Weeds A: Actin binding proteins — regulators of cell architecture and motility. *Nature (Lond)* 296: 811–816, 1983.
129. Weihing RR: The filamins: properties and functions. *Can J Biochem Cell Biol* 63: 397–413, 1985.

130. Willingham MC: An alternative fixation-processing method for preembedding ultrastructural immunocytochemistry of cytoplasmic antigens: the GBS (glutaraldehyde-borohydride-saponin) procedure. *J Histochem Cytochem* 31: 791–798, 1983.
131. Wulf E, Deboben A, Bautz FA, Faulstick H, Wieland T: Fluorescent phallotoxin, a tool for the visualization of cellular actin. *Proc Natl Acad Sci USA* 76: 4498–4502, 1979.

Author's address:
Prof. Roland M. Bagby
Department of Zoology
University of Tennessee
Knoxville, TN 37996-0810
USA

CHAPTER 3

The three-dimensional ultrastructure of intracellular organization of smooth muscle cells by scanning electron microscopy

TAKAO INOUÉ

1. Introduction

The membranous organization of smooth muscle cells is characterized by surface caveolae, sarcoplasmic reticulum, and mitochondria. Their structures are quite different from those recognized in skeletal or cardiac muscle cells. In smooth muscle cells, the surface caveolae and the sarcoplasmic reticulum are of great interest from the viewpoint of excitation–contraction coupling.

Although the fine structure of smooth muscle cells has been minutely studied by transmission electron microscopy (TEM) (1–7), the three-dimensional organization is still far from being completely understood. An ultrathin sectioning method for TEM has become one of the routine techniques for investigating ultrastructures. However, the three-dimensional architecture of the intracellular structures is not readily appreciated in two-dimensional thin sections.

In contrast, scanning electron microscopy (SEM) is useful to observe materials in three dimensions. However, it has been considered unsuitable for observing intracellular fine structures because of its low resolving power. In recent years, techniques have been reported to achieve high resolution in SEM, and recent development of specimen preparation techniques enabled us to observe intracellular organization three-dimensionally at high resolution (8, 9). In particular, an aldehyde-osmium-dimethyl sulfoxide-osmium method (an A-O-D-O method) (10) and a freeze-polishing method (11) have proved effective for observing intracellular structures of smooth muscle cells at high magnification.

A few articles have been published on the intracellular structures of smooth muscle cells by SEM (12–15), and their SEM images contain much information on the three-dimensional intracellular organization. This chapter intends to describe SEM methods for investigating intracellular structures of smooth muscle cells and to introduce some new findings obtained from the SEM studies on the small intestinal smooth muscle cells. Furthermore, the advantage of the SEM application to the intracellular investigations of smooth muscle cells will be discussed in comparison with TEM studies previously reported.

2. Specimen preparation

In specimen preparations for electron microscopy, 2%–3% glutaraldehyde is usually used for initial fixation of biological samples. Although effective for TEM studies as well as for surface observation by SEM, this fixative is not suitable for observing intracellular structures by SEM, because both cytoplasmic matrices and filamentous structures are fixed firmly, thus preventing the visualization of membranous structures. To observe the intracellular structures, either 1% osmium tetroxide or a mixture of 0.5% glutaraldehyde and 0.5% formaldehyde can be used (10, 16).

To reveal the interior of smooth muscle cells, three kinds of specimen preparations have been reported: a tearing method (12, 13), a freeze-cracking method (9, 15), and a freeze-polishing method (11). Sawada (12) first demonstrated many caveolae on the inner surface of the plasmalemma of the smooth muscle cells from guinea pig taenia coli under SEM using the tearing method (12, 13). According to his method, the tissues were fixed by perfusion with either 2% formaldehyde–2.5% glutaraldehyde in 0.1 M cacodylate buffer or with 1% formaldehyde–1% glutaraldehyde in 0.1 M cacodylate buffer. The fixed specimens were then conductive-stained, dehydrated, and critical-point dried. The dried samples were then torn to reveal the interior. By this method, many caveolae arranged in rows were clearly shown under SEM. Although sarcoplasmic reticulum and mitochondria were also demonstrated by this method, it is difficult to elucidate their three-dimensional organization. This is because such membranous structures were mostly hidden in the myofilaments of the cells.

A freeze-cracking or freeze-fracturing method is effective to expose the interior of cells and tissues. Many methods for SEM have been developed. In these methods, frozen specimens, previously treated with a cryoprotectant are fractured on a metal plate chilled with liquid nitrogen using a razor blade and a hammer. As cryoprotectants, glycerol (17), ethanol (18), and dimethyl sulfoxide (DMSO) (19) have been used. DMSO is superior among these.

Although the freeze-cracking method has been widely applied to bulk tissues, it is difficult to fracture thin materials parallel to the specimen surface. A freeze-polishing method was developed to resolve the difficulty (11). According to this method, intracellular structures are exposed by abrasing frozen specimens using a polishing film at low temperature. The internal structures of mesothelial cells and smooth muscle cells were displayed using this technique (9,11).

Since the intracellular membranous structures of the cracked or polished surfaces are usually embedded within fixed cytoplasmic matrices, they cannot be displayed without removing the excess cytoplasmic matrix. For this problem, an osmic maceration technique was developed (10), with which the excess cytoplasmic matrix can be removed with 0.1% osmium tetroxide at 20°C for three days. The membranous structures such as endoplasmic reticulum and mitochondria were unaffected by the treatment; therefore, three-dimensional architecture is clearly demonstrated under SEM. The mechanism of the extraction of the cytoplasmic matrix by the dilute osmium tetroxide was discussed by Inoué (9). The osmic maceration method was subsequently found to dissolve fixed myofilaments, enabling the three-dimensional demonstration of the sarcoplasmic reticulum of skeletal and cardiac muscle cells (20, 21). Cytoskeletal elements are also dissolved by maceration (10). However, such elements in cultured cells can be retained by shortening maceration periods (22). In smooth muscle cells, it will be possible to demonstrate myofilaments at high magnification under SEM with a suitable specimen preparation.

The method for observing intracellular membranous structures of small intestinal smooth muscle cells is here introduced. All the figures described here were obtained by the following methods.

As materials, smooth muscle cells of the mouse small intestine were used. After animals were sacrificied by cervical dislocation, a mixture of 0.5% glutaraldehyde and 0.5% formaldehyde in 1/15 M phosphate buffer (pH 7.2) was perfused from the left ventricle. After rinsing in the buffer, specimens were postfixed with 1% osmium tetroxide for one hour at room temperature, rinsed, and successively transferred to 25% and 50% DMSO solutions for 30 minutes each. Intracellular structures were then exposed either by the freeze-cracking method using DMSO (19) or by the freeze-polishing method (11). In the freeze-cracking method, they were placed and frozen on a metal plate chilled with liquid nitrogen, and were split into two pieces by a precooled razor blade and a hammer using a freeze-cracking apparatus (TF-1; EIKO Engineering Co. Ltd., Japan). In the freeze-polishing method, frozen specimens on the metal plate chilled with liquid nitrogen were abraded against a precooled polishing film (Imperial Lapping Film, grain size; 1 μm, 0.3 μm, 3M Co. Ltd., USA) using the same freeze-cracking apparatus. After exposing the interior of the specimen, they were thawed in 50% DMSO at room temperature. They were then rinsed in the buffer, treated with 1% osmium tetroxide, rinsed again, and placed in 0.1% osmium tetroxide for 72 hours at 20°C (the osmic

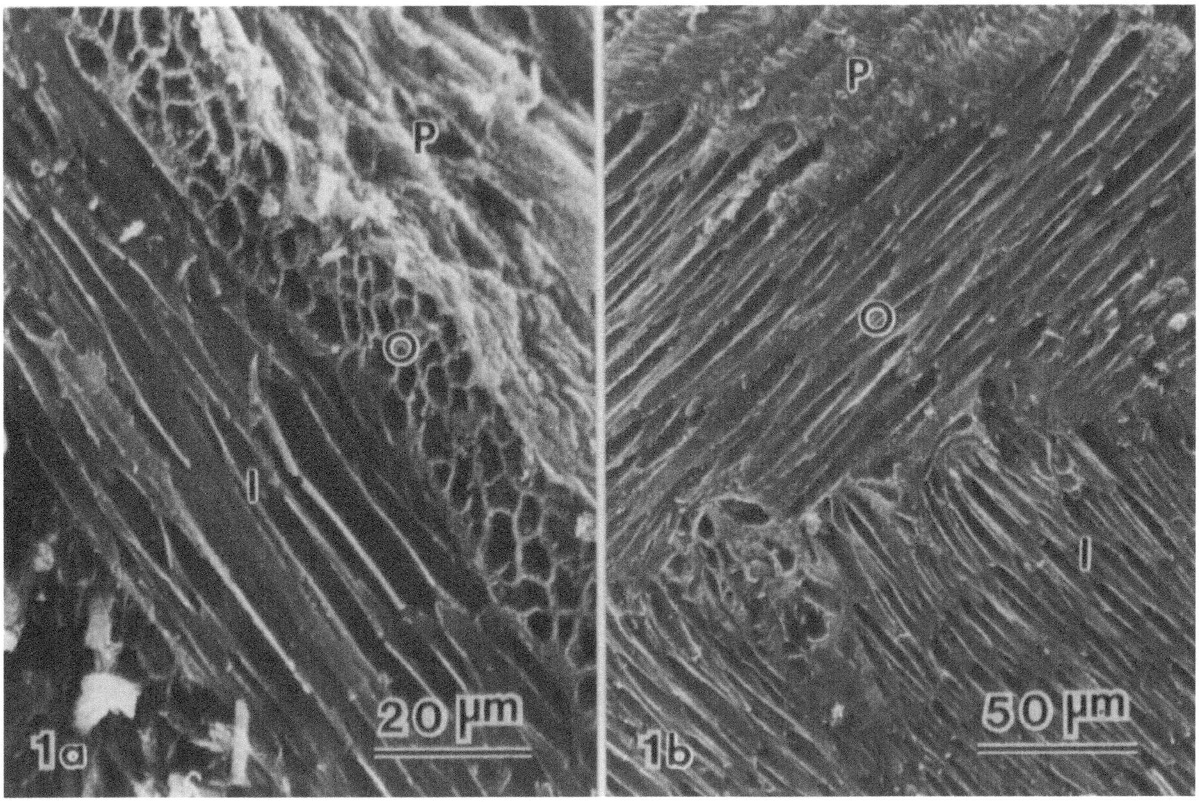

Figure 3-1. A low-magnification view of the fractured surface of a mouse small intestine exposed by a freeze-cracking method (a) and a freeze-polishing one (b). Figure 3-1a shows a cross section through the small intestine, demonstrating the outer longitudinal and the inner circular muscular layer in cross and longitudinal sections, respectively. Figure 3-1b shows a polished surface parallel to the serosal surface. Both two-muscular layers are exposed longitudinally. O: Outer muscular layer; I: Inner muscular layer; P: Peritoneal layer.

maceration procedure of the A-O-D-O method (10). They were further conductive-stained with 1% osmium tetroxide and 2% tannic acid (23), dehydrated in a graded series of ethanol, and critical-point dried using dry ice (24). The dried specimens were coated with platinum of approximately 4 nm in thickness using an ion sputter coater with a rotating stage (VX-10R, EIKO Engineering Co. Ltd., Japan), and observed with a field emission SEM (Hitachi HFS-2ST) operated at 25 kV. Stereopairs were taken at tilt angles 10°–20° apart.

3. Intracellular organelles of smooth muscle cells of the mouse small intestine

3.1. Muscular layer of the small intestine

The muscularis externa of the small intestine is composed of two distinct muscular layers: an inner circular and an outer longitudinal layer.

Figures 3-1a and 3-1b show the fractured surfaces of the muscular layers obtained by the freeze-cracking and the freeze-polishing method, respectively. In Figure 3-1a, the outer longitudinal and the inner circular muscular layer, having been cracked transversely to the long axis of the small intestine, are demonstrated in cross and longitudinal sections, respectively. In Figure 3-1b, both the outer and the inner muscular layer are revealed in longitudinal sections, since the specimen has been abraded from the serosal surface. To observe the interior of the smooth muscle cells, the longitudinal fracture is preferable to the cross fracture, because the internal structures are exposed more widely. It is evident that the ultrastructural comparison between the outer and the inner muscular layer can be easily performed in the longitudinal fracture. Ultrastructural differences between the longitudinal and circular muscle cells were reported in the guinea pig stomach (25) and the guinea pig ileum (26). In the present observations on the intracellular organelles of the mouse small intestine, significant differences between the two muscular layers have not been thus far noted.

3.2. *Surface caveolae*

In ultrathin sections cut perpendicularly to the cell surface of smooth muscle cells, the plasma membrane shows numerous oval or flask-shaped invaginations. The membrane of the invagination has a trilamellar structure, similar to the plasma membrane. The invaginations have been called pinocytotic vesicles (1,27), surface inpocketings (2), caveolae intracellulares (4,7,28–30), or surface vesicles (5,6,31). Strictly speaking, the invagination is not a spherical vesicle but a caveola, which is restricted on the surface cell membrane. For this reason, *surface caveola* is the most suitable terminology for describing the invagination. The distribution of the caveolae has been well understood by freeze-replica techniques (27,31–35). It is true that the images of the replica provide us with a three-dimensional appearance, but the surfaces exposed are not large enough when compared with SEM specimens. Furthermore, the relationship between caveolae and sarcoplasmic reticulum cannot be estimated sufficiently because the cells contain a large amount of myofilaments. Without removing or dissolving them, it would be difficult to investigate such membranous system adequately, even if a deep-etching and rotary shadowing technique is introduced. Under SEM, the arrangement of the surface caveolae was first demonstrated by Sawada (12,13), who described many caveolae arranged in five or six rows parallel to the longitudinal axis of the smooth muscle cells from guinea pig taenia coli. He also exposed the true outer surface of the cell by incubation with 0.2% pronase at 37°C for 30 minutes prior to fixation, and demonstrated many openings of the caveolae on its surface under SEM.

On the cytoplasmic side of the plasma membrane of the smooth muscular layer from the mouse small intestine, many vesicular structures that correspond to surface caveolae are observed (Fig. 3-2). They are usually arranged in ordered linear aggregates separated from each other by intervening flat areas (Fig. 3-2, 3-4–3-6), but are occasionally distributed randomly (Fig. 3-2). The discrepancy in the caveolae distribution seems to reflect the regional difference in the cell. The random distribution of the caveolae is usually observed in the vicinity of the perinuclear region, while the regular row arrangement is commonly seen in the peripheral region far from the nucleus. The rows of the caveolae are 2 to 12 vesicles wide (0.2–0.6 μm in width). The flat clear spaces between the rows of caveolae are approximately 0.1–0.3 μm wide. The rows of the clear spaces between the caveolae correspond to the areas where myofilamentous bundles or dense bodies have been located before the osmic maceration procedure. Dense bodies observed in thin sections (5,6) or in freeze-replicas (27) have not been observed by SEM. The linear arrangement of the aggregation of surface caveolae in smooth muscle cells has been reported from thin-sectioned images (4,6,29) and freeze-replica images (27,31,34). Such a regular arrangement is not noted in skeletal and cardiac muscles.

Most of the individual caveolae recognized in the mouse small intestinal muscle cells appear spherical or oval in shape, and measure 60–70 nm in diameter. When viewed stereoscopically, the caveolae appear to have a narrow neck just beneath the plasma membrane (Fig. 3-3). Often, neighboring caveolae appear fused to each other, forming double-vesiculated caveolae (Fig. 3-4) or multivesiculated ones (Fig. 3-10). Several kinds of such membranous invaginations have been described in turtle oviduct smooth muscle cells: flask-shaped vesicles, tubular ones, and multilobed ones (5). The flask-shaped invagination is the most common type in the surface caveolae recognized in the small intestinal smooth muscle cells. The multilobed vesicles described by Somlyo et al. (5) correspond to multivesiculated caveolae shown in this study. In the smooth muscle cells of the mouse small intestine, the tubular invagination was unrecognized under SEM. All the caveolae demonstrated under SEM appear to be uncoated with clathrin basket on their surfaces, although Riley (29) reported that

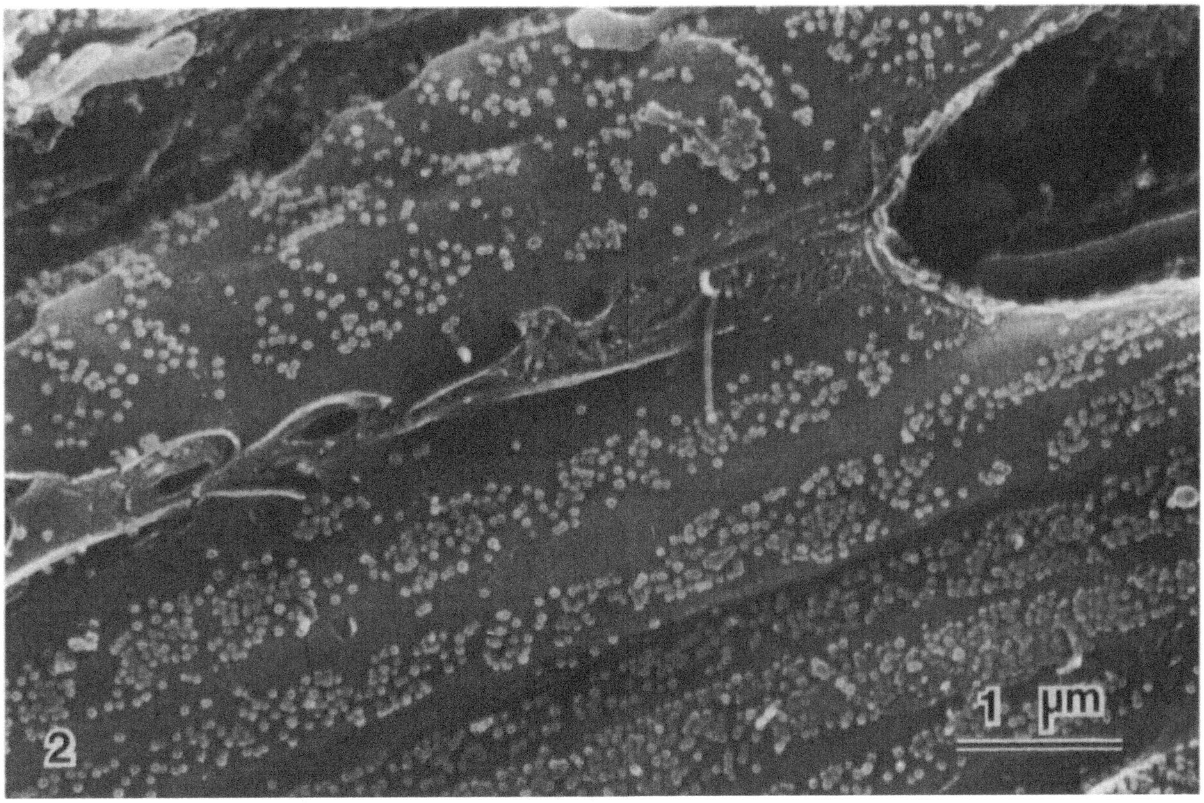

Figure 3-2. A fractured surface of mouse small intestinal smooth muscle cells, demonstrating the cytoplasmic side of the plasma membranes. Since intracellular organelles and filamentous elements have been removed during the specimen preparation, the cytoplasmic side of the plasma membrane is revealed. Many surface caveolae are observed underneath the plasma membrane. In this micrograph, the cytoplasmic sides of two different smooth muscle cells (the upper and the lower of the micrograph) are shown. Most of the surface caveolae are arranged in ordered linear aggregates as shown in the lower part of the micrograph, but some are randomly distributed as shown in the upper part.

coated caveolae are occasionally seen in guinea pig taenia coli smooth muscle cells. This is because the clathrin framework of coated vesicles is dissolved during the osmic maceration procedure (Inoué, unpublished).

It is of interest whether or not muscular contraction changes the number, distribution, or contour of surface caveolae. In freeze-replica studies comparing relaxed and contracted smooth muscle cells, Watanabe and Yamamoto (27) reported that no differences were detected either in the width of the rows of the caveolae or in the center-to-center distances of adjacent vesicles. In contrast, Gansler (36) and Kelly and Rice (3) described an increase in the number of the caveolae in smooth muscle cells during contraction. No attempts have been made to clarify such structural changes between contraction and relaxation by SEM.

3.3. Sarcoplasmic reticulum

Three-dimensional pictures of the sarcoplasmic reticulum in skeletal or cardiac muscle cells have been described based on the intensive studies of the ultrathin sections (37, 38) or on the stereoscopical investigations of thick sections previously stained with heavy metals (39). On the other hand, in smooth muscle cells few pictures of the sarcoplasmic reticulum have been described (40). This may be due to the structural complexity of sarcoplasmic reticulum in smooth muscle cells.

When TEM was first introduced to study the ultrastructure studies of smooth muscle cells, it was generally accepted that sarcoplasmic reticulum was poorly developed in smooth muscle cells, especially when compared with striated muscles (1, 18). Many studies, however subsequently confirmed the occurrence of a relatively

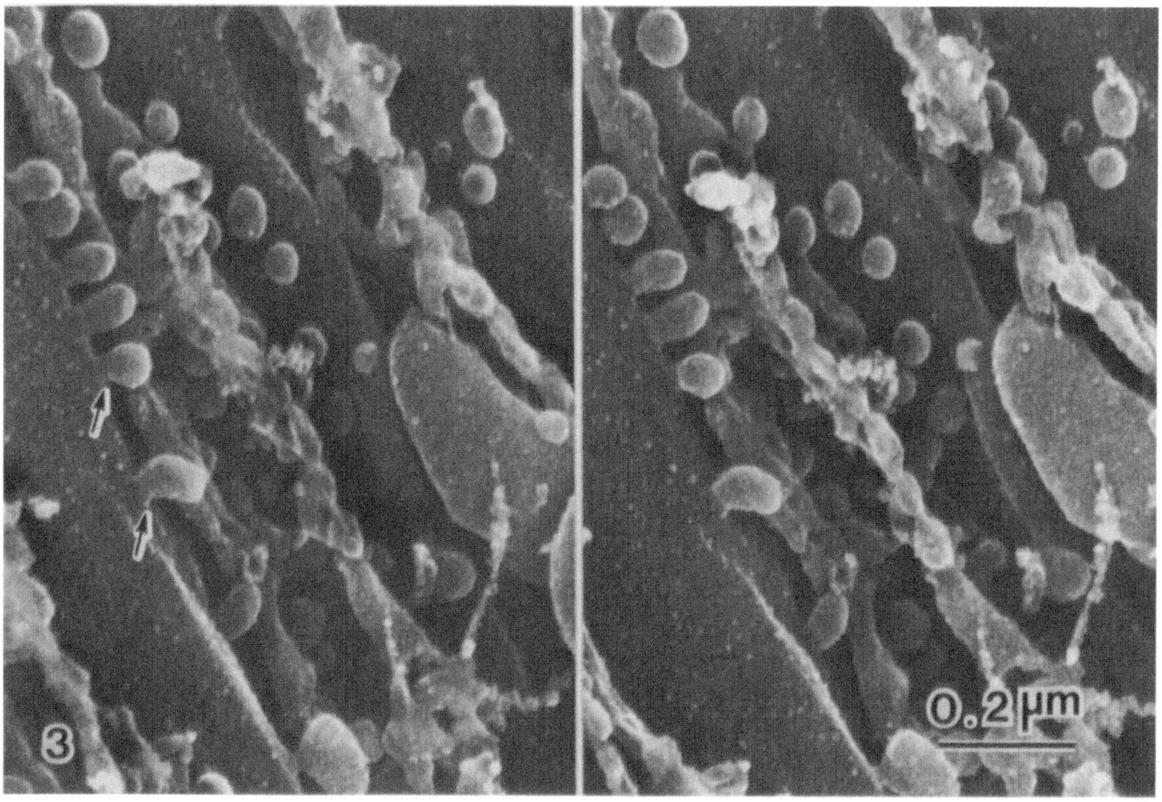
3
0.2 µm

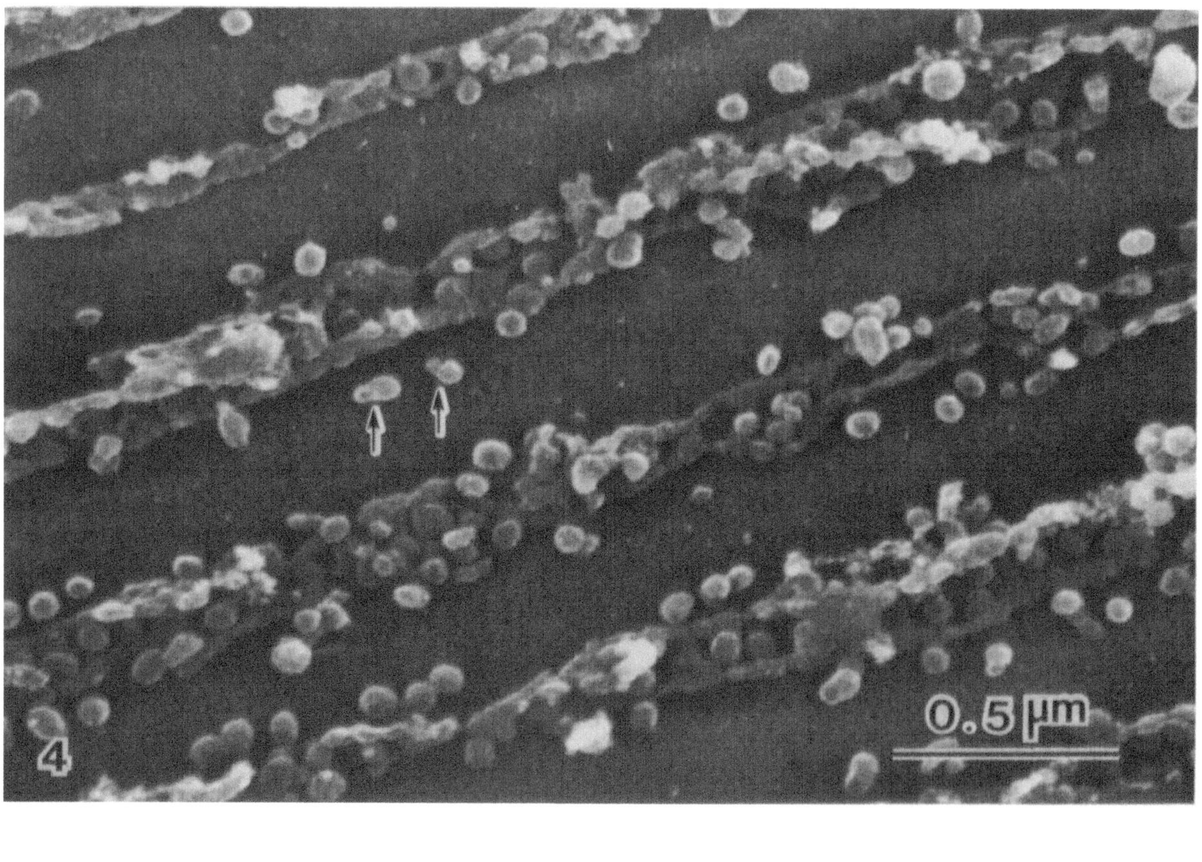
4
0.5 µm

abundant sarcoplasmic reticulum (4–6, 31, 41). Thus far, the morphology of sarcoplasmic reticulum has been studied mainly by ultrathin sections (2, 4–6, 29, 30), and the close association between sarcoplasmic reticulum and surface caveolae has been demonstrated. In a tangential section through the peripheral portion of a smooth muscle cell, a lacelike network of sarcoplasmic reticulum encircled surface caveolae (4, 6). Such spatial relationship has received great attention from the viewpoint of excitation–contraction coupling (4, 6). Under SEM, Sawada (12) first demonstrated sarcoplasmic reticulum as well as surface caveolae in guinea pig taenia coli. His results, however, were unsatisfactory from the three-dimensional analysis of the membranous system by SEM, because the sarcoplasmic reticulum was embedded within the large amount of myofilaments as well as within the fixed cytoplasmic matrix. When specimens were prepared with an osmic maceration treatment (10), which can dissolve both cytoplasmic matrix and myofibrils, the sarcoplasmic reticulum was clearly demonstrated in three dimensions under SEM (15). In such specimens, the relationship between sarcoplasmic reticulum and other membranous elements (e.g., surface vesicles and mitochondria) was clearly displayed.

As for the three-dimensional structure of the sarcoplasmic reticulum in a smooth muscle cell, the diagram of Popescu and Bruijn (40) is the only one available, as far as this author knows. They observed the intracellular topography of the sarcoplasmic reticulum stained by a potassium-oxalate method (potassium oxalate is a specific chemical prefixation of calcium), and classified the topography of the sarcoplasmic reticulum into three types: peripheral, intermediate, and central. According to their findings, the peripheral sarcoplasmic reticulum lies beneath the plasma membrane, both across and along the longitudinal axis of the cell, forming a network among the caveolae. This peripheral sarcoplasmic reticulum is tubular and occasionally is in close contact with the plasmalemma (junctional sarcoplasmic reticulum). The intermediate sarcoplasmic reticulum is radially arranged, connecting the peripheral sarcoplasmic reticulum with the central sarcoplasmic reticulum. The central sarcoplasmic reticulum is located deeply in the central sarcoplasmic axis, among the myofilaments.

The three-dimensional topography demonstrated under SEM is fundamentally the same as that proposed by Popescu and Bruijn (40) or described from ultrathin sections (1–6), but it differs in some points and involves some new findings. Observations by SEM have confirmed that all types of sarcoplasmic reticulum are connected to each other, forming a continuous system. In this chapter, we have classified the sarcoplasmic reticulum of smooth muscle cells into three types from our SEM findings: peripheral, perinuclear, and connecting.

3.3.1. Peripheral sarcoplasmic reticulum. A well-developed sarcoplasmic reticulum is commonly found underneath a plasma membrane or underneath a surface caveolae, spreading in close relationship with the caveolae (Figs. 3-4–3-7). We refer to such sub-surface sarcoplasmic reticulum as *peripheral.* The sarcoplasmic reticulum is usually accompanied with the ordered linear aggregation of the surface caveolae and is not recognized in the flat clear area where no surface caveolae are present. Three types of the sarcoplasmic reticulum are distinguishable from their morphology; tubular, fenestrated, and netty.

The tubular sarcoplasmic reticulum is observed along the linear aggregation of the caveolae partially skirting one to four vesicles (Fig. 3-4). This tubular sarcoplasmic reticulum usually occurs

Figure 3-3. A stereomicrograph of the cytoplasmic side of the plasma membrane of a mouse small intestinal smooth muscle cell. When viewed stereoscopically, the narrow necks of the surface cavolae are clearly seen (arrows). Peripheral sarcoplasmic reticulum skirting the surface caveolae is continuous with the overlying sarcoplasmic reticulum.

Figure 3-4. A higher-magnification view of the cytoplasmic side of the plasma membrane of a mouse small intestinal smooth muscle cell, showing the peripheral sarcoplasmic reticulum and the surface caveolae. Most of the caveolae are spherical or oval, but some appear to be fused to each other, forming double-vesiculated caveolae (arrows). In this micrograph, the linear aggregation of the surface caveolae is 4–5 vesicles wide and is accompanied with the tubular sarcoplasmic reticulum. Ribosomes are not visible on the surface of the tubular sarcoplasmic reticulum.

along caveolae aggregation less than five vesicles wide.

When the rows of the caveolae are more than six vesicles wide, the sarcoplasmic reticulum shows either the flat fenestrated type (Fig. 3-5, 3-6, 3-8) or the netty type (Fig. 3-7). The former has many fenestrations on its surface, like a sieve plate, and usually covers the surface caveolae from the cytoplasmic side. When the fenestrated sarcoplasmic reticulum is viewed from the cytoplasmic side in a stereomicrograph, the convex undulation of the sarcoplasmic reticulum is visible in three dimensions (Fig. 3-6). Both edges of the undulated sarcoplasmic reticulum appear to contact the plasma membrane. Gabella (7) observed in thin sections cut perpendicularly to the cell surface that the peripheral sarcoplasmic reticulum frequently forms a kind of gutter for a row of caveolae: the cisterna gets close to the cell membrane with both edges and encloses the caveolae. The undulations observed by the SEM may correspond to the gutter. Since this type of fenestrated cisternal sarcoplasmic reticulum is usually located between surface caveolae and mitochondria, it is impossible to observe the sarcoplasmic reticulum without eliminating the overlying mitochondria. In the specimens thus far prepared by the present method, during which mitochondria are removed, the surface of the intervening sarcoplasmic reticulum is successfully exposed, as shown in Figures 3-5 and 3-6. From the margin of the fenestrated cisternal sarcoplasmic reticulum, tubular sarcoplasmic reticulum extends to surround the overlying mitochondria (Fig. 3-5, 3-10).

The netty sarcoplasmic reticulum underlying a plasma membrane is not so common compared with the fenestrated type. It consists of both a tubular portion and a flat cisternal area, spreading as a two-dimensional network (Fig. 3-7). The tubular network of the sarcoplasmic reticulum is partially skirting one to two surface caveolae. A fenestrated convex area is visible in the sarcoplasmic reticulum, which appears to cover a underlying surface caveola (Fig. 3-7).

Each type of sarcoplasmic reticulum cited above frequently has ribosomes attached to its surface (Figs. 3-7, 3-8). They are arranged in rows, loops, or spirals to form polysomes. The polysomal arrangement is evident on the fenestrated or netty sracoplasmic reticulum. Gabella (7) reported from his ultrathin sectioning study that the peripheral sarcoplasmic reticulum is smooth but on occasion may have ribosomes attached. In bovine tracheal smooth muscle cells, some rough-surfaced sarcoplasmic reticulum was found underneath the plasma membrane, although the sarcoplasmic reticulum is mainly of the smooth type (30).

Most of the peripheral sarcoplasmic reticulum is clearly separated from the surface caveolae. Experiments using extracellular markers such as ferritin and lanthanum have indicated that there is no communication between the sarcoplasmic reticulum and the surface caveolae (6, 31). In our observation by SEM, however, some of the surface caveolae infrequently communicated with the sarcoplasmic reticulum, as shown in Figure 3-8. It has not clearly been demonstrated whether the surface caveolae have pinocytotic activity or not. The SEM micrograph shown in Figure 3-8 suggests that the caveolae may be pinched off from the surface plasma membrane and incorporated into the sarcoplasmic reticulum.

3.3.2. Perinuclear sarcoplasmic reticulum. The perinuclear sarcoplasmic reticulum is located among the accumulation of mitochondria at both poles of the nucleus. It is tubular in shape and forms a complex three-dimensional network. On its surface, many ribosomes are studded. In the specimen in which the nuclear surface is successfully exposed, the continuity between the perinuclear sarcoplasmic reticulum and the nuclear envelope is clearly shown (Fig. 3-9). The continuity of the sarcoplasmic reticulum with the Golgi complex has not been demonstrated yet in small intestinal smooth muscle cells, although the continuity was reported in smooth muscle cells of the rat esophageal lamina muscularis mucosae (14).

3.3.3. Connecting sarcoplasmic reticulum. Connecting sarcoplasmic reticulum links the peripheral sarcoplasmic reticulum with the perinuclear one (Fig. 3-11), corresponding to the intermediate sarcoplasmic reticulum described by Popescu and Bruijn (40). It is tubular in shape, and its surface is smooth.

In addition to the sarcoplasmic reticulum

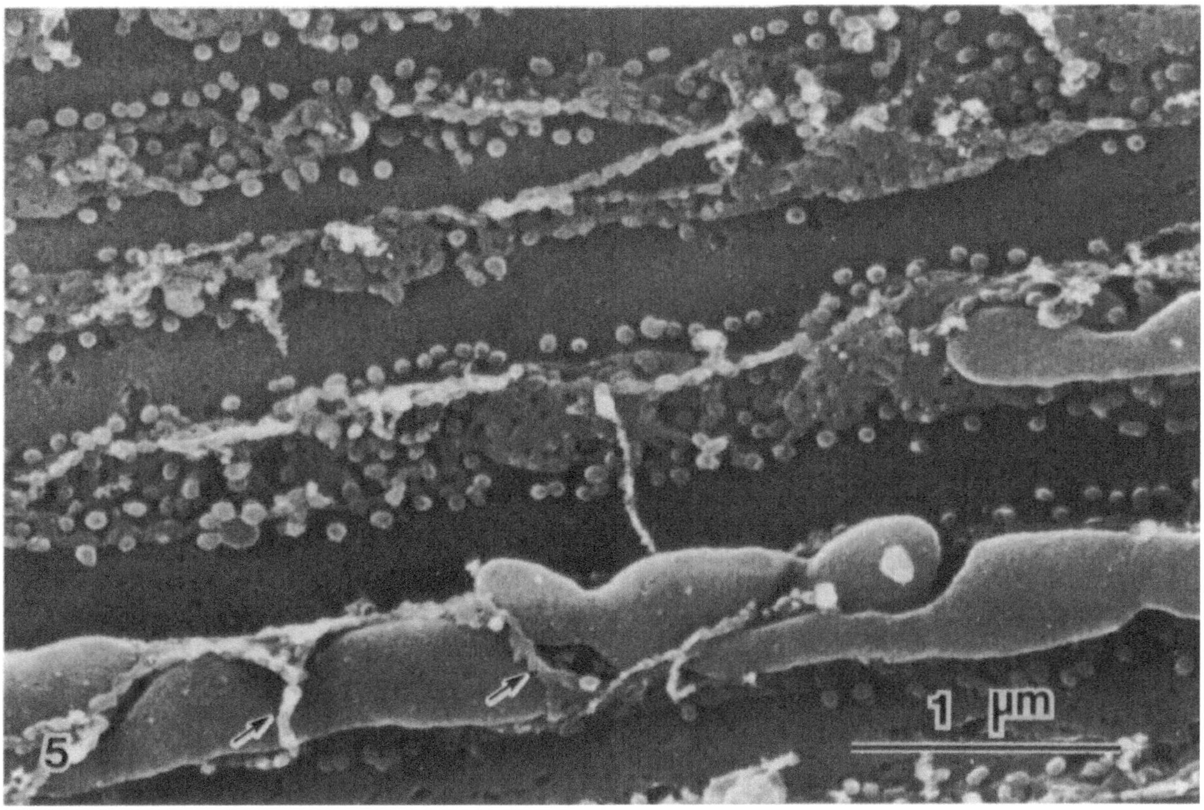

Figure 3-5. A cytoplasmic side of the plasma membrane of a mouse small intestinal smooth muscle cell, showing the surface caveolae, peripheral sarcoplasmic reticulum, and mitochondria. In this micrograph, linear aggregation of the surface caveolae is 6–12 vesicles wide and is accompanied with the fenestrated sarcoplasmic reticulum located between the surface caveolae and the mitochondria. At the upper part of the micrograph, mitochondria having been partially removed during the specimen preparation, the intervening sarcoplasmic reticulum is exposed. From the edges of the intervening fenestrated sarcoplasmic reticulum, tubular sarcoplasmic reticulum is extended surrounding the adjacent mitochondria (arrows).

mentioned above, another type of sarcoplasmic reticulum is certainly located deeply in the sarcoplasm, among the myofibrils. In the SEM specimen, however, this sarcoplasmic reticulum loses its support by myofilaments during the osmic maceration procedure and is mostly eliminated from the cracked surface during the specimen preparation. Further studies are need to clarify the three-dimensional topography of such sarcoplasmic reticulum.

3.4. Ribosomes

Ribosomes are the site of protein synthesis and are often associated in clusters to form polysomes. According to TEM studies, two types of polysomes are known; free polysomes and polysomes attached on the membranous structures such as the endoplasmic reticulum or the nuclear envelope. The polysomes attached on the membranes are preserved after the osmic maceration procedures, while free polysomes that have been removed during the procedure cannot be observed under SEM in this preparation. Since it is difficult to disclose an *en face* view of the polysomes by an ultrathin sectioning method, it has not been clarified whether the sarcoplasmic reticulum in smooth muscle cells, especially the peripheral sarcoplasmic reticulum, has polysomes or not. However, in the SEM micrographs in Figure 3-7 and 3-8, the ribosomal attachment is clearly shown. Some ribosomes are arranged in spirals and others in loops to form polysomes. Underneath the plasma membrane, the polysomes are observed more frequently on the fenestrated or netty sarcoplasmic reticulum than on the tubular sarcoplasmic reticulum. On the perinuclear tubular sarcoplasmic reticulum, many ribosomes are also present, but most of them are not organized into the typical polysomal arrangement.

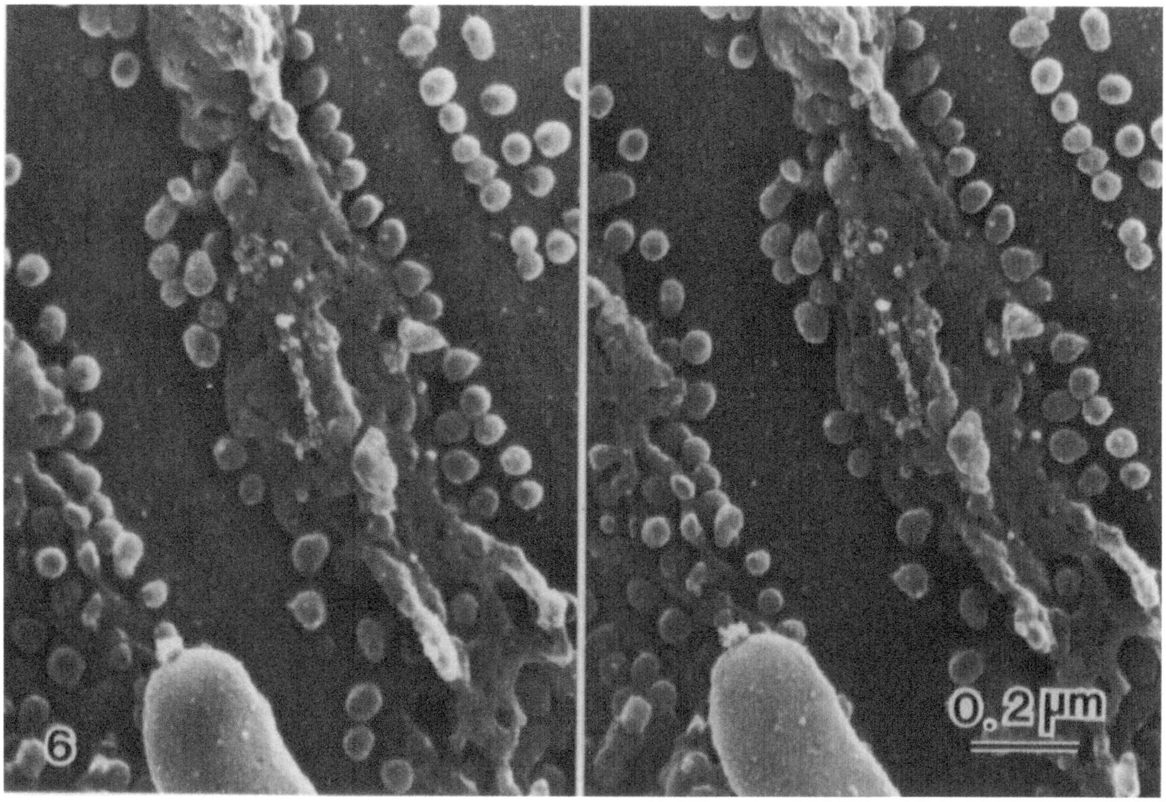
6
0.2 µm

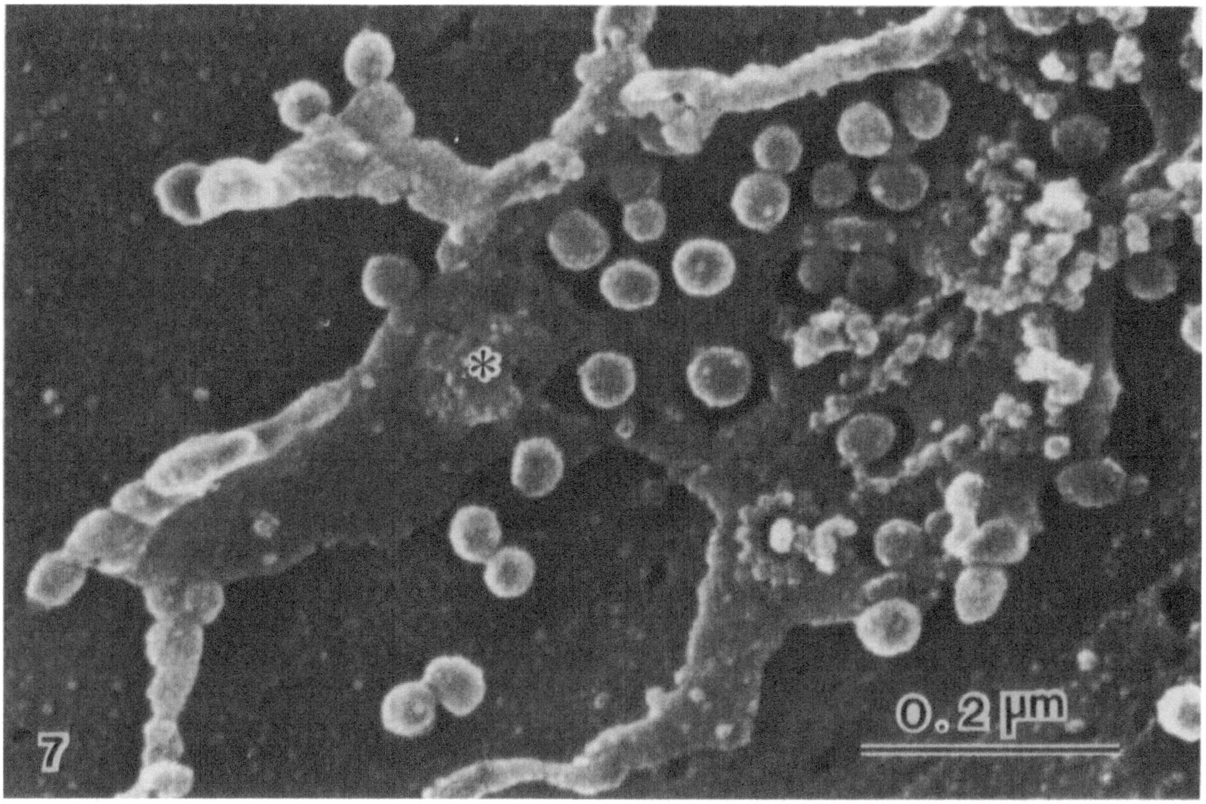
7
0.2 µm

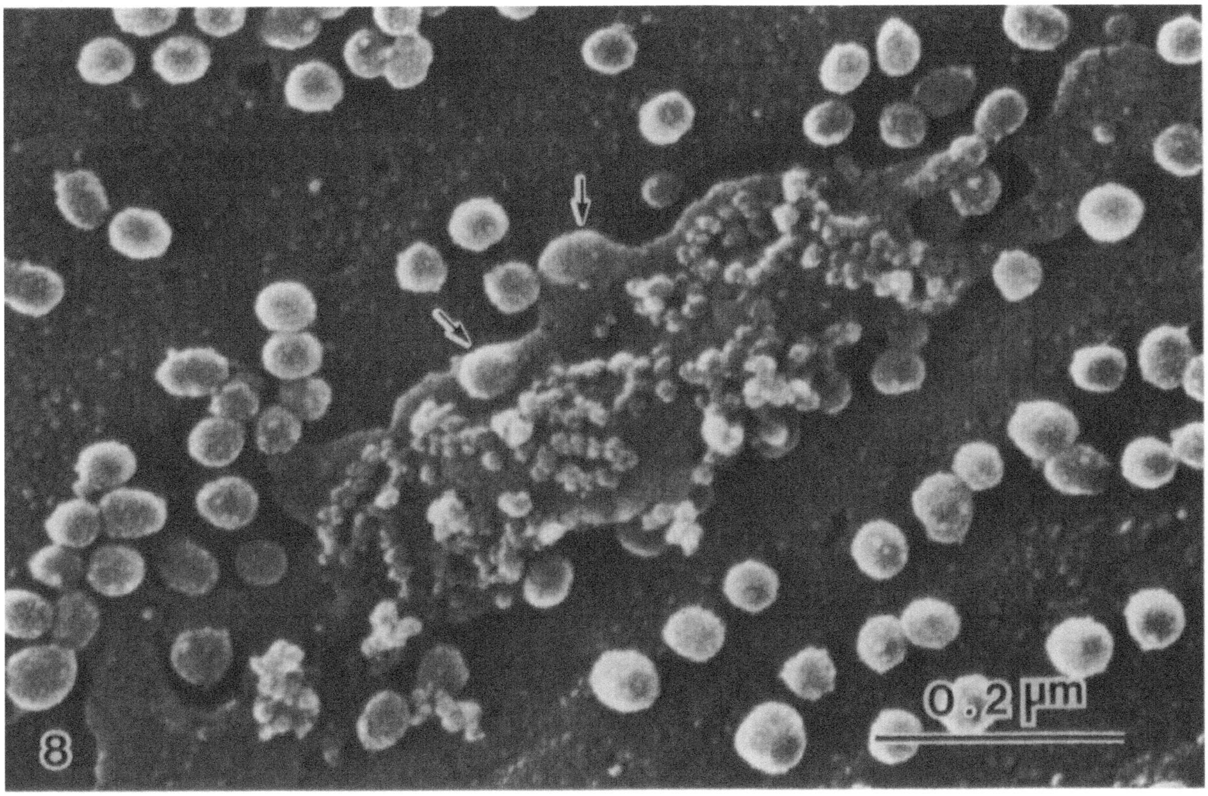

Figure 3-8. A higher-magnification view of the cytoplasmic side of the plasma membrane of a mouse small intestinal smooth muscle cell. The flat sarcoplasmic reticulum with many ribosomes is visible. Some surface caveolae appear to be incorporated into the sarcoplasmic reticulum (arrows).

It is known that smooth muscle cells in their early development contain well-developed ribosomes (42). Regarding the aggregation of ribosomes, Yamauchi and Burnstock (42) described the appearance in 6–12 days postnatal mice of prominent ribosomal rosettes in the vas deferens smooth muscle cells, which later became less marked.

3.5. Mitochondria

Mitochondira of smooth muscle cells are mainly situated either at the perinuclear area or beneath the plasma membrane. The shape and size of the mitochondria differ in their locations. Since myofilaments have been dissolved by the osmic maceration procedure, intermyofilamentous mitochondria cannot be retained. For this reason, most of the mitochondria situated among the myofibrils cannot be observed in this study. Here, two types of the mitochondria are described.

3.5.1. Peripheral mitochondria. Several rows of mitochondria are observed in the vicinity of the plasma membrane (Fig. 3-5, 3-10). The mitochondria are located along the linear arrangement of the surface caveolae and are unrecognizable in the flat area without the caveolae. All of the peripheral mitochondria show elongated forms parallel to the long axis of the cell. They are

←

Figure 3-6. A stereomicrograph of the cytoplasmic side of a mouse small intestinal smooth muscle cell. A convex undulation of the fenestrated sarcoplasmic reticulum covering surface vesicles is seen in three dimensions.

Figure 3-7. A high-magnification view of the sarcoplasmic side of the plasma membrane of a mouse small intestinal smooth muscle cell, showing the netty sarcoplasmic reticulum. The sarcoplasmic reticulum consists of both a tubular part and a flat cisterna. The tubules of the sarcoplasmic reticulum skirt one to two caveolae. On the flat cisterna, ribosomes are seen forming spirally arranged polysomes. A fenestrated convex area is visible in the sarcoplasmic reticulum, which appears to cover an underlying surface caveola (asterisk).

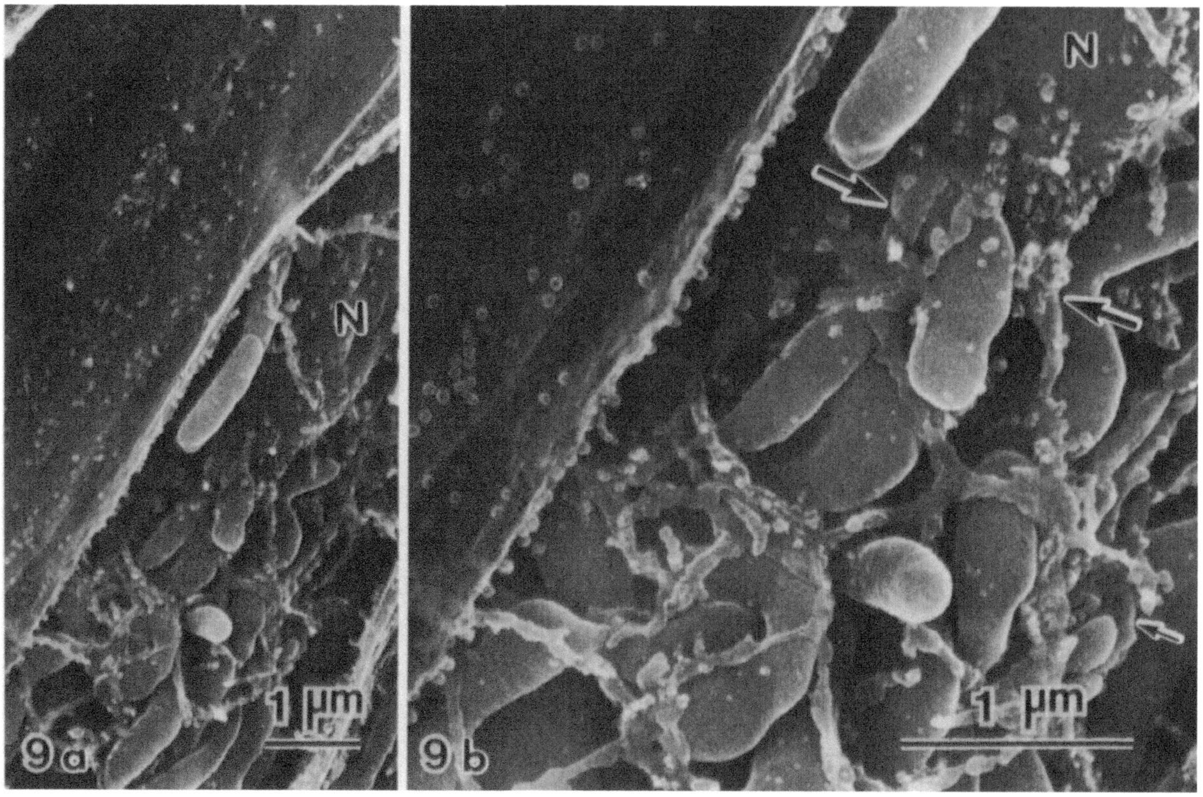
N
1 µm
9a
N
1 µm
9b

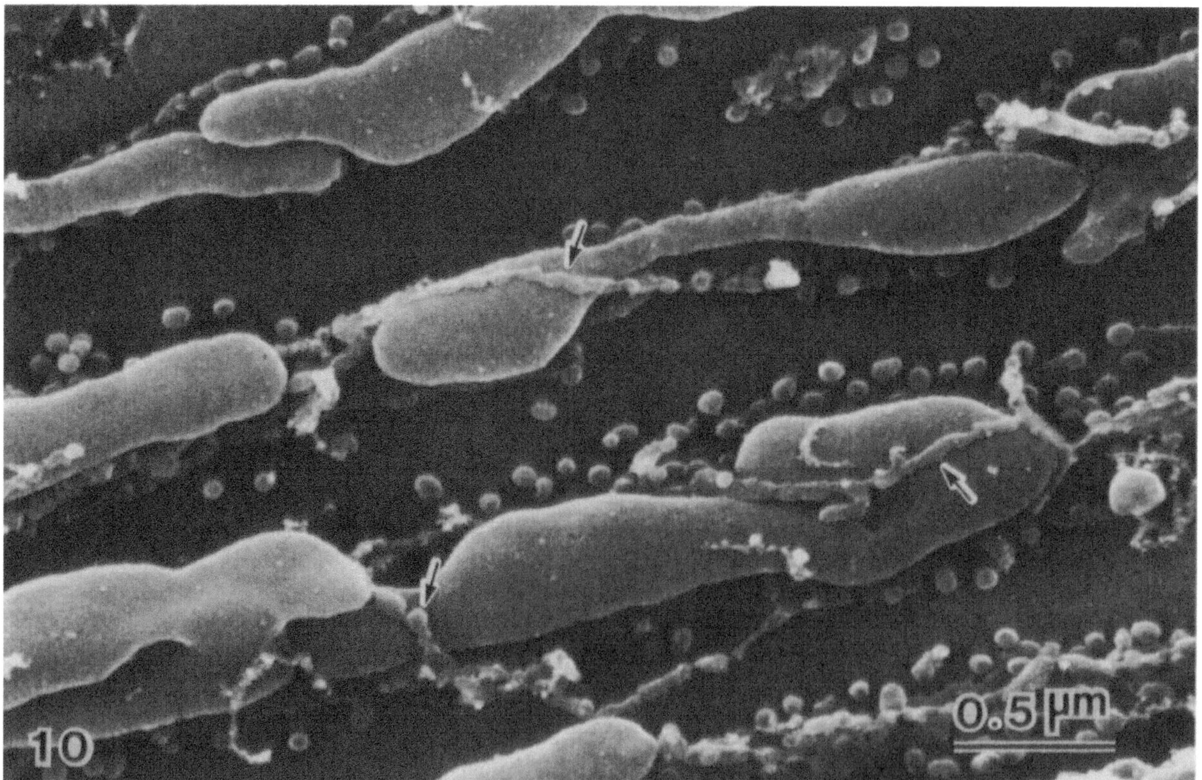
0.5 µm
10

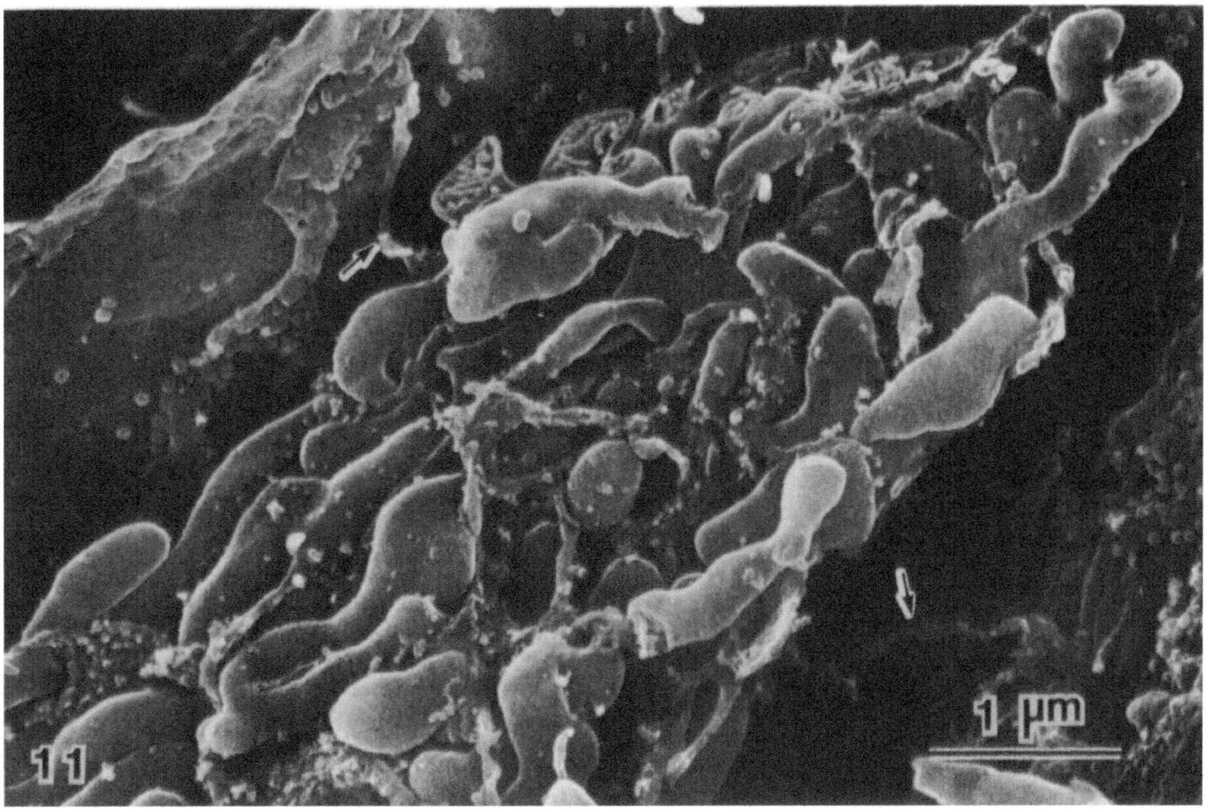

Figure 3-11. Perinuclear region of a mouse small intestinal smooth muscle cell, showing the perinuclear sarcoplasmic reticulum and the accumulation of mitochondria. The perinuclear sarcoplasmic reticulum is tubular in shape, forming a complex three-dimensional network. The mitochondria are interwoven in a remarkably complex pattern. Smooth tubules of the connecting sarcoplasmic reticulum are visible between the peripheral sarcoplasmic reticulum and the perinuclear sarcoplasmic reticulum (arrows).

0.2–0.4 μm in width and 2–5 μm in length. Most of the mitochondria show rodlike appearance without branching, but some are bifurcated or curved showing J- or H-shapes (Fig. 3-10).

3.5.2. Perinuclear mitochondria. In the perinuclear region, an accumulation of the mitochondria was observed (Fig. 3-9, 3-11). According to Bloom and Fawcett (43), the juxtanuclear sarcoplasm contains long slender mitochondria. In fact, however the mitochondria in the juxtanuclear region are interwoven in a remarkably complex pattern (Fig. 3-11). The complexity of this labyrinthine pattern is not readily appreciated by TEM.

3.6. *Golgi complex*

The Golgi complex of smooth muscle cells is located at the perinuclear region together with the accumulation of numerous mitochondria. Its development has been considered to be poor. In

←

Figure 3-9. A low-magnification (a) and high-magnification (b) view of the perinuclear region of a mouse small intestinal smooth muscle cell. An accumulation of the mitochondria and the nuclear envelope (N) are visible. A perinuclear sarcoplasmic reticulum is tubular in shape and is situated together with the accumulation of mitochondria, forming a threedimensional complex network. Ribosomal granules are visible on the surface, but the typical formation of polysomes is not seen. The tubular perinuclear sarcoplasmic reticulum protrude from the nuclear envelope, and the continuity between the sarcoplasmic reticulum and the nuclear envelope is clearly demonstrated (large arrows). The fenestrated *cis*-cisternae of the Golgi complex is partially seen (small arrow).
Figure 3-10. A higher-magnification view of the cytoplasmic side of the plasma membrane of a mouse small intestinal smooth muscle cell. Longitudinally extended mitochondria (M) are observed on the linear aggregation of the surface vesicles. Some mitochondria are bifurcated or curved showing J- or H-shapes. The mitochondria are partially surrounded by the tubules protruding from the underlying sarcoplasmic reticulum (arrows).

our observations in small intestinal smooth muscle cells, only the fenestrated surface of the Golgi complex is visualized (Fig. 3-9). Yokoyama (14) observed by SEM the intracellular structures of smooth muscle cells in the rat esophageal lamina muscularis mucosae and reported the three-dimensional architecture of the Golgi complex. According to his study, the Golgi complex consisted of three to eight Golgi cisternae, Golgi vesicles, and Golgi vacuoles, and the Golgi cisternae were continuous with the rough endoplasmic reticulum. The continuity between the Golgi cisternae and the endoplasmic reticulum was also reported in the rat lacrimal glandular cells under SEM (44).

4. Conclusions

As described above, the architecture of intracellular structures of smooth muscle cells is three-dimensionally demonstrated at high magnifications under SEM. Although the morphology of the sarcoplasmic reticulum obtained by SEM is fundamentally the same as that thus far reported by TEM, the present SEM study provides new findings. All membranes of the sarcoplasmic reticulum in a cell appear to be connected to each other, forming a continuous system. The continuity between the nuclear envelope and the sarcoplasmic reticulum is discerned under SEM. In addition, the morphology of the polysomes attached on the sarcoplasmic reticulum is clearly shown, which indicates that the peripheral sarcoplasmic reticulum as well as the perinuclear one is a site of active protein synthesis.

The osmic maceration technique which can dissolve the myofilaments of muscle cells, has proved effective for ultrastuctural studies on the three-dimensional architecture of the membranous system. In particular, the topography of the surface caveolae and sarcoplasmic reticulum demonstrated here cannot be appreciated by the previous electron microscopic techniques. Thus, high-resolution SEM has opened new possibilities to clarify intracellular structures of smooth muscle cells in three dimensions. With further progress in specimen preparations, as well as further SEM applications to various kinds of smooth muscle cells, the intracellular organization of smooth muscle cells will be more precisely understood.

References

1. Caesar R, Edwards GA, Ruska H: Architecture and nerve supply of mammalian smooth muscle tissue. *J Biophys Biochem Cytol* 3: 867–878, 1957.
2. Rhodin JAG: Fine structure of vascular walls in mammals with special reference to smooth muscle component. *Phys Rev* 42 *(Suppl)*: 48–81, 1962.
3. Kelly RE, Rice RV: Ultrastructural studies on the contractile mechanism of smooth muscle. *J Cell Biol* 42: 683–694, 1969.
4. Gabella G: Caveolae intracellulares and sarcoplasmic reticulum in smooth muscle. *J Cell Sci* 8: 601–609, 1969.
5. Somlyo AP, Devine CE, Somlyo AV, North SR: Sarcoplasmic reticulum and the temperature-dependent contraction of smooth muscle in calcium-free solutions. *J Cell Biol* 51: 722–741, 1971.
6. Devine CE, Somlyo AV, Somlyo AP: Sarcoplasmic reticulum and excitation–contraction coupling in mammalian smooth muscles. *J Cell Biol* 52: 690–718, 1972.
7. Gabella G: The arrangement of sarcoplasmic reticulum in smooth muscle. *Experientia* 28: 948–949, 1972.
8. Tanaka K: Demonstration of intracellular structures by high resolution scanning electron microscopy. *Scanning Electron Microsc* 2: 1–8, 1981.
9. Inoué T: High resolution scanning electron microscopic cytology — Specimen preparation and intracellular structures observed by scanning electron microscopy. In: Science of Biological Specimen Preparation. M Müller et al. (eds), Chicago: SEM Inc., p 245–256, 1986.
10. Tanaka K, Mitsushima A: A preparation method for observing intracellular structures by scanning electron microscopy. *J Microsc* 133: 213–222, 1984.
11. Inoué T, Osatake H: Freeze-polishing method for observing intracellular structures by scanning electron microscopy. *J Electron Microsc* 33: 356–362, 1984.
12. Sawada H: Scanning electron microscopy of guinea pig taenia coli. *Biomed Res 2 (Suppl)*: 153–158, 1981.
13. Sawada H: Three-dimensional observation on muscular tissues. *Scanning Electron Microsc* 4: 7–15, 1981.
14. Yokoyama M: Scanning electron microscopic study on the smooth muscle cells. *J Yonago Med Assoc* 36: 259–269 (in Japanese with English abstract), 1985.
15. Inoué T, Osatake H: Three-dimensional architecture of the sarcoplasmic reticulum in smooth muscle cells observed by scanning electron microscopy. Proc XIth Int Cong Electron Microsc Kyoto, Japan, 1986, p 3115–3116.
16. Tanaka K, Naguro T: High resolution scanning electron microscopy of cell organelles by a new specimen preparation method. *Biomed Res* 2 (Suppl): 63–70, 1981.
17. Nemanic MK: Critical point drying, cryofracture, and serial sectioning. *Scanning Electron Microsc* 297–304, 1972.
18. Humphreys WJ, Spurlock BO, Johnson JS: Critical point drying of ethanol-infiltrated, cryofractured biological specimens for scanning electron microscopy. *Scanning Electron Microsc* 275–282, 1974.
19. Tokunaga J, Edanaga M, Fujita T, Adachi K: Freeze cracking of scanning electron microscope specimens. A study of the kidney and spleen. *Arch Histol Jpn* 37: 165–182, 1974.

20. Ohmori T: Three-dimensional architecture of sarcotubules of rat skeletal and heart muscle cells observed by scanning electron microscopy. *J Yonago Med Assoc* 35: 241–251 (in Japanese with English abstract), 1984.
21. Yoshikane H, Nihei T, Morinaga K: Three-dimensional observation of intracellular membranous structures in dog heart muscle cells by scanning electron microscopy. *J Submicrosc Cytol* 18: 629–636, 1986.
22. Inoué T, Katsumoto T, Osatake H, Tanaka K: Three-dimensional observations of intracellular structures of cultured cells by scanning electron microscopy. In: Proceedings of the 3rd Asia-Pacific Conference on Electron Microscopy. MF Chung (ed), Singapore: Applied Research Corporation, p 395–396, 1984.
23. Murakami T: A revised tannin-osmium method for non-coated scanning electron microscope specimens. *Arch Histol Jpn* 36: 189–193, 1974.
24. Tanaka K, Iino A: Critical point drying method using dry ice. *Stain Technol* 49: 203–206, 1974.
25. Moriya M, Miyazaki E: Structural analysis of functionally different smooth muscles. *Cell Tissue Res* 202: 337–341, 1979.
26. Gabella G: Intercellular junctions between circular and longitudinal intestinal muscle layers. *Z Zellforsch* 125: 191–199, 1972.
27. Watanabe H, Yamamoto T: Freeze-etch study of smooth muscle cells from vas deferens and taenia coli. *J Anat* 117: 553–564, 1974.
28. Yamada E: The fine structure of the gall bladder epithelium of the mouse. *J Biophys Biochem Cytol* 1: 445–458, 1955.
29. Riley DA: Silver staining the caveolae intracellularis of smooth muscle. *J Anat* 123: 819–825, 1977.
30. Cameron AR, Bullock CG, Kirkpatrick CT: The ultrastructure of bovine tracheal smooth muscle. J Ultrastruc Res 81: 290–305, 1982.
31. Devine CE, Simpson FO, Bertaud WS: Surface features of smooth muscle cells from the mesenteric artery and vas deferens. *J Cell Sci* 8: 427–443, 1971.
32. Wells GS, Wolowyk MW: Freeze-etch observations on membrane structure in the smooth muscle of guinea-pig taenia coli. *J Physiol* 218: 11P–13P, 1971.
33. Muggli R, Baumgartner HR: Pattern of membrane invaginations at the surface of smooth muscle cells of rabbit arteries. Experientia 28: 1212–1214, 1972.
34. Devine CE, Rayns DG: Freeze-fracture studies of membrane systems in vertebrate muscle. II. Smooth muscle. *J Ultrastruct Res* 51: 293–306, 1975.
35. Gabella G, Blundell D: Effect of stretch and contraction on caveolae of smooth muscle cells. *Cell Tissue Res* 190: 255–271, 1978.
36. Gansler H: Struktur und Funktion der glatten Muskulatur. II. Licht- und elektronenmikroskopishe Befunde an Hohlorganen von Ratte, Meerschweinchen und Mensch. *Z Zellforsch mikrosk Anat* 55: 724–762, 1961.
37. Fawcett DW, McNutt NS: The ultrastructure of the cat myocardium. I. Ventricular papillary muscle. *J Cell Biol* 42: 1–45, 1969.
38. Peachey LD: The sarcoplasmic reticulum and transverse tubules of the frog's sartorius. *J Cell Biol* 25: 209–231, 1965.
39. Segretain D, Rambourg A, Clermont Y: Three dimensional arrangement of mitochondria and endoplasmic reticulum in the heart muscle fiber of the rat. *Anat Rec* 200: 139–151, 1981.
40. Popescu LM, de Bruijn WC: Calcium in the sarcoplasmic reticulum of smooth muscle. X-ray microanalysis of oxalate-treated muscle fibers. Proc 10th Int Cong Electron Microsc Hamburg. *Electron Microsc* 3: 385–386, 1982.
41. Popescu LM, Diculescu I, Zelck U, Ionescu N: Ultrastructural distribution of calcium in smooth muscle cells of guineapig taenia coli. *Cell Tissue Res* 154: 357–378, 1974.
42. Yamauchi A, Burnstock G: Post-natal development of smooth muscle cells in the mouse vas deferens. A fine structural study. *J Anat* 104: 1–5, 1969.
43. Bloom W, Fawcett DW: A Textbook of Histology, 10th ed. Philadelphia: WB Saunders Company, 1975.
44. Tanaka K, Mitsushima A, Fukudome H, Kashima Y: Three-dimensional architecture of the Golgi complex observed by high resolution scanning electron microscopy. *J Submicrosc Cytol* 18: 1–9, 1986.

Author's address:
Prof. Takao Inoué
Department of Anatomy
Tottori University School of Medicine
Yonago 683
Japan

CHAPTER 4

Ultrastructure of smooth muscle cells in culture

GORDON R. CAMPBELL & JULIE H. CAMPBELL

1. Smooth muscle cells express a spectrum of phenotypic states

Various cell types can alter their character when the environment changes. These alterations in character are called modulations of the differentiated state and involve reversible interconversions between phenotypes. Modulations in phenotype may occur as a result of cell interactions or alterations of the extracellular matrix, or in response to other signals such as hormones.

The smooth muscle cell is capable of expressing a range of phenotypes (1). At one end of the spectrum of phenotypes is the cell whose function is almost exclusively that of contraction (we have termed this cell as being in the *contractile state*). This function is reflected structurally, with 80% to 90% of the cell volume occupied with contractile apparatus (2). Organelles such as rough endoplasmic reticulum (ER), Golgi, and free ribosomes are few in number and are located in the perinuclear region. Cells of the taenia coli, vas deferens, circular muscle of the ileum, and smaller muscular arteries express this phenotype. These smooth muscle tissues contain relatively little connective tissue; for example, the volume of extracellular space is about 30% in taenia coli and 10% to 15% in the circular muscle of the ileum. In visceral muscle tissues, much of the extracellular matrix is synthesized by constituent fibroblasts, and the smooth muscle cells express minimal synthetic function. At the opposite end of the spectrum of phenotypic expression is the muscle cell whose function is almost exclusively that of synthesis (we have termed this cell as being in the *synthetic state*). In line with other cell types actively engaged in production of extracellular matrix (such as fibroblasts), the cytoplasm contains few filament bundles but large amounts of rough ER, Golgi, and free ribosomes (3).

It must be emphasized that the contractile and synthetic states as described above represent the extreme ends of a continuous spectrum of phenotypes, with most smooth muscle expressing intermediate morphology. For instance, the volume of the connective tissue containing extracellular space in large mammalian elastic arteries is 50% to 60%, and smooth muscle is the only cell type present (4–6). This cell type must therefore be responsible for not only contraction/relaxation but also the normal turnover of extracellular matrix components. This dual function is reflected structurally, with only 60% to 70% of the cell volume occupied with myofilaments in the adult animal (7, 8).

2. Modulation of smooth muscle phenotype in vivo

2.1. During development

Initially in the development of most visceral smooth muscle organs, undifferentiated mesenchymal cells surround the newly formed epithelium. These soon develop a typical fibroblast appearance, with their cytoplasm containing a large number of organelles, particularly free ribosomes, rough ER, mitochondria, and Golgi (9–13). With increasing age, there is a progressive reduction in the nucleus/cytoplasm ratio and the appearance of bundles of thin filaments with associated dark bodies. With further time, filament bundles increase in size, thick filaments appear, and there is a concomitant decrease in the number of synthetic organelles. Other characteristic features of smooth muscle, such as dense areas along the cell membrane, plasmalemmal vesicles, and a basal lamina, appear at about the same time or a little later than thick myofilaments (11, 14).

Blood vessels develop in the embryo from the mesenchyme. Firstly, a budding network of small endothelial-lined channels is formed (15). These channels are soon ensheathed by extracellular matrix and later become surrounded by locally derived irregularly shaped mesenchymal cells (16–18). At the stage when elastic lamellae and other extracellular matrix components are first produced, the mesenchymal cells resemble fibroblasts (17, 19). But with time, as the elastic lamellae in large arteries become more identifiable, the muscle cells take on a more characteristic appearance, although they do not do so at the same rate across the wall since with further development new lamellae are added onto the adventitial aspect (5). At parturition most arteries appear to have developed their adult number of lamellar units (20), for after this stage the number of layers in the wall does not increase and medial thickening is due to the production of connective tissue. In the newborn rat aorta, myofilaments occupy 7.7% of the volume of smooth muscle cells and are usually confined to the periphery of the cell. Golgi and rough ER constitute about 30% of the cell volume (7). Over the 8 to 12 weeks following birth, the amount of elastin increases from 6% to 35% and collagen increases from 8% to 26% dry weight of the media, which are the approximate adult values. At about the same time as these adult extracellular matrix values are reached, the volume fraction of smooth muscle cytoplasm occupied by myofilaments reaches the adult level of 70%, with rough ER occupying 7.2% and Golgi 2.4% (7).

2.2. *Injury and repair*

Smooth muscle cells with a low-volume fraction of myofilaments and large amounts of synthetic organelles (synthetic state) have been widely reported in areas of regeneration and repair after damage to visceral smooth muscle tissues (21–25). These cells appear to be smaller than their neighboring unaffected cells (26). These synthetic-state cells are actively engaged in synthesis of extracellular matrix and/or proliferation. Although several reports have shown that some vascular and visceral smooth muscle cells are capable of division while contractile (27–30), the vast majority of smooth muscle cells observed in mitosis are at least partially modulated towards the synthetic state (22, 31, 32).

Studies of direct damage to the wall of a blood vessel show that arterial medial cells respond in a similar manner to damaged visceral smooth muscle (33–41). Poole et al. (37) wrote the following in their description of injured arterial media:

> On looking at cells in the tunica media further and further away from the site of injury, it was seen that there was a continuous gradient in cell morphology from normal smooth muscle cells of the tunica media (which had presumably not been injured) to the cells showing great lack of differentiation nearer to the silk suture. Mitoses were seen among these cells.

Many studies have been made of the effects of removal of blood vessel endothelium, since the fibromusculoelastic intimal thickenings that occur as a result of this procedure have been proposed as an accelerated model for the events leading to the formation of atherosclerotic plaques (42–44). Injury and removal of the endothelium has been caused experimentally by a variety of traumata such as painting with acid (45), balloon catheterization (46–48), other mechanical methods (42, 49), and air drying (50, 51). If the damage is of sufficient size, smooth muscle cells from the media migrate to the intima where they subsequently proliferate, forming a neo-intima of longitudinally orientated smooth muscle cells. Autoradiographic studies have shown that thymidine indices reach a maximum in the neo-intima during the first week following endothelial denudation (50, 52–55) and return to the baseline by eight weeks after the intima is re-endothelialized (56). The volume fraction of myofilaments (V_v myo) (see 57) in smooth muscle cells of the neo-intima formed in the rabbit carotid artery two weeks after endothelial denudation is significantly less (37%) than that in control medial smooth muscle (68%). Six weeks after injury, the volume density rises to 54%, and by 26 weeks after injury it has returned to 70% (see 58). These data demonstrate that in vivo smooth muscle phenotypic modulation is a reversible phenomenon.

3. Modulation of smooth muscle phenotype in primary culture

3.1. Smooth muscle outgrowth from explants

Kasai and Pollack (59) were among the first to study smooth muscle cells in primary culture. They examined the cellular outgrowth from rabbit arterial wall explants and suggested that fibroblasts appeared within 3 to 5 days and smooth muscle cells within 8 to 10 days. Similar observations were made on explants of human aorta in culture (60). However, light microscope stains (such as Pollack's trichrome) are inadequate to distinguish the spectrum of phenotypes that smooth muscle cells express; the electron microscope is far more appropriate for this task. Using this technique, Daoud, Fritz, Jarmolych, and colleagues (61, 62) described the presence of four cells types in outgrowth from pig aortic media explants. These were termed "*primitive cells*", *fibroblastlike cells*, *modified smooth muscle cells*, and *mature smooth muscle cells*, according to the number of filaments and the concomitant increase or decrease in the number of synthetic organelles present. They suggested that mature smooth muscle cells dedifferentiated in the first few days in culture to modified smooth muscle cells, then to fibroblastlike cells, then finally to primitive cells, where they rapidly proliferated. Peak proliferation (as determined by ^{3}H-thymidine incorporation into DNA) occurred between 9 and 14 days in culture, whereas production of extracellular matrix was minimal at 7 to 9 days, but then increased up to 21 days. The primitive cells subsequently redifferentiated back to smooth muscle (see also 63).

3.2. Enzyme-dispersed smooth muscle cells

With phase contrast microscopy, the morphological appearance of enzyme-dispersed smooth muscle cells in primary culture varies with the tissue of origin and the age and species of the donor animal. It also varies with the length of time that the cell has been in culture. Generally, however, a smooth muscle cell that has been taken from a postnatal animal and that has been grown in culture for less than five days has a ribbon or spindle shape (100–200 μm × 10–15 μm) with an oval or sausage-shaped nucleus containing two or more nucleoli. The cytoplasm is phase-dense and homogeneous and contains few visible inclusions (32, 64–69). These cells do not migrate to any extent, and only a very small percentage undergo mitosis in the presence of whole blood serum. Enzyme-isolated visceral smooth muscle cells from many tissues and species contract spontaneously at rates of contractions 1–8 per minute, while vascular smooth muscle cells, although usually not spontaneously contractile, can be induced to contract with mechanical stimulation and the application of drugs such as angiotensin II or norepinephrine (70). We thus refer to these smooth muscle cells as being in a contractile functional state (32, 69). With time in culture (and this also varies according to factors such as the species and age of animal), the cells spontaneously undergo a modulation of phenotype. They become broader (100–200 μm × 20–30 μm), flatter, and more polyhedral in shape, are less phase-dense, and have a large nucleus. It is at this stage that the cells proliferate in the presence of serum mitogens.

The smooth muscle cells also change in ultrastructural appearance with time in culture. Within the first few days, the enzymatically isolated cells resemble those of the intact tissue from which they were taken. As can be seen from previous sections and other chapters, their appearance varies considerably (particularly with respect to the cytoplasmic volume occupied by myofilaments) according to the species, the age of the animal, and whether we are dealing with

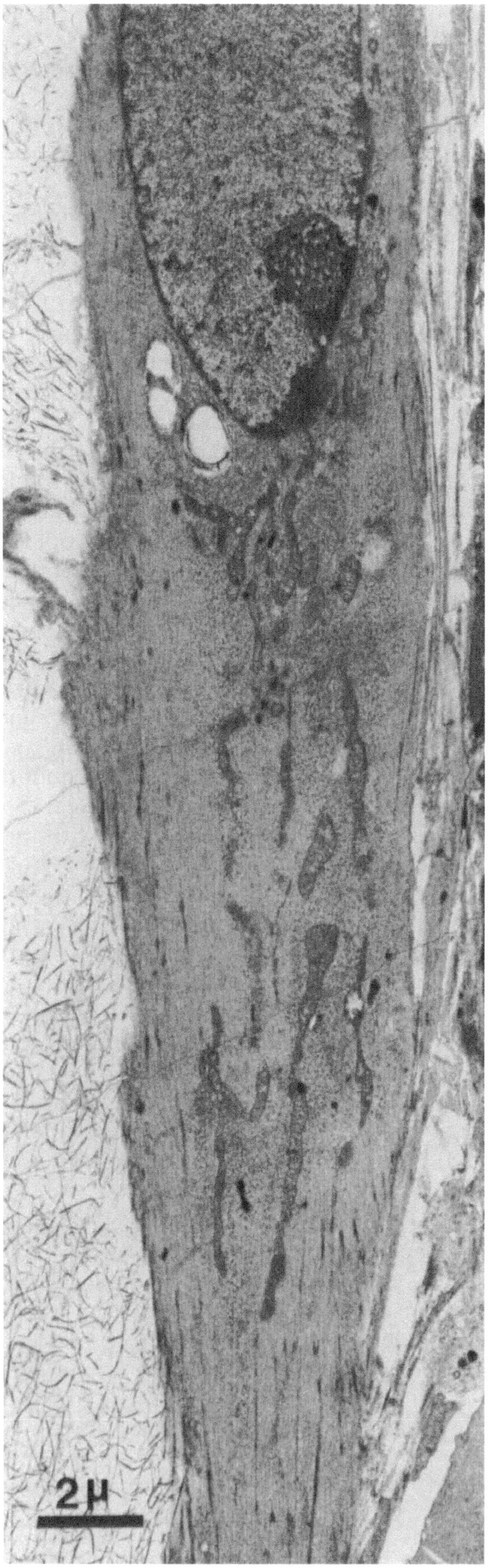

vascular or visceral tissue. However, in general the cytoplasm of the cells is largely occupied by tracts of myofilament bundles with associated dark bodies (Fig. 4-1). In visceral smooth muscle, both thick (120–180 A) and thin (60–80 A) myofilaments can often be observed in these bundles (32, 64, 68, 71–73) (Fig. 4-2). However, in cultured vascular smooth muscle the thick myofilaments are inconsistently observed (32, 70, 74). This may be due to differences in myosin from the different tissues. Intermediate filaments (100 A) are also present within these myofilament bundles, often in association with the dark bodies (71, 75). They can also be seen inserting into dense bands along the cell membrane. Mitochondria and small amounts of rough ER and free ribosomes are located between the tracts of myofilaments and towards the periphery of the cell. The vast majority of organelles such as rough ER, free ribosomes, Golgi apparatus, lysosomes, and mitochondria are poorly developed and are located in the perinuclear region (3, 32, 76–81). The cell membrane contains clusters of plasmalemmal vesicles interspersed with dense bands (Figs. 4-3 and 4-4). Little basal lamina is present around the smooth muscle cells in the first few days in culture. This layer has presumably been lost due to the enzyme dispersal treatment (Figs. 4-3 and 4-4).

Over the next few days in culture (the exact time varies again due to the species, age of animal, and whether the tissue is vascular or visceral in origin), the response of the smooth muscle cells is in many respects analogous to that which is seen in injury and repair (see previous section). That is, the cells undergo a process of phenotypic modulation (3, 32, 64, 67–70, 72, 73, 76–81) in response to the differing functional demands placed upon them.

Ultrastructurally, the phenotypically modulated smooth muscle cells have a number of features in common with fibroblasts. They can,

Figure 4-1. Spindle-shaped smooth muscle cell from newborn guinea pig vas deferens four days in primary culture. Cells have been seeded onto a rat-tail-collagen-coated coverslip and sections cut parallel to the coverslip. Myofilament bundles with associated dark bodies extend throughout the cytoplasm. A number of small lysosomes are present surrounded by ribosomes and elongate mitochondria. Centrioles are present in the perinuclear region.

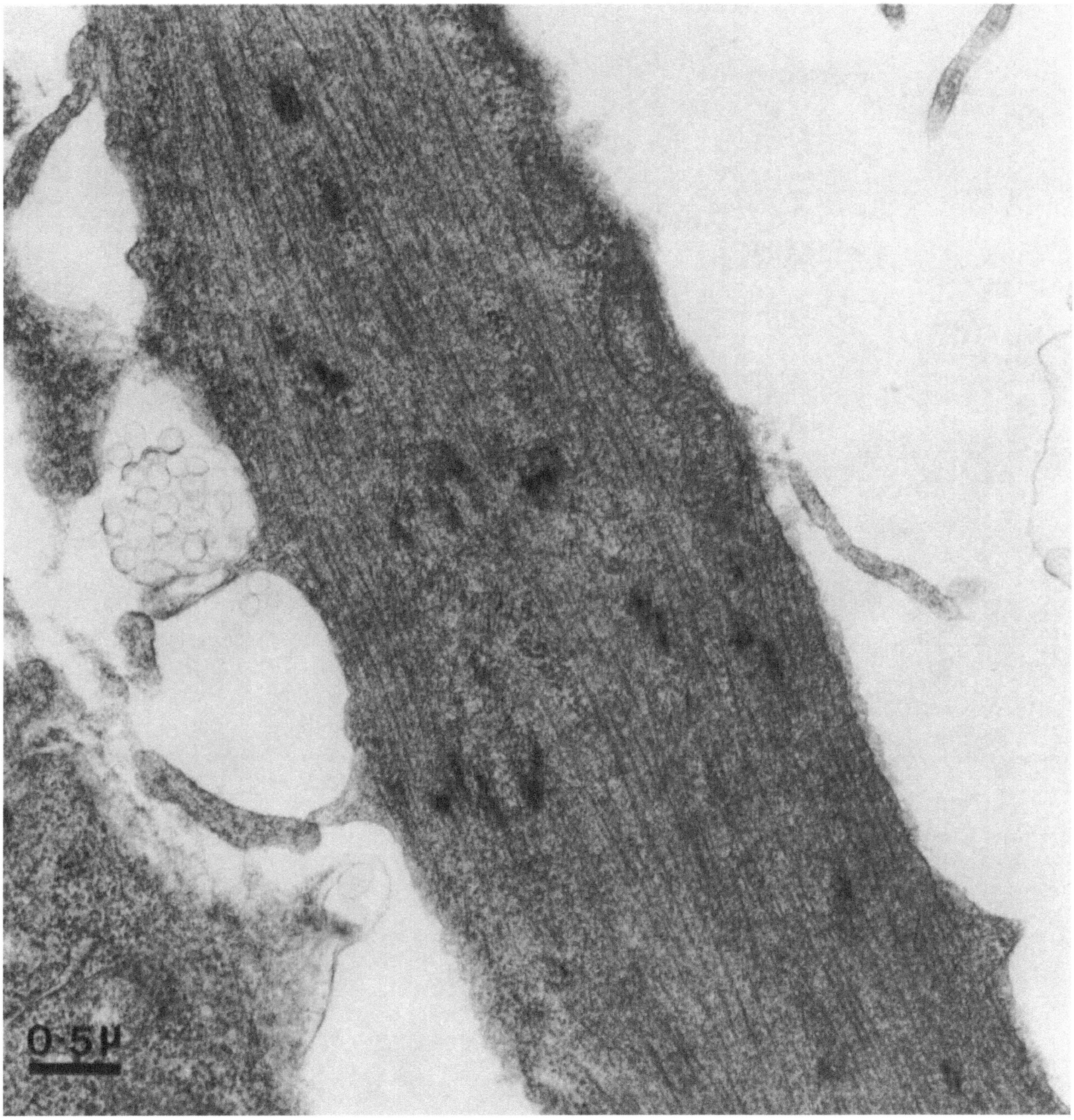

Figure 4-2. Smooth muscle cell enzymatically isolated from the thoracic aorta of a one-year-old Rhesus monkey and grown in primary culture for four days. Cytoplasm in this region contains both thick and thin myofilaments. Note the fingerlike projections extending from the cell. These are often present on cells at this stage in culture. From Chamley JH, Campbell GR, McConnell JD, Groschel-Stewart U: *Cell Tissue Res* 177: 503–522, 1977.

however, be easily distinguished from these cells by the use of labeled specific antibodies (82–89). As the process of phenotypic modulation occurs, there is a general loss of filamentous material, which is largely replaced by rough ER cisternae, free ribosomes, and Golgi (Figs. 4-5 and 4-6). Thus, the phenotypically modulated smooth muscle cell contains fewer bundles of myofilaments (32, 68, 70, 73, 76, 78–80). These bundles with associated dark bodies are located generally towards the periphery of the cell and are particularly prominent at the bottom of the cell where it is attached to the substratum. Thick myofilaments have not been detected in these cells. However, some myosin is present as shown by antibody staining, but it is of a different isoform

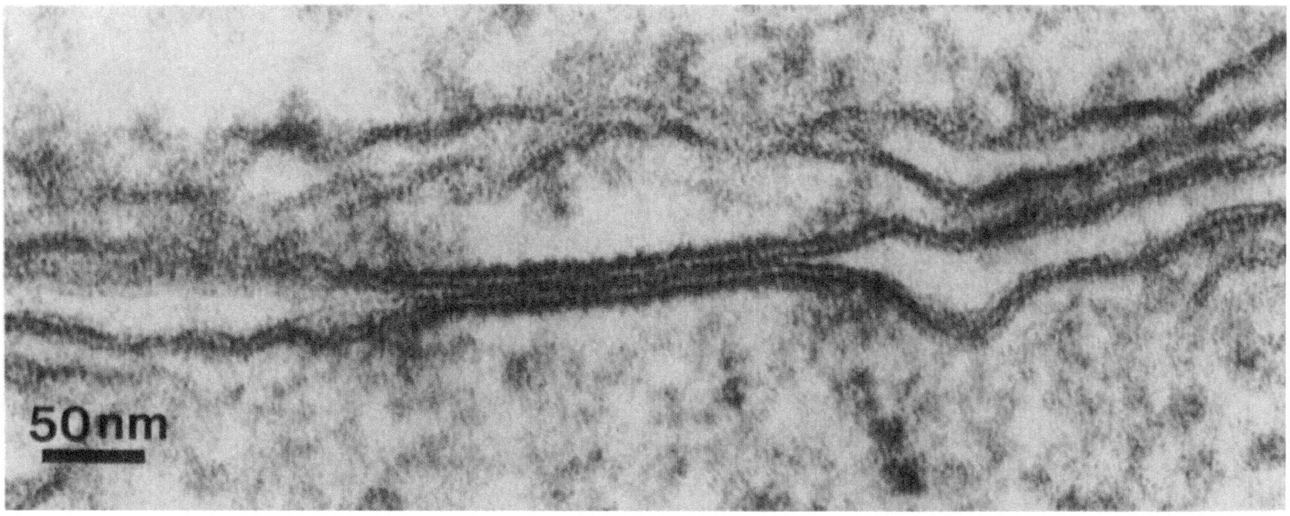
50nm

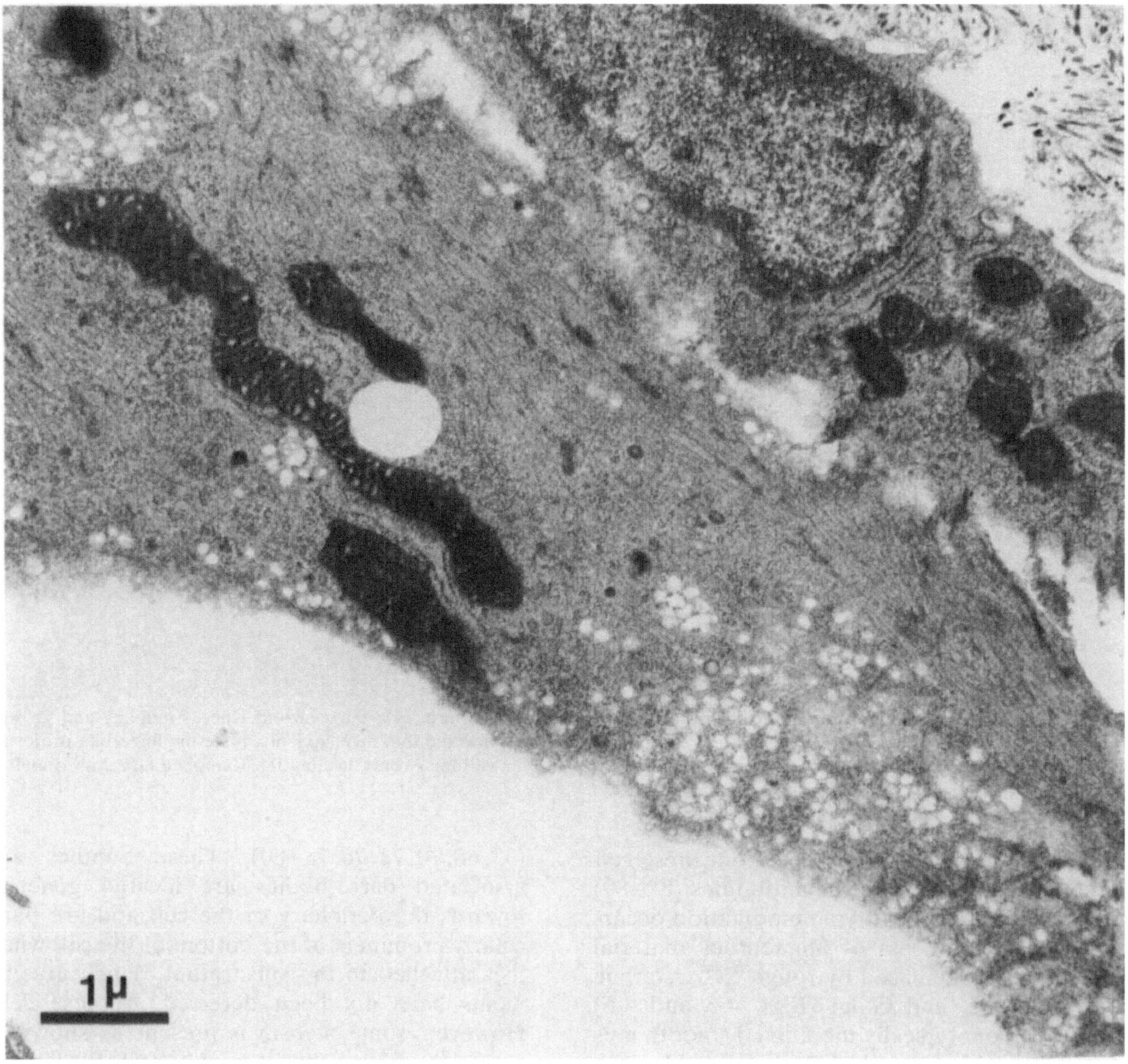
1µ

(91,92) from most of that present in contractile cells. Since these phenotypically modulated cells are not capable of contraction, this myosin of different isoform is probably involved in cell motility. Intermediate filaments are prominent within these cells, and more lysosomes and vesicles are also present (Fig. 4-7). The cell membrane contains a few plasmalemmal vesicles, and dense bands although present tend to be smaller and are often located at the cell–substratum interface. Gap junctions are often observed between cells in clumps (32,68,93) (Fig. 4-3). The cell is often surrounded by an incomplete basal lamina.

These changes in phenotype are demonstrated clearly by ultrastructural morphometric studies. Thyberg et al. (94) has shown that in freshly isolated cells from the eight-month old rat aorta, myofilaments occupy 60.32% of the cytoplasmic volume; rough ER, 5.33%; Golgi cisternae, 1.79%; Golgi vesicles, 8.61%; lysosomes, 3.8%; and mitochondria, 8.59%. On day 2 after isolation, the cytoplasmic volume of the cultured cells occupied by myofilaments has dropped to 42.42% and by mitochondria to 8.34%; however, the volume occupied by rough ER has risen to 9.84%; Golgi cisternae, 2.6%; Golgi vesicles, 10.13%; and lysosomes, 7.35%. The same trends continue on day 4 with myofilaments occupying 5.34% of the cytoplasmic volume; rough ER, 23.77%; Golgi cisternae, 5.5%; Golgi vesicles, 5.77% lysosomes, 3.54%; and mitochondria, 8.05%. By days 7–8, confluence is achieved, accompanied by a slight increase in the volume occupied by myofilaments such that on day 10 they occupy 8.72% of the cytoplasmic volume. At that time, rough ER occupies 24.39%; Golgi cisternae, 5.29%; Golgi vesicles, 4.55%; lysosomes, 6.53%; and mitochondria, 7.15% (94).

4. Factors affecting smooth muscle phenotype in primary cell culture

4.1. Cell seeding density

4.1.1. Moderate seeding density. Smooth muscle cells from the nine-week rabbit aorta seeded in primary culture at $3.03 \pm 0.09 \times 10^5$ cells/dish have a seeding efficiency of 72%, leaving $2.18 \pm 0.08 \times 10^5$ cells attached to each dish on day 1. The cells remain quiescent until day 6, when logarithmic growth commences. Proliferation continues until confluency ($7.80 \pm 0.29 \times 10^5$ cells/dish) on day 9, after which time there is no significant increase in number and the cells remain in monolayer formation (95).

By ultrastructural morphometry, smooth muscle cells in the aorta of nine-week-old rabbits have a V_v myo of $39.50 \pm 1.20\%$. When the aorta is dispersed into single cells and then pelleted by centrifugation, the V_v myo falls to $35.37 \pm 1.51\%$. This does not change after one day in primary culture ($34.55 \pm 2.28\%$), but decreases gradually over day 2 ($30.32 \pm 0.78\%$), day 3 (26.93 ± 2.79), and day 4 ($22.48 \pm 2.30\%$), falling sharply to $11.52 \pm 1.56\%$ on day 5, one day prior to the onset of logarithmic growth. The V_v myo remains low over the next two or three days, then begins to rise once confluency is reached on day 9 ($21.93 \pm 1.20\%$). Two days after confluency (day 11), the V_v myo increases to $30.55 \pm 0.64\%$ and on day 12 is $32.02 \pm 2.45\%$, indicating that the cells have almost regained their original complement of myofilaments (95). That is, at this moderate seeding density, the process of phenotypic modulation is reversible, just as it is in injured tissue.

4.1.2. Dense seeding density. Cells seeded at $9.20 \pm 0.16 \times 10^5$ cells/dish have a seeding efficiency of 73%, leaving $6.70 \pm 0.20 \times 10^5$ cells attached to each dish on day 1. The cells remain quiescent until day 7, when the cell number increases slightly but not significantly ($7.01 \pm 0.25 \times 10^5$ cells/dish). Confluency is attained on day 9 ($8.26 \pm 0.32 \times 10^5$ cells/dish) and maintained on day 12 with no further increase ($8.42 \pm 0.35 \times 10^5$ cells/dish).

The V_v myo of the same cells as above falls from $35.37 \pm 1.51\%$ on day 0 ($39.50 \pm 1.2\%$ intact media) to $32.78 \pm 1.26\%$ on day 5 and $33.08 \pm 0.89\%$ on day 7, rising to $37.62 \pm 2.49\%$ on day 12. Thus the change in the complement of myofilaments of the smooth muscle cell popu-

←

Figure 4-3. Gap junction formed between two enzymatically isolated smooth muscle cells from the 10-day chick embryo gizzard five days in culture. From Campbell GR, Uehara Y, Mark G, Burnstock G: *J Cell Biol* 49: 21–34, 1971.

Figure 4-4. Newborn guinea pig vas deferens smooth muscle cell four days in primary cell culture. Note the presence of thick and thin myofilaments, numerous plasmalemmal vesicles, lipid droplet, and the elongate mitochondrion.

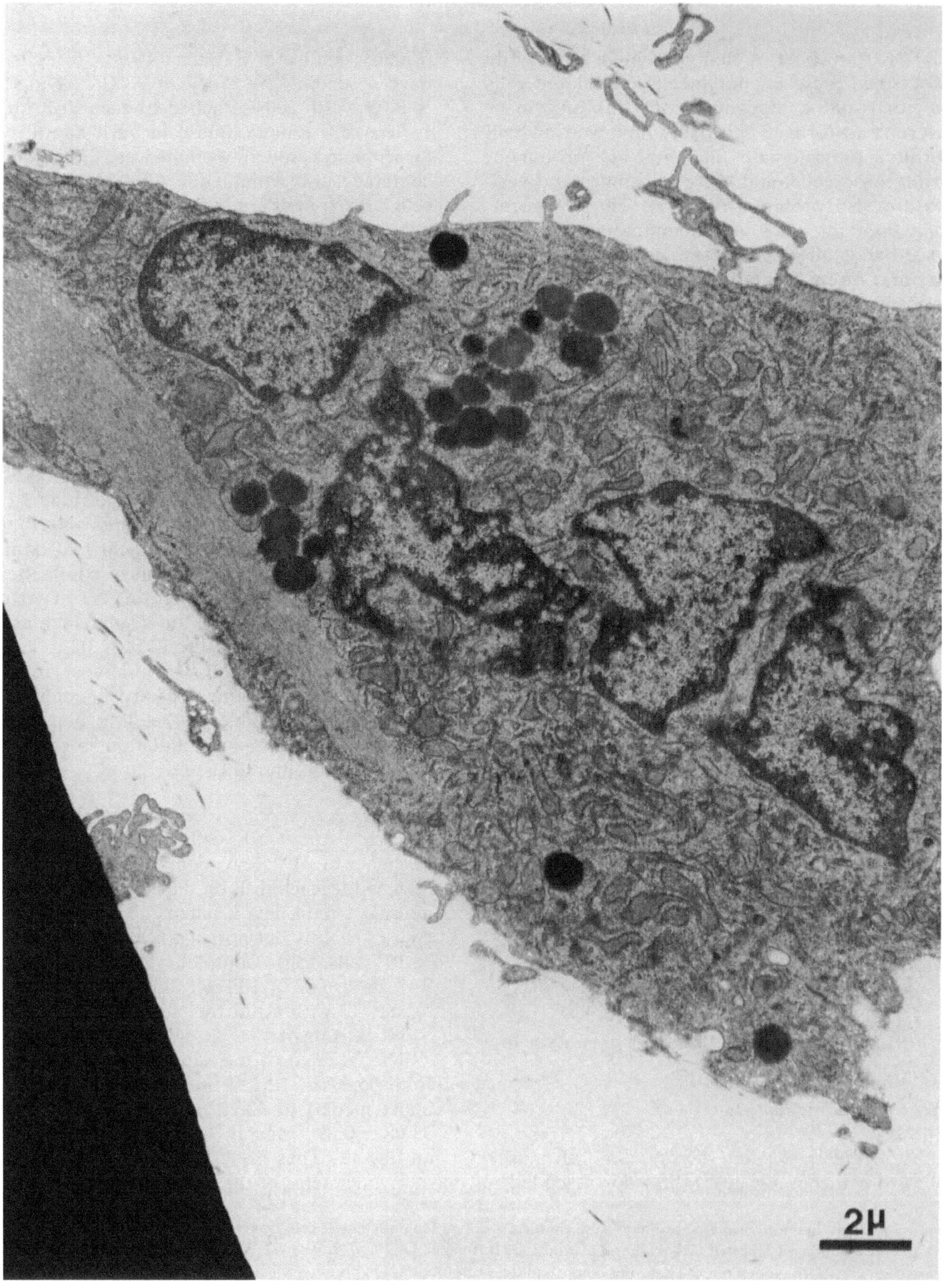
2μ

lations as a whole is very small and completely reversible (95). That is, if the cells are seeded at a high density from the beginning of culture, they do not undergo a process of phenotypic modulation.

4.1.3. Sparse seeding density. Rabbit aortic smooth muscle cells seeded sparsely in primary culture at $0.30 \pm 0.02 \times 10^5$ cells/dish have a seeding efficiency of 66%, leaving $0.20 \pm 0.02 \times 10^5$ cells/dish on day 1. Logarithmic growth commences on day 6 and continues until confluency on day 19 ($7.70 \pm 0.42 \times 10^5$ cells/dish), after which the cell number remains constant (day 24: $8.25 \pm 0.36 \times 10^5$ cells/dish).

The V_v myo of the same population of cells as above decreases to 10.26 ± 0.21% on day 5, then remains low throughout the culture period, including five days after confluency (day 24) when the V_v myo is 8.06 ± 1.24% (95). Thus the process of phenotypic modulation under these circumstances is not reversible, with the cells remaining in a functionally synthetic phenotype indefinitely (96).

4.2. Co-culture with endothelium or smooth muscle

Spontaneous phenotypic modulation of sparsely seeded smooth muscle from the contractile to synthetic phenotype in primary cell culture is prevented if the cells are grown in co-culture with a confluent monolayer of endothelial cells (68, 96, 97). The two cell layers do not have to be in contact, but must be bathed by the same nutrient medium. This occurs in modified Rose chambers where the test and feeder cell layers are grown on opposite coverslips (96). A feeder layer of confluent, contractile smooth muscle cells (which is above the critical cell density and does not undergo the spontaneous phenotypic change) also prevents the test, sparsely seeded, contractile smooth muscle cells from spontaneously modulating their phenotype. Co-culture with confluent adventitial fibroblasts, confluent subcultured synthetic state smooth muscle cells, or subconfluent proliferating endothelial cells does not prevent the spontaneous phenotypic change of contractile smooth muscle (96).

Thus confluent smooth muscle cells and endothelial cells release inhibitors for smooth muscle phenotypic modulation. The approximate Mr of this inhibitory substance or substances is 10,000–15,000 as determined by insertion of spectropor wet dialysis membranes of different molecular weight cutoff between the test and feeder layers of cells (97). A glycosaminoglycan extract of Mr ≈ 12,000 from the artery wall inhibits smooth muscle phenotypic change (96, 97). Treatment of this aortic glycosaminoglycan extract with 4 units/ml heparinase from *Flavobactrium heparinum* for 6 hours at 37°C destroys the active factor, and addition of sodium heparin to culture medium also inhibits smooth muscle phenotypic change (96, 97). These results suggest that the active factor produced by endothelium and contractile smooth muscle which inhibits smooth muscle phenotypic change is a glycosaminoglycan related to heparin.

Karnovsky and colleagues found that heparin inhibits myointimal proliferation after endothelial injury in vivo, and that the addition of anticoagulant or nonanticoagulant heparin to culture medium inhibits proliferation of smooth muscle in vitro. The active inhibitory component of heparin is a pentasaccharide fragment with a 3-0-sulphate group in the internal glucosamine residue (98). Further studies indicate that endothelial cells exert their inhibitory effect on smooth muscle growth by the release of a heparinlike molecule from the basal lamina of the endothelium (97, 99), which then acts on the smooth muscle. Postconfluent smooth muscle cells also produce an antiproliferative heparin sulphate species (100). A serum factor is required for release of the heparinlike inhibitory factor, and has been identified as the endoglycosidase heparitinase (101) found in platelet lysosomes (102).

The mechanism by which heparinlike molecules exert their antiproliferative action is poorly understood. Heparin binds to the surface of smooth muscle cells via specific, high-affinity

←

Figure 4-5. Enzymatically isolated smooth muscle cell from the nine-week rabbit thoracic aortic media six days in primary culture. Note the presence of large amounts of dilated rough ER, free ribosomes, and mitochondria. Plasmalemmal vesicles are present along the cell membrane, as are small fingerlike projections. A few osmiophilic lipid droplets are also present in the cytoplasm.

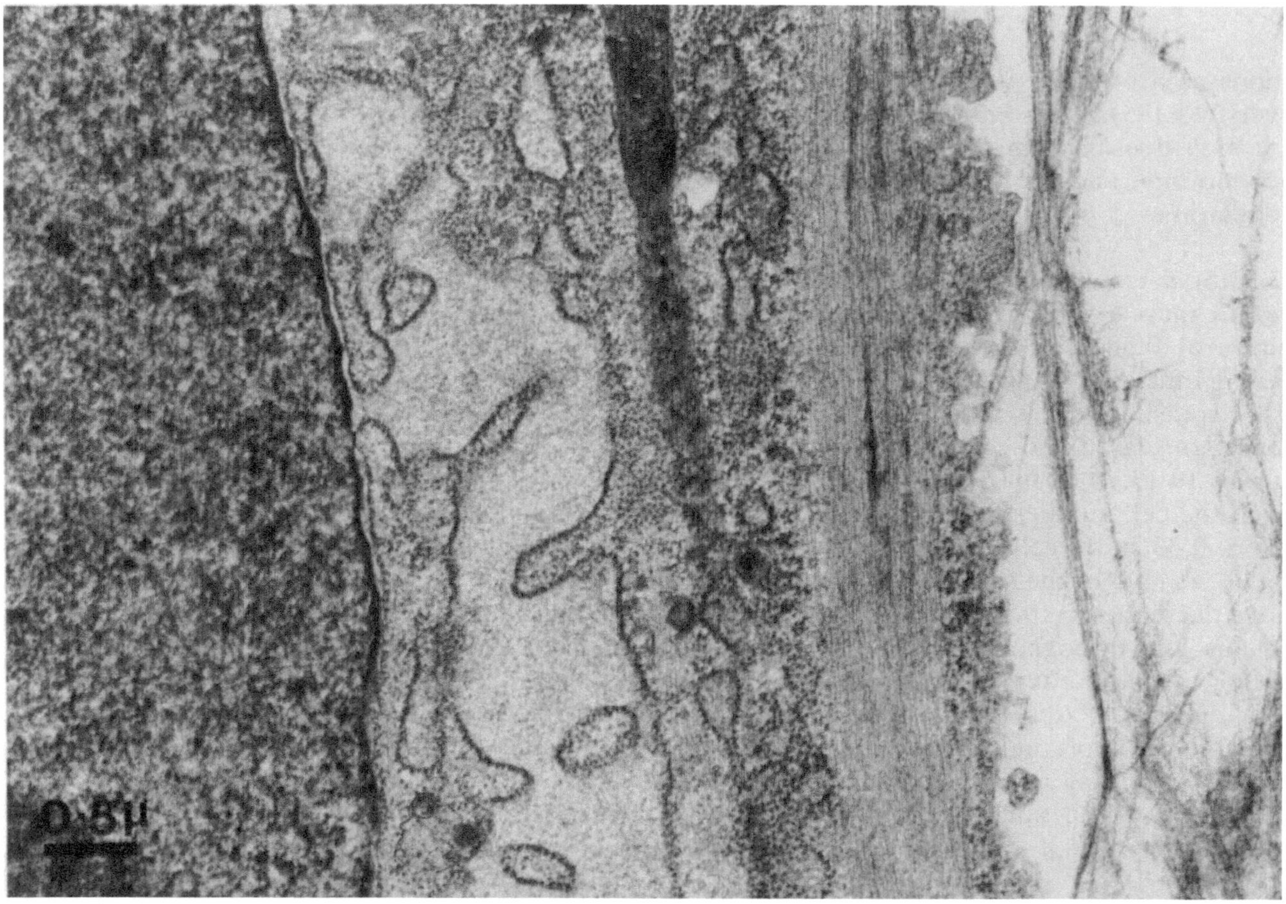
0·5 μ

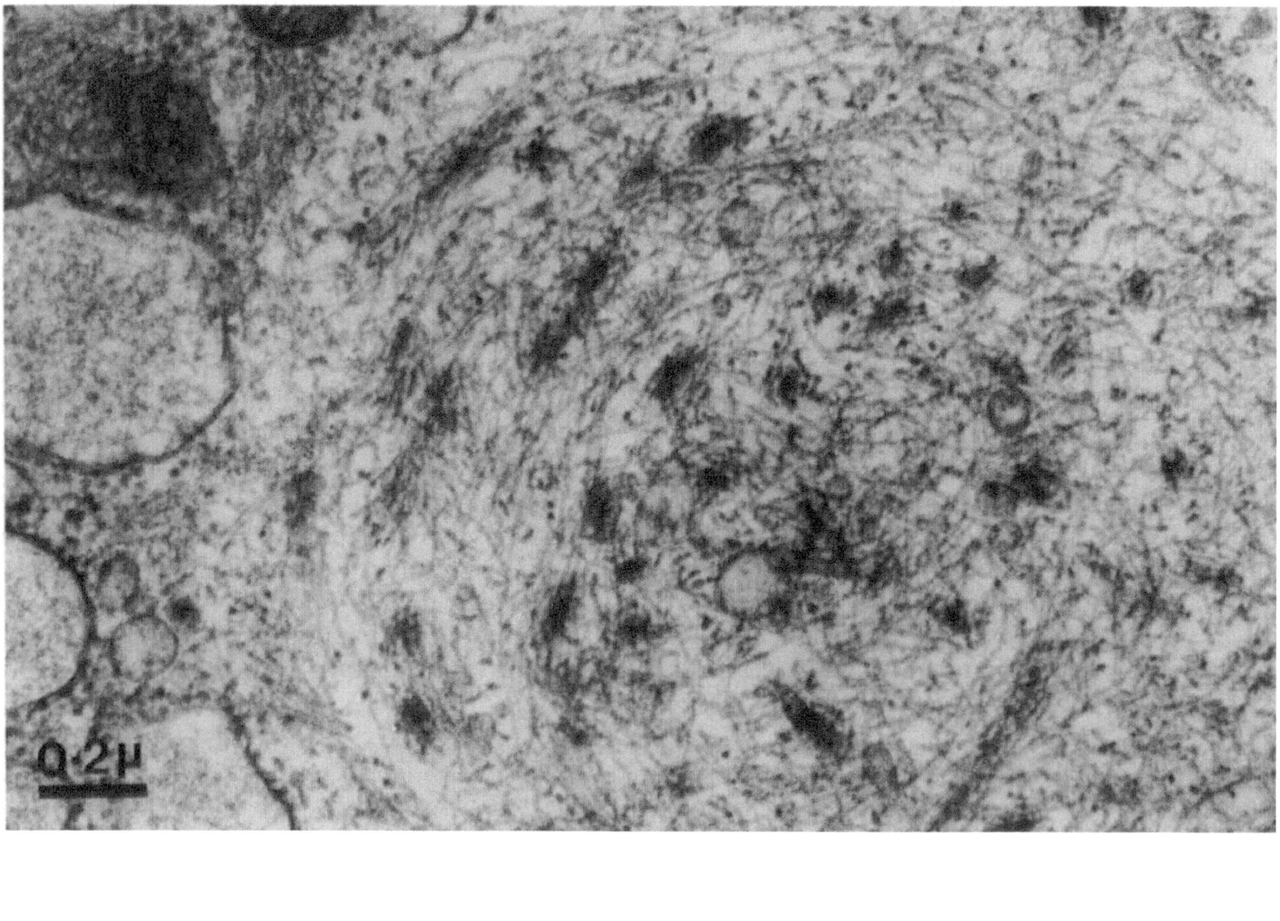
0·2 μ

binding sites and is subsequently internalized by a mechanism consistent with a receptor-mediated endocytotic pathway (103). In addition, the glycosaminoglycan retains its complete antiproliferative ability when assayed in medium depleted of all heparin-binding proteins (104). Thus, heparin may exert its effects at specific cellular or intracellular sites rather than in the extracellular environment. Heparin does not exert its action indirectly by binding the smooth muscle mitogen platelet-derived growth factor (PDGF), nor does it act by blocking the PDGF receptors on smooth muscle (104). However, the antiproliferative effects of heparin are reversed by epidermal growth factor (EGF), opening the possibility that heparin exerts its antiproliferative effects by interfering with the response of smooth muscle to EGF-like mitogens of platelet origin (105). This notion is consistent with the work of Majack and Bornstein (106–108), which suggests that thrombospondin (a glycoprotein component of the smooth muscle cell extracellular matrix in vitro) plays an important role in the growth response of these cells. Thrombospondin synthesis by smooth muscle cells is regulated by PDGF (109) at the mRNA level (100). Once synthesized, the thrombospondin is bound to the cell surface, where it facilitates the response to EGF (108). Heparin inhibits the binding of thrombospondin to the smooth muscle cell surface (109) and prevents thrombospondin/EGF-mediated mitogenesis (108, 111).

The observation that vessel wall cells can produce a connective tissue molecule able to maintain smooth muscle in the contractile phenotype and to inhibit proliferation suggests a mechanism for releasing cells from the quiescent state. Platelets are known to contain a heparan sulphate-degrading endoglycosidase that could theoretically digest the extracellular matrix, removing its inhibitory effect and thereby allowing the cells to replicate (112, 113). Certainly, incubation of endothelial cells with a crude platelet enzyme preparation, or with a partially purified preparation of heparan-sulphate-degrading endoglycosidase from the same source, causes a marked release of cell-surface heparan sulphate, which appears in the incubation medium as oligosaccharides. The platelet heparitinase cuts the heparinlike species at the relatively rare glucuronsyl-glycosamine bonds outside the highly sulphated regions (102). Castellot et al. (101) proposed that, following endothelial denudation or injury, platelets are deposited on the subendothelium, releasing heparitinase, platelet factor 4, and PDGF. The heparitinase cleaves heparinlike substances on the endothelium and smooth muscle into fragments that diffuse away, with additional inactivation of the substance by platelet factor 4 (114). With the heparinlike substance removed, smooth muscle cells may undergo phenotypic changes from the contractile to synthetic state (115) and may also be released from growth inhibition. PDGF and other mitogens can then act on the cells to stimulate their proliferation.

4.3. Factors from sympathetic nerves

Chamley and Campbell (64, 66–68, 72, 116) have demonstrated that when smooth muscle cells from the newborn guinea pig vas deferens are enzymatically dispersed into single cells and grown in culture, they maintain a similar phenotype to the in situ tissue for approximately five days before undergoing the process of phenotypic modulation. However, the presence of sympathetic nerve fibers in association with these single isolated smooth muscle cells inhibits their phenotypic modulation. The addition of sympathetic chain homogenate has a similar inhibitory effect (Fig. 4-8), while the neurotransmitters acetylcholine or noradrenaline have little or no effect (64, 116). The presence of nerve fibers also accelerates smooth muscle bundle formation and the presence of gap junctions between cells (68).

←

Figure 4-6. Smooth muscle cell from the newborn guinea pig vas deferens after seven days in vitro. The myofilament bundle contains only thin (60–80A) filaments with associated dark bodies. The rough ER is continuous with the nuclear envelope and is dilated, containing an electron-dense flocculent material. From Chamley JH, Campbell GR, Burnstock G: *J Embryol Exp Morph* 32: 297–323, 1974.

Figure 4-7. Network of intermediate filaments with associated dark bodies found in a smooth muscle cell from the ten-day chick embryo gizzard enzymatically isolated and grown in culture for five days. From Campbell GR, Uehara Y, Mark G, Burnstock G: *J Cell Biol* 49: 21–34, 1971.

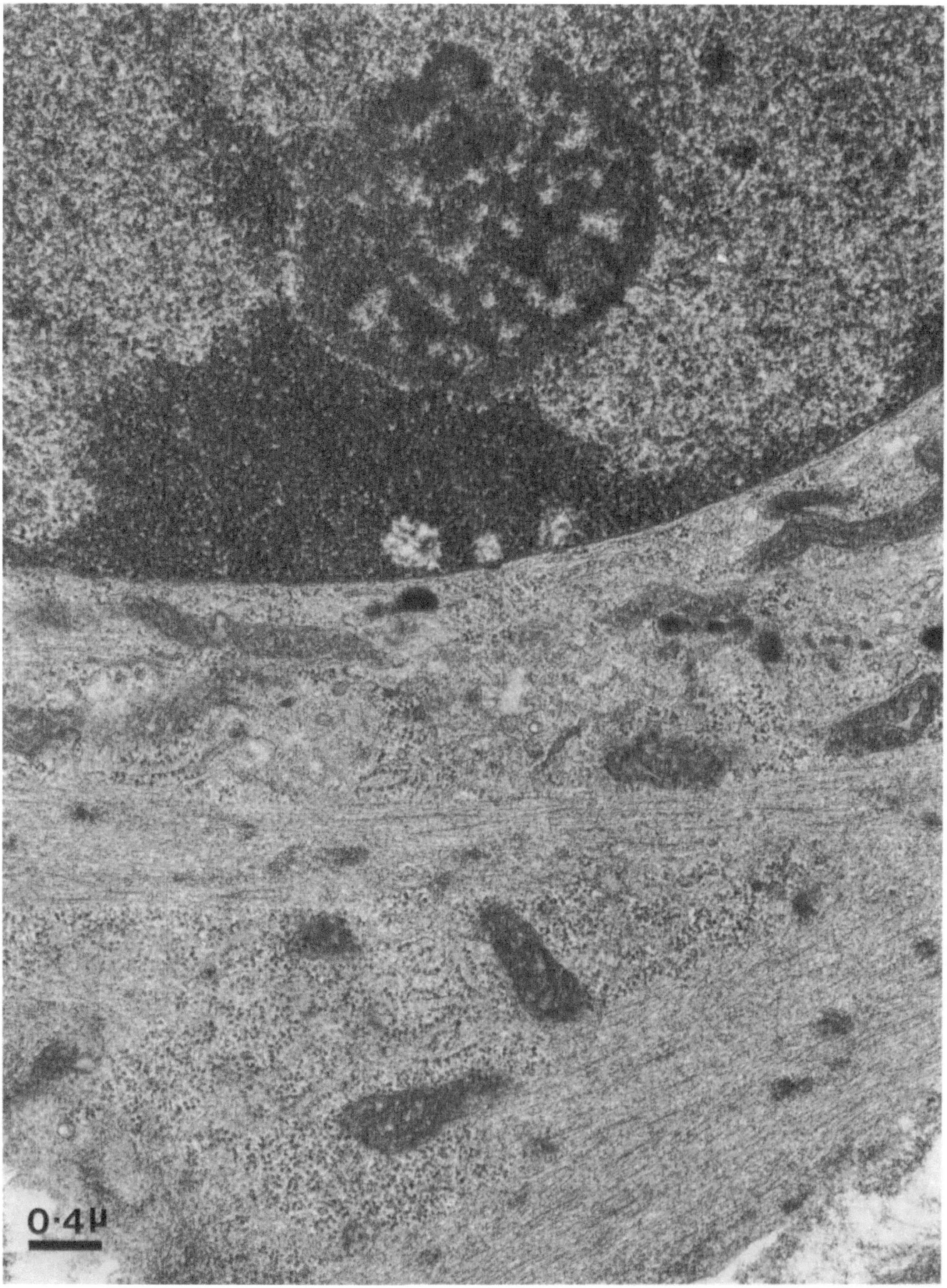
0·4μ

4.4. Dibutyryl cyclic AMP

Dibutyryl cyclic AMP (N^6, 0^6-dibutyryl adenosine 3′:5′-cyclic monophosphoric acid) or theophylline (a cyclic AMP phosphodiesterase inhibitor) added to the culture medium maintains sparsely seeded smooth muscle cells in a phenotype similar to that of the tissue of origin (64). Even after eight to ten days in culture, the cytoplasm of guinea pig vas deferens cells is almost completely occupied by thick and thin myofilaments with associated dark bodies (Fig. 4-9). Plasmalemmal vesicles are numerous, as are dense areas along the cell membrane. Organelles such as free ribosomes, mitochondria, and Golgi are few in number and are usually confined to the perinuclear region.

4.5. Co-culture with macrophages

The effect of macrophages on rabbit vascular smooth muscle phenotype and proliferative ability has recently been examined (117, 118). With ultrastructural morphometry the volume fraction of myofilaments (V_v myo) in smooth muscle cells from nine-week-old rabbit aorta in vivo is 39.5 ± 1.2%. After seeding the enzymatically isolated cells at 4×10^5 cells/ml in primary culture, the V_v myo is 38.9 ± 1.2% on day 3, dropping to 29.9 ± 2.0% by day 5. On day 6, the V_v myo is 29.2 ± 1.8%, and the cells begin to proliferate. Confluency is reached after less than 24 hours proliferation, and the V_v myo rises abruptly on day 7 to 36.9 ± 1.9%. When the cells are co-cultured with macrophages, the V_v myo falls to 31.2 ± 0.9% on day 3 and to 25.9 ± 0.5% on day 5, at which time cells commence proliferation. Confluency occurs on day 6, but the V_v myo does not rise throughout the rest of the culture period (27.4 ± 1.8% and 26.9 ± 1.3% on days 7 and 9, respectively) and the cells, unlike the controls, continue to proliferate becoming multilayered (118).

Measurement of proliferation by cell counts and tritiated thymidine autoradiography shows that macrophages stimulate smooth muscle cells in primary culture to proliferate at a significantly greater rate than control cells grown alone in 5% whole blood serum. Proliferation of subcultured smooth muscle cells co-cultured with macrophages is also stimulated. Prior loading of macrophages with lipid or macrophages activated with concanavalin A (ConA) at low seeding densities does not alter the degree of stimulation. However, when high seeding densities of macrophages activated with ConA are present, smooth muscle proliferation is inhibited (118).

These results suggest that macrophages, as well as being a source of lipid-laden foam cells in atherosclerosis, may play other important roles in this disease, such as initiating a change in smooth muscle phenotype and influencing their proliferative response and their pattern of growth.

4.6. Plasma fibronectin

Recent studies have shown that plasma fibronectin is a determinant of the phenotype of rat arterial medial cells (119). When seeded on a human plasma fibronectin-coated substrate and cultured in a defined, serum-free medium, these cells more rapidly modulate to the synthetic phenotype than control freshly isolated cells. Also, the cells seeded on the plasma fibronectin-coated substrate do not synthesize DNA and divide until stimulated with PDGF or serum (119).

5. Subcultured smooth muscle cells

5.1. General features

Subcultured smooth muscle cells are usually obtained by cutting the tissue into 1 mm^3 pieces and placing the explants in a culture flask (see 120, 121). Outgrowth from the explants reaches confluency in two to three weeks. The cells are then detached from the substrate and placed in culture dishes at a known concentration (sub-

←

Figure 4-8. Newborn guinea pig vas deferens smooth muscle cell after eight days in vitro with sympathetic ganglion extract plus ascorbic acid added to the medium (see 64). Myofilament bundles contain both thick and thin filaments. Note the nucleous and the small lysosomes and microtubules in the perinuclear region.

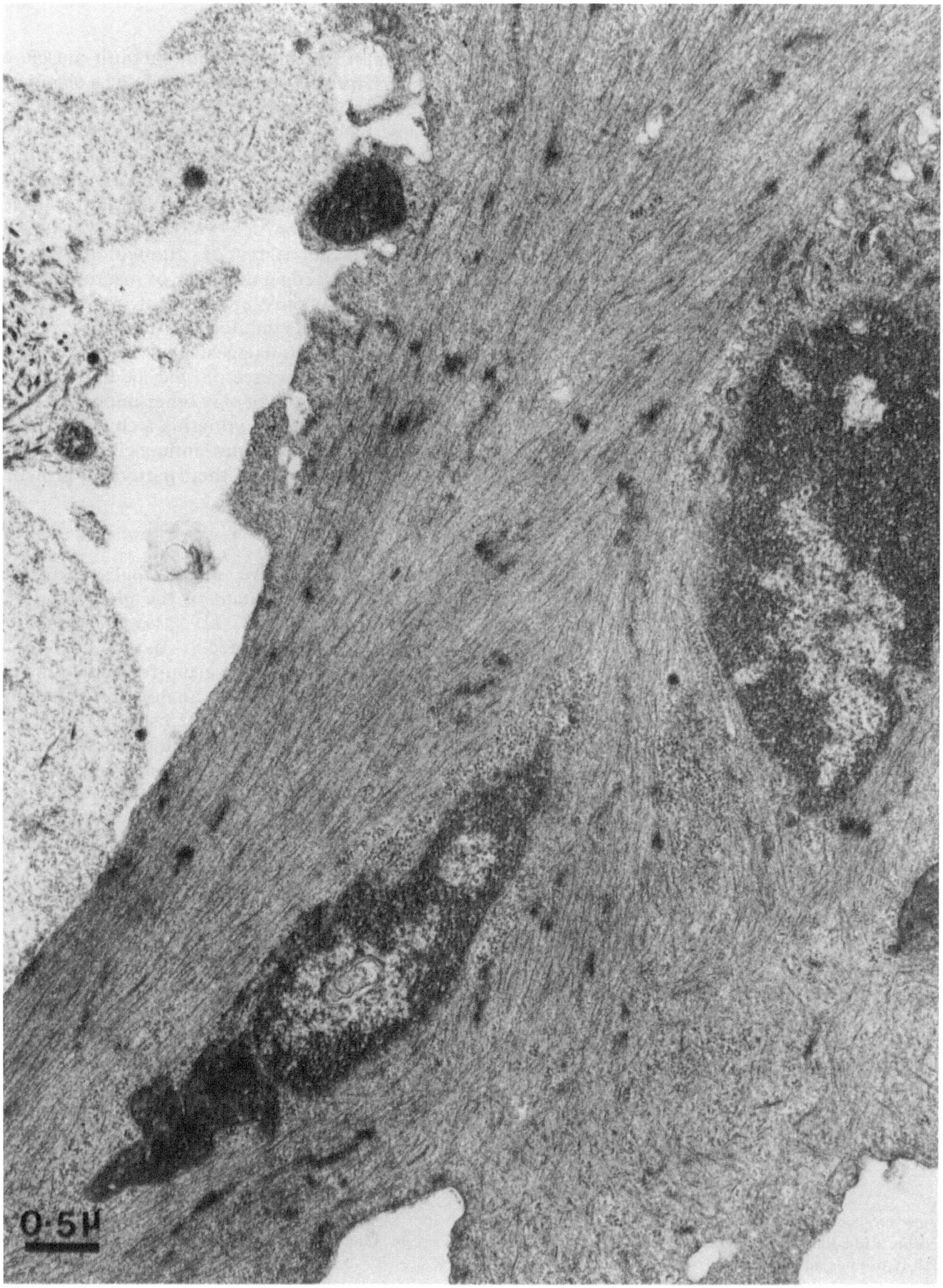
0·5μ

culture). When these cells proliferate to reach confluency, they are again detached to form further subcultures (passaging). The size and shape of the passaged cells vary and depend on culture conditions and density of cell seeding (32, 70, 120–122). The origin of the cells also appears to be important in early passages of subcultured cells (123). The perinuclear region of the cells is usually granular and surrounded by a broad expanse of clear cytoplasm containing a series of prominent parallel lines. Some cells have long, narrow cytoplasmic processes that contact adjacent cells. Ultrastructurally, the cells appear to have primarily a synthetic function with thin filament bundles interspersed with large areas of free ribosomes and polysomes, dilated rough ER, mitochondria, lysosomes, and prominent Golgi complexes. Dark bodies, or attachment plaques, are found throughout the bundles of thin filament, which are usually located on the bottom of the cell adjacent to the substratum. No thick myofilaments have been seen under a variety of fixation conditions. Plasmalemmal vesicles are occasionally observed, as is material reminiscent of a basal lamina. More 100-A filaments appear to be present in these smooth muscle cells than those of primary culture.

In the presence of the standard 5%–10% fetal calf serum, subcultured smooth muscle cells grow logarithmically in overlapping layers until they reach a certain density. In the presence of the same concentration of homologous serum, the cells grow to the same or higher density but the pattern is different in that they tend to grow in a series of hills and valleys. The hills contain cells that have piled upon one another to form as many as 10–15 cell layers, whereas the valleys may contain no cells or 1–3 layers. Gap junctions are sometimes present between cells in these hills (124–126). The cells behave in the same manner with each subsequent passage, except that their doubling time increases and they grow to lower population densities. Cultures of either growing or confluent cells stain only very weakly with fluoresceinated antibodies to smooth muscle myosin (70), and do not contract spontaneously or in response to drugs such as angiotensin II, norepinephrine, epinephrine, serotonin, creatinine sulphate, and histamine, or to electrical or mechanical stimulation (70, 127, 128).

In 1977, Fowler et al. (129) biochemically compared subcultured smooth muscle cells with those of the calf aortic media. They found that in the subcultured cells there was a ninefold increase in 5′-nucleotidase (plasma membranes), a fourfold increase in neutral α-glucosidase (lysosomes and microsomes), a sevenfold increase in cytochrome oxidase (mitochondria), a 21-fold increase in acid cholesteryl esterase (lysosomes), a 26-fold increase in β-galactosidase (lysosomes), a 5.5-fold increase in N-acetyl-β-glucosaminidase (lysosomes), and a 4.5-fold increase in cathepsin C (lysosomes). These increases in enzymatic activity are indicative of the increase in organelles (particularly lysosomes) within subcultured smooth muscle cells at the expense of myofilaments (129–131). These lysosomes, while having a similar K^+/Na^+ concentration ratio to that in the cytoplasm (132), have a higher sulphur concentration, and many have an unusual tubular structure (133).

5.2. *Morphometry*

Mazurkowitz et al. (134) morphometrically analyzed changes in organelle content in subcultured rabbit and calf smooth muscle cells with time in culture. They found large changes in cytoplasmic volume content of particular components depending upon the time in culture. For example, in seond-passage rabbit aortic arch medial cells, myofilaments constitute approximately 48% of the cytoplasmic volume by seven days in culture. This rises to just over 60% by 21 days, then drops to approximately 25% by 78 days in culture. However, lysosomes constitute 10%–15% of the volume composition during the first 21 days in culture, then rise significantly to make up al-

←

Figure 4-9. Enzymatically isolated smooth muscle cell from newborn guinea pig vas deferens eight days in primary culture in the presence of medium 199 with 5×10^{-4} g/ml 3′ : 5′ dibutyryl cyclic AMP + 5×10^{-4} g/ml theophylline. Under these conditions, the cells maintain a phenotype similar to that in vivo and when first placed in culture. The cytoplasm of the cell here is almost completely filled with thick and thin myofilaments and associated dark bodies. X 24,000. From Chamley JH, Campbell GR: *Cell Tissue Res* 161: 497–510, 1975.

most 65% of the cytoplasmic volume by 78 days. Ribosomes and rough ER volume also decrease substantially by 78 days. Further passaging of the cells (particularly beyond passage 3) also leads to significant reduction in the myofilament volume and increases in lysosomal volume (134).

The effects of ascorbate on cultured smooth muscle cellular organelle content have also been determined morphometrically (134). It has been shown in fibroblast cultures that underhydroxylated collagen is not secreted as readily as that which is fully hydroxylated (a process requiring ascorbate) (135, 136). Second-passage rabbit aortic arch medial cells grown without ascorbate develop large rough ER cisternae by 14 days that constitute almost 20% of the cytoplasmic volume at this time. In contrast, ascorbate-fed rabbit cells have smaller rough ER that constitutes just over 10% of the cytoplasmic volume (134).

5.3. *Effect of cyclic stretching*

Subcultured rabbit aortic cells, when grown on a cyclically stretched purified bovine aortic elastic membrane, increase their synthesis of collagen and certain acid mucopolysaccharides without affecting their proliferative rate (137, 138). Quantitation of the organelles within these stretched cells reveals that rough ER profiles are five times more abundant in stretched than in nonstretched cells, and these appear to increase with the duration of cyclic stretching. That is, cells stretched for 56 hours have 25% more rough ER than those stretched for eight hours. There appeared to be a reciprocal relationship between the cytoplasmic volume of myofilaments and rough ER (139).

6. Development of smooth muscle cells in primary culture

There are two ultrastructural reports of the progressive development of embryonic smooth muscle cells in culture.

When gizzards from ten-day-old chick embryos are dispersed into single cells, they attach to a substrate and flatten within a few hours. About 40% of these isolated immature muscle cells are polyhedral, while the remaining 60% are spindle-shaped (140). Intense proliferation immediately takes place in both the polyhedral and spindle-shaped muscle cells and in fibroblasts, forming a confluent monolayer after 24–36 hours. The polyhedral cells do not contract spontaneously, and during the first three days they gradually elongate and narrow. The spindle-shaped cells contract at a rate of about once per minute and gradually elongate to become ribbon-spindle-shaped by day 3. The muscle cells that are polyhedral early in culture become ribbon-spindle-shaped by day 6 and begin to contract synchronously in large sheets. The contractions are strong and at a rate of about two per minute. The cells that early in culture are spindle-shaped become ribbon-shaped by day 6. By day 11 all muscle cells have become ribbon-shaped and cease spontaneous contractions. By day 14 they have elongated further to about 280 μm and are fusiform in shape. Ultrastructurally, the cultured cells of the gizzard pass through stages closely resembling normal in vivo development (141). In addition, isolated smooth muscle cells from gizzards of 8-, 10-, 12-, 17-, and 19-day-old chick embryos, when first in culture, have a polyhedral, spindle, ribbon-spindle, ribbon, or fusiform shape, respectively, which is the same progression that cells from the ten-day-old chick undergo during development in culture. This suggests that, during development in vivo, smooth muscle cells may progress through the same changes in shape before reaching their mature fusiform shape (140). The presence of spontaneous contractions in only the spindle-shaped and ribbon-spindle-shaped cells of the gizzard in culture may reflect a particular developmental stage at which they have both a well-developed contractile apparatus and resting potentials sufficiently low to be within the zone of firing (142), since cells of the adult gizzard are not spontaneously active (143).

Wight et al. (144) examined the outgrowth of cells from explants of 18-day-old pigeon embryos. They found that during subsequent periods of culture (5–12 days), various stages of smooth muscle cell development occur, similar to the stages characteristic of developing smooth muscle cells in vivo (see previous sections).

7. Conclusions

Enzyme-dispersed smooth muscle cells in primary culture closely resemble their in vivo counterparts in the first few days of primary culture. After this time, their ultrastructure and biology (phenotype) depends on their initial seeding density. Embryonic cells, seeded densely, undergo normal development and differentiation. Adult cells, seeded densely, remain unchanged with a high volume fraction of myofilaments. Adult cells, seeded less densely, undergo a change in phenotype after a few days in culture such that they develop a low volume fraction of myofilaments and a high volume fraction of synthetic organelles. These cells respond to mitogens present in whole blood serum and proliferate to confluency. If the cells undergo more than five population doublings, they regain their full complement of myofilaments. However, cells that are moderately seeded and undergo fewer than five population doublings return to their original phenotypic state upon confluency.

Similar phenotypic changes occur in vivo under conditions of injury and repair, and modulation of smooth muscle phenotype is a characteristic feature of some pathological conditions such as atherosclerosis. Cell culture is thus a useful technique to study these phenomena and to determine factors that control smooth muscle phenotypic expression.

Acknowledgments

The authors wish to thank Ms. Fabian Bowers for her patient typing of the manuscript. This work was supported by grants from the National Heart Foundation of Australia and the National Health and Medical Research Council.

References

1. Campbell JH, Campbell GR: Chemical stimuli of the hypertrophic response in smooth muscle. In: Hypertrophic Response in Smooth Muscle. CL Seidel, NW Weisbrodt (eds), Boca Raton, FL: CRC Press, 153–192, 1987.
2. Gabella G: Structural apparatus for force transmission in smooth muscles. *Physiol Rev* 64: 447–455, 1984.
3. Campbell GR, Chamley-Campbell JH, Burnstock G: Differentiation and phenotypic modulation of arterial smooth muscle cells. In: Structure and Function of the Circulation, Vol 3. CJ Schwartz, NT Werthessen, S Wolf (eds), New York: Plenum 357–399, 1981.
4. Pease DC, Paule WJ: Electron microscopy of elastic arteries. The thoracic aorta of the rat. *J Ultrastruct Res* 3: 469–483, 1960.
5. Karrer HE: An electron microscope study of the aorta in young and aging mice. *J Ultrastruct Res* 5: 1–27, 1961.
6. Paule WJ: Electron microscopy of the newborn rat aorta. *J Ultrastructure Res* 8: 219–235, 1963.
7. Gerrity RG, Cliff WJ: The aortic tunica media of the developing rat. I. Quantitative stereologic and biochemical analysis. *Lab Invest* 32: 585–600, 1975.
8. Olivetti G, Anversa P, Melissari M, Loud AV: Morphometry of medial hypertrophy in the rat thoracic aorta. *Lab Invest* 42: 559–565, 1980.
9. Yamamoto I: An electron microscope study on development of uterine smooth muscle. *J Electron Microsc (Tokyo)* 10: 145–160, 1961.
10. Leeson TS, Leeson CR: The rat ureter. Fine structural changes during its development. *Acta Anat* 62: 60–79, 1965.
11. Bennett T, Cobb JLS: Studies on the avian gizzard: the development of the gizzard and its innervation. *Z Zellforsch Mikrosk Anat* 98: 599–621, 1969.
12. Imaizumi M, Kuwabara T: Development of the rat iris. *Invest Ophthalmol* 10: 733–744, 1971.
13. Hoyes AD, Ramus NI, Martin BGH: Differentiation of the muscle of the human fetal bladder: an ultrastructural study. *Micron* 3: 414–419, 1972.
14. Yamauchi A, Burnstock G: Post-natal development of smooth muscle cells in the mouse vas deferens. A fine structural study. *J Anat* 104: 1–16, 1969.
15. Sethi N, Brookes M: Ultrastructure of the blood vessels in the chick allantois and chorioallantois. *J Anat* 109: 1–15, 1971.
16. Manasek FJ: The ultrastructure of embryonic myocardial blood vessels. *Dev Biol* 26: 42–54, 1971.
17. De Simone-Santoro I, Renda T: Recherches ultrastructurales, histochimiques et histoenzymologiques sur la paroi aortique pendant sa morphagenese chez l'embryon de poulet. *Ann Histochim* 16: 171–181, 1971.
18. *Blatt JH*: Uber die Entwichlung der Coronararterien bei der Ratte Licht-und electronmikroskopische Untersuchungen. *Z Anat Entwicklungsgesch* 142: 53–64, 1973.
19. Gonzalez-Crussi F: Vasculogenesis in the chick embryo. An ultrastructural study. *Am J Anat* 130: 441–460, 1971.
20. Wolinsky H, Glagov S: A lamellar unit of aortic medial structure and function in mammals. *Circ Res* 20: 99–101, 1967.
21. Dilley RJ, McGeachie JK, Prendergast FJ: A review of the proliferative behaviour, morphology and phenotypes of vascular smooth muscle. *Atherosclerosis* 63: 99–107, 1987.
22. Campbell GR, Uehara Y, Malmfors T, Burnstock G: Degeneration and regeneration of smooth muscle trans-

plants in the anterior eye chamber. An ultrastructural study. *Z Zellforsch Mikrosk Anat* 117: 155–175, 1971.
23. Kiviat MD, Ross R, Ansell JS: Smooth muscle regeneration in the ureter. Electron microscopic and autoradiographic observations. *Am J Pathol* 72: 403–412, 1973.
24. McGeachie JK: Smooth muscle regeneration. A review and experimental study. *Monogr Dev Biol* 9: 1–190, 1975.
25. Dalley BK, Bartone FF, Gardner PJ: Smooth muscle regeneration in swine ureters. A light and electron microscope study. *Invest Urol* 14: 104–110, 1976.
26. Yokota R, Burnstock G, Jones R, Brown JD: An ultrastructural study of regeneration of minced smooth muscle in the vas deferens of the guinea-pig. *Cell Tissue Res* 481–493, 1978.
27. Florentin RA, Nam SC, Lee KT, Thomas WA: Increased mitotic activity in aortas of swine after 3 days of cholesterol feeding. *Arch Pathol* 88: 463–469, 1969.
28. Cobb JLS, Bennett T: An ultrastructural study of mitotic division in differentiated gastric smooth muscle cells. *Z Zellforsch Mikrosk Anat* 108: 177–189, 1970.
29. Scott RF, Jarmolych J, Fritz KE, Imai H, Kim DN, Morrison ES: Reactions of endothelial and smooth muscle cells in the atherosclerotic lesion. *Atherosclerosis* 2: 50–58, 1970.
30. Chamley JH, Campbell GR: Mitosis of contractile smooth muscle cells in tissue culture. *Exp Cell Res* 84: 105–110, 1974.
31. Gabella G: Fine structure of smooth muscle. I. Cellular structures and electrophysiological behaviour; fine structure of smooth muscle. *Philos Trans R Soc London B* 265: 7–16, 1973.
32. Chamley-Campbell J, Campbell GR, Ross R: The smooth muscle cell in culture. *Physiol Rev* 59: 1–61, 1979.
33. Thomas WA, Jones R, Scott RF, Morrison E, Goodale F, Imai H: Production of early atherosclerotic lesions in rats is characterised by proliferation of "modified smooth muscle cells". *Exp Mol Pathol* 1 (Suppl): 40–61, 1963.
34. Scott RF, Jones R, Daoud AS, Zumbo O, Coulston F, Thomas WA: Experimental atherosclerosis in Rhesus monkeys. II. Cellular elements of proliferative lesions and possible role of cytoplasmic degeneration in pathogenesis as studied by electron microscopy. *Exp Mol Pathol* 7: 34–57, 1967.
35. Thomas WA, Florentin RA, Nam SC, Kim DN, Jones RM, Lee KT: Preproliferative phase of atherosclerosis in swine fed choelsterol. *Arch Pathol* 86: 621–643, 1968.
36. Imai H, Lee KJ, Lee SK, Lee KT, O'Neal RM, Thomas WA: Ultrastructural features of aortic cells in mitosis in control and cholesterol-fed swine. *Lab Invest* 23: 401–415, 1970.
37. Poole JCF, Cromwell SB, Benditt EP: Behavior of smooth muscle cells and formation of extracellular structures in the reaction of arterial walls to injury. *Am J Pathol* 62: 391–414, 1971.
38. Stary HC: Proliferation of arterial cells in atherosclerosis. *Adv Exp Med Biol* 43: 59–81, 1974.
39. Glagov S, Ts'ao CH: Restitution of aortic wall after sustained necrotizing transmural ligation injury: role of blood cells and artery cells. *Am J Pathol* 79: 7–30, 1975.
40. Kamio A, Huang WY, Imai H, Kummerow FA: Mitotic structures of aortic smooth muscle cells in swine and in culture: paired cisternae. *J Electron Microsc (Tokyo)* 26: 29–40, 1977.
41. Taura M: Origin and fate of paired cisternae in mitotic aortic cells of swine. *J Electron Microsc (Tokyo)* 27: 283–291, 1978.
42. Bjorkerud S, Bondjers G: Arterial repair and atherosclerosis after mechanical injury. Part 5. Tissue response after induction of a large superficial transverse injury. *Atherosclerosis* 18: 235–255, 1973.
43. Stemerman MB, Spaet TH, Pitlick F, Cintron J, Lejnieks I, Tiell ML: Intimal healing. The pattern of reendothelialization and intimal thickening. *Am J Pathol* 87: 125–142, 1977.
44. Ross R: Smooth muscle cells and atherosclerosis. In: Vascular Injury and Atherosclerosis. S Moore (ed), New York: Marcel Dekker, 53–60, 1981.
45. Veress B, Kadar A, Jellinek H: Ultrastructural elements in experimental intimal thickening. I. Electron microscopic study of the development and cellular elements of intimal proliferation. *Exp Mol Pathol* 11: 200–211, 1969.
46. Baumgartner HR, Studer A: Consequences of vessel catheterization in normo- and hypercholesterolaemic rabbits (German). *Pathol Microbiol* 29: 393–405, 1966.
47. Stemerman MB, Ross R: Experimental arteriosclerosis. I. Fibrous plaque formation in primates, an electron microscope study. *J Exp Med* 136: 769–789, 1972.
48. Schwartz SM, Stemerman MB, Benditt EP: The aortic intima. II. Repair of the aortic lining after mechanical denudation. *Am J Pathol* 81: 15–42, 1975.
49. Knieriem H-J, Bondjers G, Bjorkerud S: Electron microscopy of intimal plaques following induction of large superficial mechanical injury (transverse injury) in the rabbit aorta. *Virchows Arch A* 359: 267–282, 1973.
50. Fishman JA, Ryan GB, Karnovsky MJ: Endothelial regeneration in the rat carotid artery and the significance of endothelial denudation in the pathogenesis of myointimal thickening. *Lab Invest* 32: 339–351, 1975.
51. Van Pelt-Verkuil E, Van Pelt W, Jense D: Morphometry of air-drying-induced arteriosclerosis in rat carotid artery. Effect of air-flow rate. *Atherosclerosis* 3: 441–451, 1983.
52. Burns ER, Spaet TH, Stemerman MB: Response of the arterial wall to endothelial removal: an autoradiographic study. *Proc Soc Exp Biol Med* 159: 473–477, 1978.
53. Hassler O: The origin of the cells constituting arterial intimal thickening: an experimental autoradiographic study with the use of H^3-thymidine. *Lab Invest* 22: 286–293, 1970.
54. Webster WS, Bishop SP, Geer JC: Experimental aortic intimal thickening. I. Morphology and source of intimal cells. *Am J Pathol* 76: 245–264, 1974.
55. Goldberg ID, Stemerman MB, Ransil BJ, Fuhro RL: In vivo aortic muscle cells growth kinetics: differences

between thoracic and abdominal segments after intimal injury in the rabbit. *Circ Res* 47: 182–189, 1980.
56. Clowes AW, Reidy MA, Clowes MM: Kinetics of cellular proliferation after arterial injury. I. Smooth muscle growth in the absence of endothelium. *Lab Invest* 49: 327–333, 1983.
57. Mosse PRL, Campbell GR, Wang Z-L, Campbell JH: Smooth muscle phenotypic expression in human carotid arteries. I. Comparison of cells from diffuse intimal thickenings adjacent to atheromatous plaques with those of the media. *Lab Invest* 53: 556–562, 1985.
58. Campbell GR, Campbell JH, Ang AH, Campbell IL, Horrigan S, Manderson JA, Mosse PRL, Rennick RE: Phenotypic changes in smooth muscle cells of human atherosclerotic plaques. In: Evolution of the Human Atherosclerotic Plaque. S Glagov, W Newman, SA Schaeffer (eds), Berlin: Springer-Verlag, in press.
59. Kasai T, Pollack OJ: Smooth muscle cells in aortic cultures of untreated and cholesterol-fed rabbits. *Z Zellforsch Mikrosk Anat* 62: 743–752, 1964.
60. Pollack OJ, Adachi M: Human and rabbit arterial cells compared in tissue cultures. *Prog Biochem Pharmacol* 4: 294–304, 1968.
61. Jarmolych J, Daoud AS, Landau J, Fritz KE, McElvene E: Aortic media explants. Cell proliferation and production of mucopolysaccharides, collagen, and elastic tissue. *Exp Mol Pathol* 9: 171–188, 1968.
62. Fritz KE, Jarmolych J, Daoud AS: Association of DNA synthesis and apparent dedifferentiation of aortic smooth muscle cells *in vitro*. *Exp Mol Pathol* 12: 354–362, 1970.
63. Rossi GL, Alroy J, Rothernmund S: Morphological studies of cultured swine aorta media explants. *Virchows Arch B* 12: 133–144, 1973.
64. Chamley JH, Campbell GR: Trophic influences of sympathetic nerves and cyclic AMP on differentiation and proliferation of isolated single smooth muscle cells in culture. *Cell Tissue Res* 161: 497–510, 1975.
65. Campbell GR, Chamley JH: Ultrastructure of differentiating vascular smooth muscle. In: Vascular Neuroeffector Mechanisms. JA Bevan, G Burnstock, B Johansson, RA Maxwell, OA Nedergaard (eds), Basel: Karger, p 1–9, Second International Symposium, Odense, 1976.
66. Chamley JH, Campbell GR: Tissue culture: interaction between sympathetic nerves and vascular smooth muscle. In: Vascular Neuroeffector Mechanisms. JA Bevan, G Burnstock, B Johansson, RA Maxwell, OA Nedergaard (eds), Basel: Karger, p 10–18, Second International Symposium, Odense, 1976.
67. Chamley JH, Campbell GR, Burnstock G: An analysis of the interactions between sympathetic nerve fibers and smooth muscle cells in tissue culture. *Dev Biol* 33: 344–361, 1973.
68. Chamley JH, Campbell GR, Burnstock G: Dedifferentiation, redifferentiation and bundle formation of smooth muscle cells in tissue culture: the influence of cell number and nerve fibres. *J Embryol Exp Morph* 32: 297–323, 1974.
69. Campbell JH, Campbell GR, (eds): Vascular Smooth Muscle in Culture, Vols I, II. Boca Raton, FL: CRC Press, p 1–339, 1987.
70. Chamley JH, Campbell GR, McConnell JD, Groschel-Stewart U: Comparison of vascular smooth muscle cells from adult human, monkey and rabbit in primary culture and in subculture. *Cell Tissue Res* 177: 503–522, 1977.
71. Campbell GR, Uehara Y, Mark G, Burnstock G: Fine structure of smooth muscle cells grown in tissue culture. *J Cell Biol* 49: 21–34, 1971.
72. Chamley-Campbell JH, Campbell GR, Burnstock G: Contraction and innervation of smooth muscle cells in tissue culture. In: Structure and Function of the Circulation, Vol III. CJ Schwartz, NT Werthessen, S Wolf (eds), New York: Plenum, p 401–425, 1971.
73. Palmberg L, Thyberg J: Uterine smooth muscle cells in primary culture. Alterations in fine structure, cytoskeletal organization and growth characteristics. *Cell Tissue Res* 246: 253–262, 1986.
74. Gunther S, Alexander RW, Atkinson WJ, Gimbrone MA Jr: Functional angiotensin II receptors in cultured vascular smooth muscle cells. *J Cell Biol* 92: 289–298, 1982.
75. Uehara Y, Campbell GR, Burnstock G: Cytoplasmic filaments in developing and adult vertebrate smooth muscle. *J Cell Biol* 50: 484–497, 1971.
76. Campbell GR, Campbell JH: Phenotypic modulation of smooth muscle cells in primary culture. In: Vascular Smooth Muscle in Culture. JH Campbell, GR Campbell (eds), Boca Raton, FL: CRC Press, p 39–56, 1987.
77. Nilsson J, Thyberg J: Fine structure of the arterial smooth muscle cells cultured in the presence of whole blood serum or plasma-derived serum. *Cell Tissue Res* 223: 87–99, 1982.
78. Sjolund M, Nilsson J, Palmberg L, Thyberg J: Phenotype modulation in primary cultures of arterial smooth-muscle cells. Dual effect of prostaglandin E_1. *Differentiation* 27: 158–162, 1984.
79. Thyberg J, Nilsson J, Palmberg L, Sjolund M: Adult human arterial smooth muscle cells in primary culture. Modulation from contractile to synthetic phenotype. *Cell Tissue Res* 239: 69–74, 1985.
80. Sjolund M, Madsen K, Von der Mark K, Thyberg J: Phenotype modulation in primary cultures of smooth-muscle cells from rat aorta. Synthesis of collagen and elastin. *Differentiation* 32: 173–180, 1986.
81. Sjolund M, Hedin U, Sejersen T, Heldin C-H, Thyberg J: Arterial smooth muscle cells express platelet-derived growth factor (PDGF) A chain mRNA, secrete a PDGF-like mitogen, and bind exogenous PDGF in a phenotype- and growth state-dependent manner. *J Cell Biol* 106: 403–413, 1988.
82. Groschel-Stewart U, Chamley JH, Campbell GR, Burnstock R: Changes in myosin distribution in dedifferentiating and redifferentiating smooth muscle cells in tissue culture. *Cell Tissue Res* 165: 13–22, 1975.
83. Chamley JH, Groschel-Stewart U, Campbell GR, Burnstock G: Distinction between smooth muscle, fibroblasts and endothelial cells in culture by the use of fluoresceinated antibodies against smooth muscle actin. *Cell*

Tissue Res 177: 445–457, 1977.
84. Chamley-Campbell JH, Campbell GR, Groschel-Stewart U, Burnstock G: FITC-labelled antibody staining of tropomyosin-containing fibrils in smooth, cardiac and skeletal muscle cells, prefusion myoblasts, fibroblasts, endothelial cells and 3T3 cells in culture. *Cell Tissue Res* 183: 153–166, 1977.
85. Campbell GR, Chamley-Campbell JH, Groschel-Stewart U, Small JV, Anderson P: Antibody staining of 10 nm (100 A) filaments in cultured smooth, cardiac and skeletal muscle cells. *J Cell Sci* 37: 303–322, 1979.
86. Burkl B, Mahlmeister C, Groschel-Stewart U, Chamley-Campbell J, Campbell GR: Production of specific antibodies to contractile proteins and their use in immunofluorescence microscopy. III. Antibody against human uterine muscle myosin. *Histochemistry* 60: 135–143, 1979.
87. Gown AM, Vogel AM, Gordon D, Lu PL: A smooth muscle-specific monoclonal antibody recognizes smooth muscle actin isozymes. *J Cell Biol* 100: 807–813, 1985.
88. Tsukada T, Tippens, D, Gordon D, Ross R, Gown AM: HHF35, a muscle-actin-specific monoclonal antibody. I. Immunocytochemical and biochemical characterization. *Am J Pathol* 126: 51–60, 1987.
89. Tsukada T, McNutt MA, Ross R, Gown AM: HHF35, a muscle-actin-specific monoclonal antibody. II. Reactivity in normal, reactive and neoplastic human tissues. *Am J Pathol* 127: 389–402, 1987.
90. Nilsson J: Growth factors and the pathogenesis of atherosclerosis. *Atherosclerosis* 62: 185–199, 1986.
91. Beckers-Bleukx G, Marechal G: Detection and distribution of myosin isozymes in vertebrate smooth muscle. *Eur J Biochem* 152: 207–211, 1985.
92. Lema MJ, Pagami Ed, Shemin R, Julian FJ: Myosin isozymes in rabbit and human smooth muscles. *Circ Res* 59: 115–123, 1986.
93. Oakes BW, Batty AC, Handley CJ, Sandberg LB: The synthesis of elastin, collagen, and glycosaminoglycans by high density primary cultures of neonatal rat aortic smooth muscle. An ultrastructural and biochemical study. *Eur J Cell Biol* 27: 34–46, 1982.
94. Thyberg J, Palmberg L, Nilsson J, Ksiazek T, Sjolund M: Phenotype modulation in primary cultures of arterial smooth muscle cells. On the role of platelet-derived growth factor. *Differentiation* 25: 156–167, 1983.
95. Campbell JH, Kocher O, Skalli O, Gabbiani G, Campbell GR: Cytodifferentiation and expression of OC-smooth muscle actin mRNA and protein during primary culture of aortic smooth muscle cells. Correlation with cell density and proliferative state. *Arteriosclerosis* 9: 633–643, 1989.
96. Chamley-Campbell JH, Campbell GR: What controls smooth muscle phenotype? *Atherosclerosis* 40: 347–357, 1981.
97. Campbell JH, Campbell GR: Cellular interactions in the artery wall. In: The Peripheral Circulation. S Hunyor, J Ludbrook, M McGrath, J Shaw (eds), New York: Elsevier North Holland, p 33–39, 1984.
98. Castellot JJ Jr, Choay J, Lormeau J-C, Petitou M, Sache E, Karnovsky MJ: Structural determinants of the capacity of heparin to inhibit the proliferation of vascular smooth muscle cells. II. Evidence for a pentasaccharide sequence that contains a 3-0-sulfate group. *J Cell Biol* 102: 1979–1984, 1986.
99. Castellot JJ Jr, Addonizio ML, Rosenberg R, Karnovsky MJ: Cultured endothelial cells produce a heparinlike inhibitor of smooth muscle cell growth. *J Cell Biol* 90: 372–379, 1981.
100. Fritze LM, Reilly CF, Rosenberg RD: An antiproliferative heparan sulfate species produced by postconfluent smooth muscle cells. *J Cell Biol* 100: 1041–1049, 1985.
101. Castellot JJ Jr, Favreau LV, Karnovsky MJ, Rosenberg RD: Inhibition of vascular smooth muscle cell growth by endothelial cell-derived heparin. Possible role of platelet endoglycosidase. *J Biol Chem* 257: 11256 –11260, 1982.
102. Oosta GM, Favreau LV, Beeler DL, Rosenberg RD: Purification and properties of human platelet heparitinase. *J Biol Chem* 257: 11249–11255, 1982.
103. Castellot JJ Jr, Wong K, Herman B, Hoover RL, Albertini DF, Wright TC, Caleb BL, Karnovsky MJ: Binding and internalization of heparin by vascular smooth muscle cells. *J Cell Physiol* 124: 13–20, 1985.
104. Reilly C, Fritze L, Rosenberg R: Heparin inhibition of smooth muscle cell proliferation. A cellular site of action. *J Cell Physiol* 129: 11–19, 1986.
105. Reilly CF, Fritze LMS, Rosenberg RD: Antiproliferative effects of heparin on vascular smooth muscle cells are reversed by epidermal growth factor. *J Cell Physiol* 131: 149–157, 1987.
106. Majack RA, Bornstein P: Biosynthesis and modulation of extracellular matrix components by cultured vascular smooth muscle cells. In: Vascular Smooth Muscle in Culture. JH Campbell, GR Campbell (eds), Boca Raton, FL: CRC Press, p 117–132, 1987.
107. Majack RA: Toward a molecular understanding of vascular smooth muscle cell growth control. *Cardiovasc Rev Rep* 7: 731–737, 1986.
108. Majack RA, Cook SC, Bornstein P: Control of smooth muscle cell growth by components of the extracellular matrix: Autocrine role for thrombospondin. *Proc Natl Acad Sci USA* 83: 9050–9054, 1986.
109. Majack RA, Cook SC, Bornstein P: Platelet-derived growth factor and heparin-like glycosaminoglycans regulate thrombospondin synthesis and deposition in the matrix by smooth muscle cells. *J Cell Biol* 101: 1059–1071, 1985.
110. Majack RA, Mildbrandt J, Dixit VM: Induction of thrombospondin messenger RNA levels occurs as an intermediate primary response to platelet-derived growth factor. *J Biol Chem* 262: 8821–8825, 1987.
111. Majack RA, Goodman LV, Dixit VM: Cell surface thrombospondin is functionally essential for vascular smooth muscle cell proliferation. *J Cell Biol* 106: 415–422, 1988.
112. Wasteson A, Hook M, Westermark B: Demonstration of a platelet enzyme, degrading heparan sulphate. *FEBS Lett* 64: 218–221, 1976.
113. Wasteson A, Glimelius B, Busch C, Westermark B, Heldin C-H, Norling B: Effect of a platelet endoglycosidase on cell surface associated heparan sulphate of human cultured endothelial and glial cells. *Thrombosis Res* 11: 309–321, 1977.
114. Handin RI, Cohen HJ: Purification and binding properties of human platelet factor four. *J Biol Chem* 251:

4273–4282, 1976.
115. Campbell GR, Campbell JH: Smooth muscle phenotypic changes in arterial wall homeostasis: Implications for the pathogenesis of atherosclerosis. *Exp Mol Pathol* 42: 139–162, 1985.
116. Chamley-Campbell JH, Campbell GR: Development of the autonomic system in culture. In: Somatic and Autonomic Nerve-Muscle Interactions. G Burnstock, G Vrbova, R O'Brien (eds), New York: Elsevier North Holland, p 35–66, 1983.
117. Campbell GR, Campbell JH, Rennick R, Wang ZL: The influence of endothelial cells and macrophages on smooth muscle phenotype and proliferation. *Atherosclerosis* 7: 389–393, 1986.
118. Rennick R, Campbell JH, Campbell GR: Vascular smooth muscle phenotype can be influenced by macrophages *in vitro*. *Atherosclerosis*, 71: 35–43, 1988.
119. Hedin U, Thyberg J: Plasma fibronectin promotes modulation of arterial smooth-muscle cells from contractile to synthetic phenotype. *Differentiation* 33: 239–246, 1987.
120. Ross R: The smooth muscle cell. II. Growth of smooth muscle in culture and formation of elastic fibers. *J Cell Biol* 50: 172–186, 1971.
121. Ross R, Kariya B: Morphogenesis of vascular smooth muscle in atherosclerosis and in cell culture. In: Handbook of Physiology, Section 2, Circulation, Vol II, Vascular Smooth Muscle. DF Bohr, AP Somlyo, Sparks HV J (eds), Bethesda, MD: American Physiological Society, p 69–91, 1980.
122. Gimbrone MA Jr, Cotran RS: Human vascular smooth muscle in culture, growth and ultrastructure. *Lab Invest* 33: 16–27, 1975.
123. Grunwald J, Wischer W: Ultrastructural morphometry of cultivated smooth muscle cells from normotensive and hypertensive rats. *Exp Pathol* 27: 91–98, 1985.
124. Grunwald J, Robenek H, Mey J, Hauss WH: *In vivo* and *in vitro* cellular changes in experimental hypertension: Electronmicroscopic and morphometric studies of aortic smooth muscle cells. *Exp Mol Pathol* 36: 164–176, 1982.
125. Blennerhassett MG, Kannan MS, Garfield RE: Functional characterization of cell-to-cell coupling in cultured rat aortic smooth muscle. *Am J Physiol* 252: C555–C569, 1987.
126. Tagami M, Nara Y, Kubota A, Sunaga T, Maezawa H, Fujino H, Yamori Y: Morphological and functional differentiation of cultured vascular smooth-muscle cells. *Cell Tissue Res* 245: 261–266, 1986.
127. Martin GM, Sprague CA: Symposium on *in vitro* studies related to atherogenesis. Life histories of hyperplastoid cell lines from aorta and skin. *Exp Mol Pathol* 18: 125–141, 1973.
128. Mauger JP, Worcel M, Tassin J, Courtois Y: Contractility of smooth muscle cells of rabbit aorta in tissue culture. *Nature* 255: 337–338, 1975.
129. Fowler S, Shio H, Wolinsky H: Subcellular fractionation and morphology of calf aortic smooth muscle cells. Studies on whole aorta, aortic explants, and subcultures grown under different conditions. *J Cell Biol* 75: 166–184, 1977.
130. Fowler S, Berberian PA, Haley NJ, Shio H: Lysosomes, vascular intercellular lipid accumulation and atherosclerosis. In: International Conference on Atherosclerosis. LA Carlson (ed), New York: Raven Press, p 19–27, 1978.
131. Yau-Young AO, Shio H, Fowler S: Growth, biochemistry, and morphology of isolated rabbit aortic smooth muscle cells maintained in the presence and absence of serum. *J Cell Physiol* 108: 461–473, 1981.
132. James Kracke MR, Sloane BF, Shuman H, Somlyo AP: Lysosomal composition in cultured vascular smooth muscle cells: Electron probe analysis. *Proc Natl Acad Sci USA* 76: 6461–6465, 1979.
133. Robinson JM, Okada T, Castellot JJ Jr, Karnovsky MJ: Unusual lysosomes in aortic smooth muscle cells: Presence in living and rapidly frozen cells. *J Cell Biol* 102: 1615–1622, 1986.
134. Mazurkowitz J, Vaughan DW, Franzblau C: A morphometric study of vascular smooth muscle cells in culture. *In Vitro* 16: 337–345, 1980.
135. Bates CJ, Prynne W, Levin CP: The synthesis of underhydroxylated collagen by 3T6 mouse fibroblasts in culture. *Biochim Biophys Acta* 263: 397–405, 1972.
136. Barnes MJ: Biological hydroxylations and ascorbic acid with special regard to collagen metabolism. *Vitam Horm* 30: 1–43, 1972.
137. Leung DYM, Glagov S, Mathews MB: Cyclic stretching stimulates synthesis of matrix components by arterial smooth muscle cells *in vitro*. *Science* 191: 475–477, 1976.
138. Leung DYM, Glagov S, Mathews MB: A new *in vitro* system for studying cell response to mechanical stimulation. *Exp Cell Res* 109: 285–291, 1977.
139. Sottiurai VS, Kollros P, Glagov S, Zarins CK, Mathews MB: Morphologic alteration of cultured arterial smooth muscle cells by cyclic stretching. *J Surg Res* 35: 490–497, 1983.
140. Campbell GR, Chamley JH, Burnstock G: Development of smooth muscle cells in tissue culture. *J Anat* 117: 295–312, 1974.
141. Bennett T, Cobb JLS: Studies on the avian gizzard: the development of the gizzard and its innervation. *Z Zellforsch Mikrosk Anat* 98: 599–621, 1969.
142. Burnstock G, Holman ME, Prosser CL: Electrophysiology of smooth muscle. *Physiol Rev* 43: 482–527, 1963.
143. Bennett T: Nerve-mediated excitation and inhibition of the smooth muscle cells of the avian gizzard. *J Physiol (Lond)* 204: 669–686, 1969.
144. Wight TN, Cooke PH, Smith SC: An electron microscopic study of pigeon aorta cell cultures. Cytodifferentiation and intracellular lipid accumulation. *Exp Mol Pathol* 27: 1–18, 1977.

Author's address:
Prof. Gordon R. Campbell
Department of Anatomy
University of Melbourne
Parkville, Victoria, 3052
Australia

CHAPTER 5

Smooth muscle cell characteristics: a computer-assisted analysis from serial sections

MARY E. TODD

1. Introduction

Accurate structural measurements of various smooth muscle cells, employing proven methodology, are relatively sparse, although some data have been provided, mainly for intestinal, uterine, and vascular cells. Morphological parameters by themselves are of only academic interest, unless their far-reaching functional significance is considered. For example, in smooth muscle cells of a given volume, if the relative proportion of surface area increases (an increase in the surface-area-to-volume ratio), then hypothetically, a greater calcium influx should occur, given that the proportion of calcium channels and all intracellular components remain constant. Conversely, if the surface-area-to-volume ratio decreases, then the reverse could be postulated. Another structural parameter, the orientation or angle of the cells within the vessel wall, will influence the plane in which the maximum force is developed. Innumerable examples of the morphofunctional aspects of smooth muscle could be given, and all these examples pose questions that can be answered. However, the role of the physiologist and pharmacologist is to incorporate structural data, to show the relevance of morphology and how it can and does affect functional properties.

Difficulties arise when two-dimensional images are translated into three dimensions, since our perceptions are influenced by the pattern information being visually transmitted to the cortex. A classic example of this misinterpretation is the dumbbell-shaped mitochondrion described by Stempak (1). In section, certainly, this was the shape, subsequently corrected to the erythocyte shape following serial sectioning (2). No biologist would conclude when seeing the same type of silhouette from a sectioned erythocyte that it was dumbbell-shaped, since the shape is known in advance. Similarly, in many vessels, vascular smooth muscle cell profiles appear to be more or less spindle-shaped in section, perpetuating the myth that the overall cell shape in all vessels is a spindle. Definitive evidence now indicates that these cells may be very irregular in shape with branching processes (3, 4, 5).

Other types, such as intestinal smooth muscle, can normally have the spindle shape, but these also become branched when hypertrophic (6, 7). Even in normal intestinal muscle, inner circular and outer longitudinal cells may have different configurations, the latter with branching terminations (8).

In random sections through tissue, there is no way to distinguish whether the profiles observed are each complete cellular units or whether some or most are only portions of cells. An example from the tail artery of the adult rat illustrates that serial sections can confirm that a profile is actually a branching process of a particular cell (Fig. 5-1). This sort of configuration may occur normally and can be misleading, when, for example, the number of cells per unit area is estimated. In other types of vascular smooth muscle, like that of the mesenteric artery (Fig. 5-2), what appears in section to be a long thin

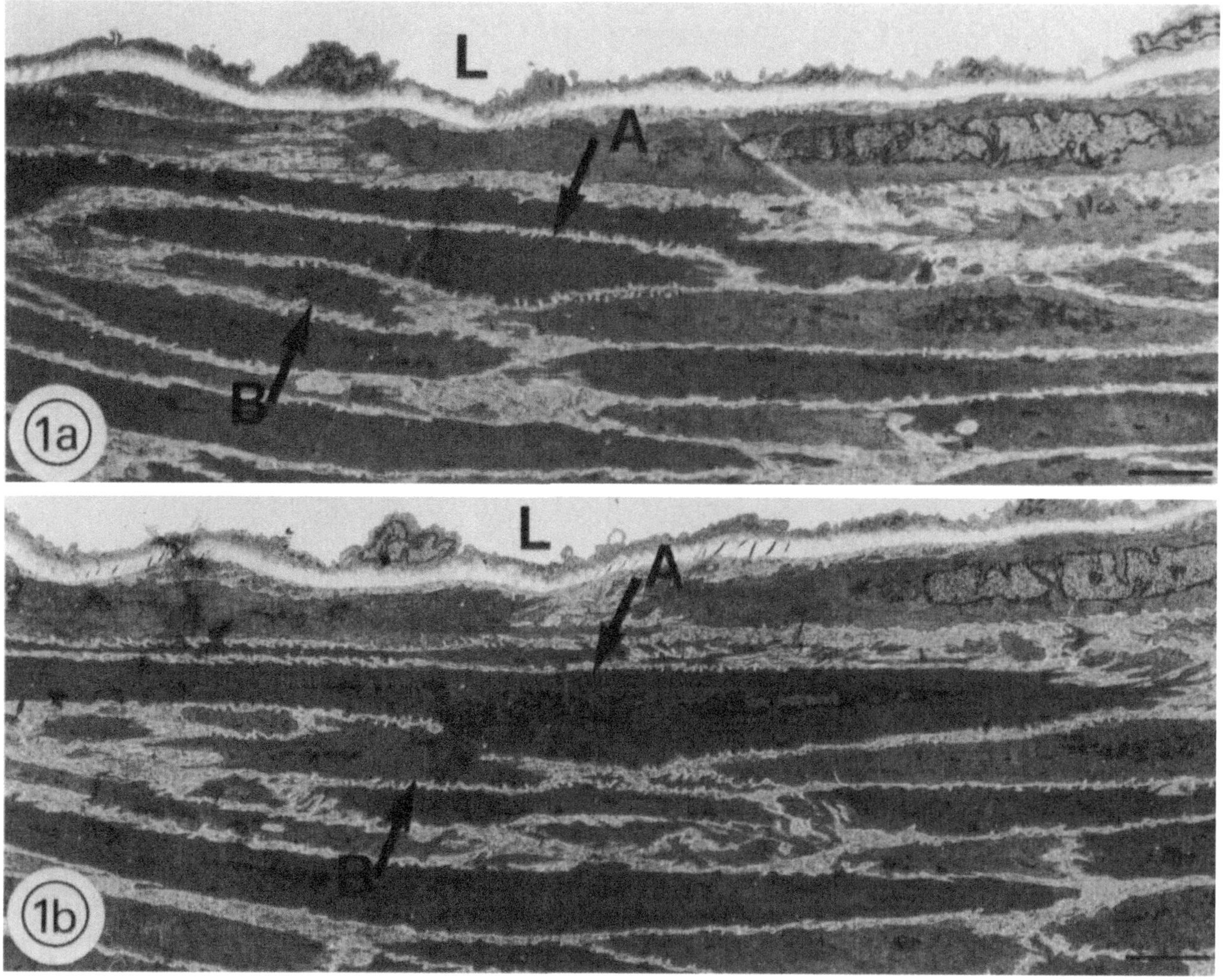
L
A
B
1a
L
A
B
1b

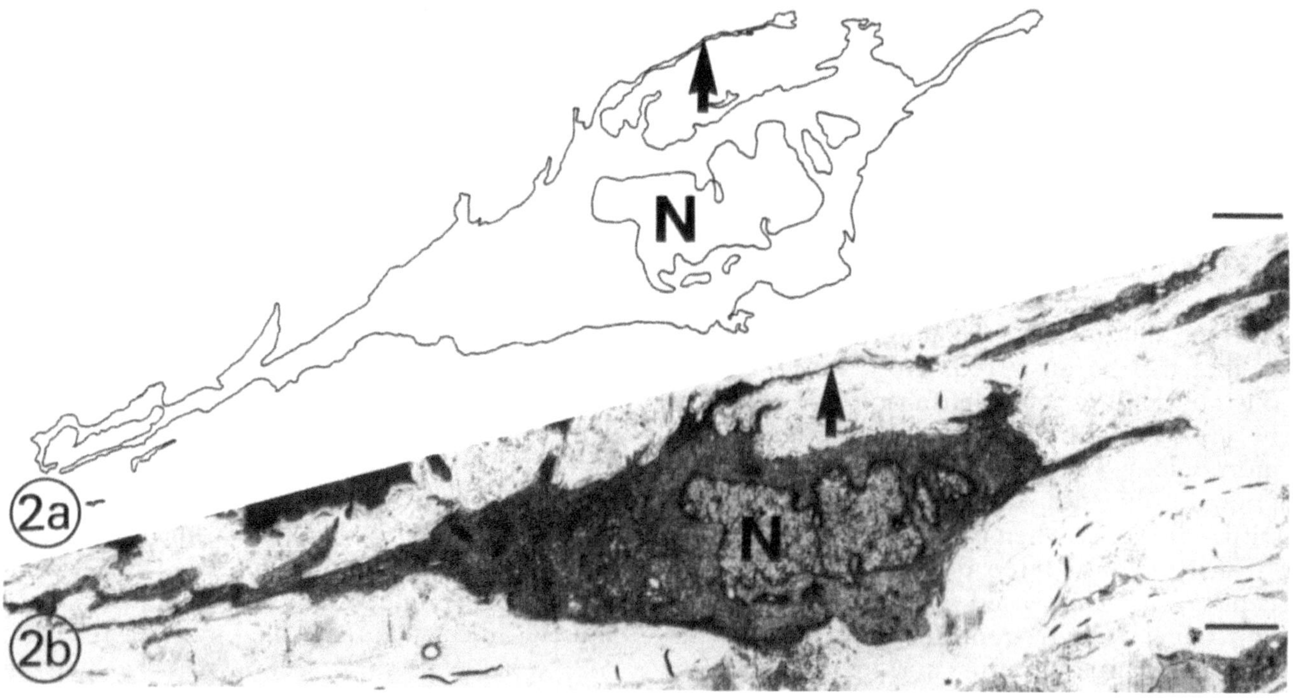
N
2a
N
2b

process is in fact part of a lamella (Fig. 5-2). Therefore, the position of the slices could not always be so fortuitous as to pass along the length of such a process. It must be part of a sheet or lamella, and in fact the one shown extends for 4.2 μm. Such a fine lamella would not be revealed by a technique using enzymatic digestion and scanning electron microscopy, since it would collapse against the cell and not be observed. Large numbers of these would significantly affect any mechanisms that depended on surface area to volume ratios.

Elias (9) has written an excellent review describing the pitfalls that await the unwary when interpreting the overall configuration from sections. He mentions the citation of the famous Scot, Lord Kelvin:

> ... when you can measure what you are speaking about and express it in numbers, you know someting about it; but when you cannot express it in numbers, your knowledge is of a meagre and unsatisfactory kind; it may be the beginning of knowledge, but you have scarcely in your thoughts advanced to the state of science.

Elias heartily disagrees with Lord Kelvin and suggests that it is futile to put numbers to an object without knowing its shape, or what kind of object it is. A reasonable compromise would probably be somewhere between these two extremes. When we try to start defining shapes, we start to run into difficulties. Williams (10) recognizes the problems in determining cell shape as being perhaps the most difficult to quantify from two-dimensional images. Simple, randomly orientated, mathematically defined shapes (spheres, cones, ellipsoids) are the easiest to quantify. The problems increase in complexity when dealing with irregular cellular shapes that may differ in size, in relative proportions, and in orientation, as well as in changes occurring in components and proportion of components within the paracellular matrix. These conditions apply to smooth muscle cells in the cardiovascular, respiratory, digestive, and genitourinary systems in different systems, within a system, in different species, in disease, or under experimentally induced conditions.

We need more than shape alone. We need to have information about the function of smooth muscle cells in order to relate to their physiological and pharmacological activities. We need to have numerical data that relate to values such as a change in surface-area-to-volume ratios that are relevant to fluid and electrolyte permeability, to contractility, and to pharmacomechanical coupling (11, 12).

Morphometric analysis of biological units commonly is obtained from stereological methods in which three-dimensional information is derived from two-dimensional measurements from sections (13). Most stereological methods, however, are based on the assumption that particles are randomly oriented and of the same known and simple shape, and that no particle in the section is part of another (14, 15). Although there are specialized methods for preferential orientation as found in skeletal muscle (13), in many cases we do not know in advance the orientation and whether or not it has altered. In the disease of hypertension, the shape and proportions of the cells may change drastically, so that in section a number of profiles all belong to a single cell (16). When interpreting only from two-dimensional images, assumptions usually have to be made that are not possible from the limited information available.

Carrying out analyses and three-dimensional reconstructions from ultrathin serial sections of biological tissue provides the most accurate method of determining the morphological characteristics. Most of the examples are from the cardiovascular system, which has the smallest smooth muscle cells (17). Due to the complexity and heterogeneity of smooth muscle within the cardiovascular system, there are numerous tech-

←

Figure 5-1. Electron micrographs of smooth muscle cells in the tail artery of an adult rat (16 weeks old). (a) In random sections, profile A could be assumed to represent a portion of an individual cell, and similarly with profile B. (b) This figure illustrates that the two profiles, followed for 33 consecutive sections, are in fact both part of one cell. L: lumen. Bar = 5 μm.

Figure 5-2. (a) Plot of a profile of a mesenteric artery smooth muscle cell from an adult rat (16 weeks old). The nucleus (N) is also plotted, and is seen to have several lobes. (b) Electron micrograph of the profile plotted in (a). The arrows indicate a thin lamella that extends through 64 sections (for 4.2 μm). Bar = 2.5 μm.

nical problems besetting anyone undertaking this course. Reconstruction has been carried out for vascular tissue by mechanical means. Sections of two arteriolar cells, one each from the rat and hamster (4), were traced onto plastic that was equivalent to section thickness, cut out, and superimposed. A similar method was used for reconstructing arteriolar cells in cat mesenteric vessels (3). This technique is obviously very time-consuming, and even with the greatest diligence, only a few cells can be reconstructed using practical considerations.

The computer expedites many analyses that otherwise would be impossible, given our allotted lifespan of three-score years and ten. There are still problems associated with serial sectioning, however. The amount of information obtained must be weighed against the labor involved in its procurement. The unique information available from serial sections will be emphasized. Thus our understanding of these extremely heterogeneous populations will be expanded by making use of the computer as a tool.

2. Techniques

Since any investigation using serial sections generally involves numerical data, a method of perfusion fixation at a physiological pressure should be carried out whenever possible. Vascular tissue would be fixed at a pressure that corresponds to in situ pressure (we chose mean blood pressure) to ensure that the dimensions represent the condition of the blood vessel and smooth muscle cells at that specific time, followed by routine plastic embedding (5).

There are a number of techniques that can utilize serial sections and help in our understanding of smooth muscle cell characteristics. Since serial sectioning per se is a standard method in classical microscopy, it is only in utilizing computer technology that new horizons are introduced. The techniques that are described are meant to be informative not about computer methodology, but rather about the means of providing the type of information that may be generated, in this particular case, about smooth muscle.

2.1. Three-dimensional analyses and reconstructions

For three-dimensional analyses, we have found that the greatest amount of information in relation to time and effort has been obtained using a combination of semithin (light microscopy, 0.5 μm thick) and thin (electron microscopy, 65 nm thick) serial sections (18). It is critical that the magnifications and section thickness be accurately determined. We have found that Small's small-fold method (19), or re-embedding of representative sections and recutting across the thickness (20), gives values that are very close to thickness estimates based on direct measurements of length of tissue cut or of interference colors. Regardless of the thickness of the sections, the principle involved in computer-assisted reconstructions and analyses is the same (5). The outline of each profile making up a cell is traced using a cursor, and converted to a series of x,y coordinates registered on a digitizing board. The resolution must be sensitive enough to record the unevenness of the perimeter (plasma membrane) of the profile. Once these coordinates have been obtained and filed, then any additional manipulation is carried out using suitable software. For anything involving the surface, either surface areas or three-dimensional reconstructions, it is essential that each successive profile is digitized in its precise relationship to the previous one, that is, in correct register, with the spacing relative to the section thickness or multiples thereof. If complete cells are being reconstructed, then the nucleus is visualized and plotted one fifth of the section thickness above the profile in which it appears. Cell organelles may be similarly incorporated. The reason for the change in plane is that the intracellular units will not show when the profile is viewed at 90° (Fig. 5-3).

A series of profiles making up a cell will produce an image than can be viewed, rotated, or plotted, at any angle of the x,y or z axes, and at any multiple of section thickness. Hidden lines can be deleted. The "wire" reconstruction of a series of lines representing individual profiles can be converted into a smoothed three-dimensional object with shading added if desired.

It is not necessary to reconstruct the cells to obtain information about volume or surface area.

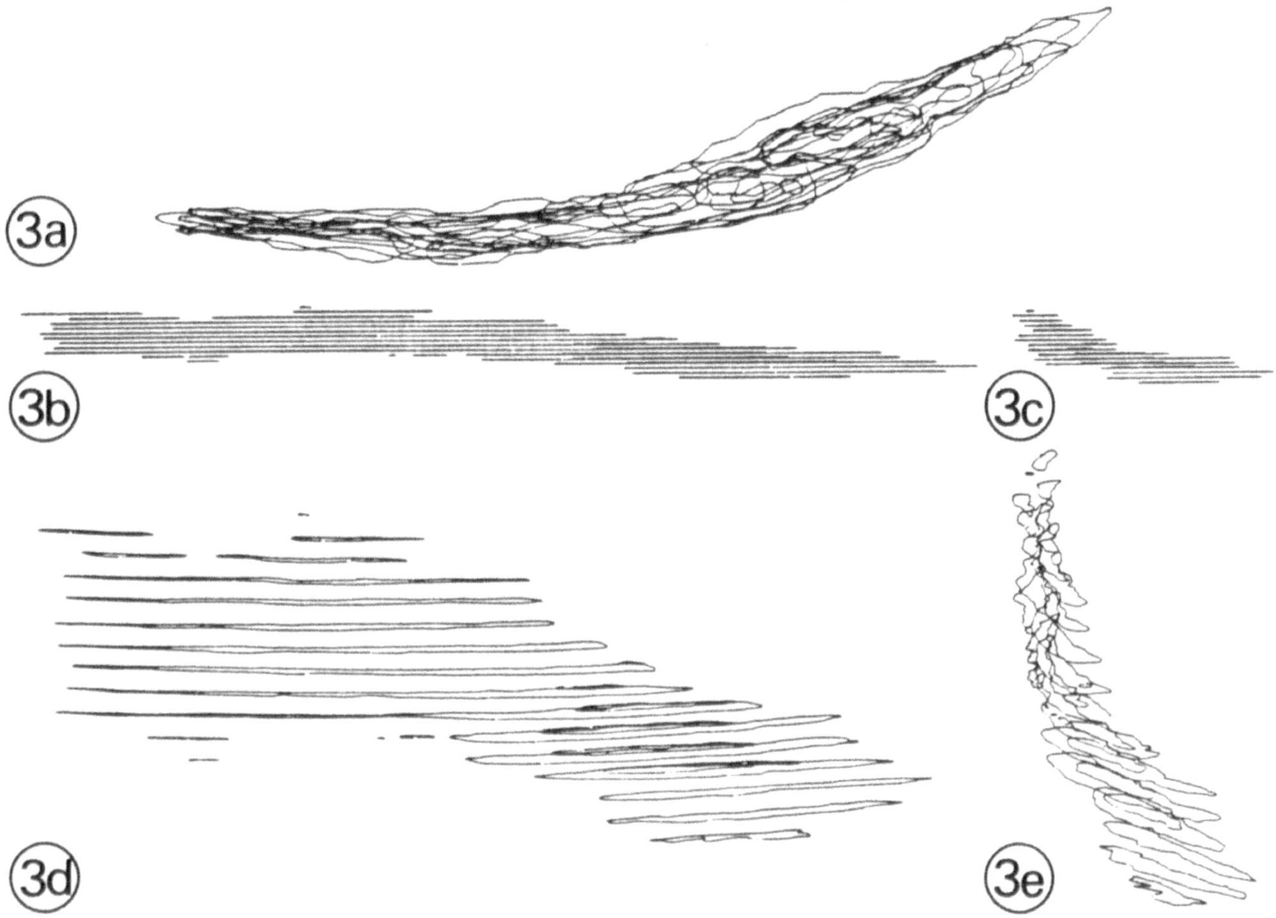

Figure 5-3. Plots of a smooth muscle cell from the proximal region of the tail artery of a two-week-old rat. These plots represent examples of the type of information about a complete cell that may be obtained if the profiles, those with and those without the nucleus, are traced. In these plots from ultrathin sections, every fifth profile was plotted. (a) x, y, and $z = 0$. These are the profile outlines as they were digitized from the serial sections, all superimposed. (b) The profiles are all tilted to 90° so that each is viewed from the x axis as if on edge. (c) The profiles, at 90°, are viewed as if from the y axis. The nucleus, at one end of the cell, is plotted one fifth of the interprofile space above the profile in which it appears. In this case, the space is proportional to 0.33 μm (five times section thickness of 65 nm). (d and e) These represent the profiles tilted to 80°, and stretched out ×5 section thickness, so that the spindle shape of the profiles can be seen. Any angle between 0° and 90° may be chosen. This cell has a very low clockwise pitch (4° from $x = 90°$) and veers toward the adventitia of the vessel (from $y = 90°$). Examples of cells that veer toward the lumen are illustrated in Figure 5-7.

Values for volume are calculated from the area of each profile times section thickness, with all summated. This gives a reliable estimation of volume even at low magnifications (13, 18). This also means that at the ultrastructural level, not every serial profile needs to be digitized to obtain volume measurements. To confirm this, following serial reconstruction, every nth profile only from the computer file was used to calculate the volume (Fig. 5-4). The most extreme case had a gap of five sections following every section, and still was within ± 5% of the volume. The program estimates the area(s) of the missing profile(s) from the measurements of profiles on either side of the gap. No matter how skillfully serial sets are prepared, sections will invariably be lost, folded, or in some way be unsuitable for digitizing. As long as the first and last profiles are present, up to 10% may be missing without significantly affecting the estimate of cell dimensions (excluding surface area). Naturally this represents an extreme case, and effort is made to avoid gaps.

Surface area values, however, require much more elaborate procedures. Our initial assumption for ultrathin sections was that profile peri-

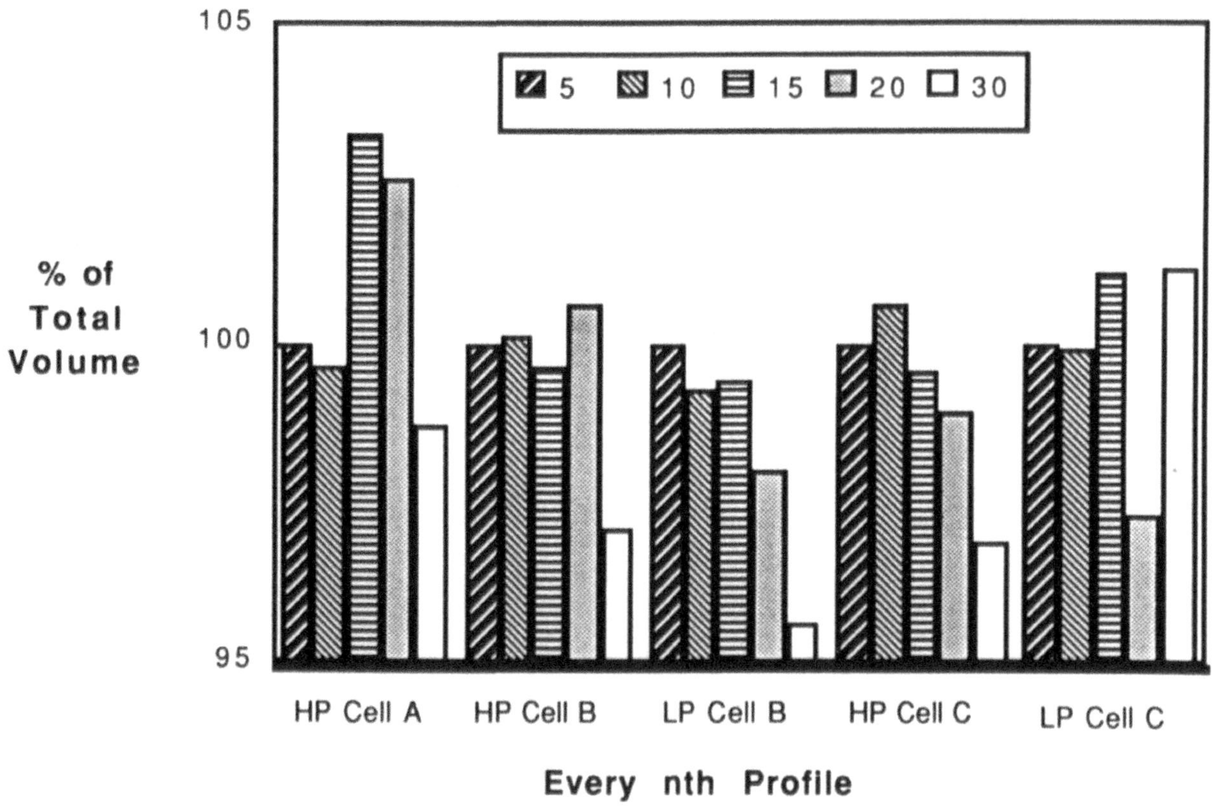

Figure 5-4. The total cell volume was calculated from several smooth muscle cells from the tail artery (adult, 16 weeks old). Volume calculations using every fifth profile were taken as representing 100% of the total volume, and then volumes were calculated using every *n*th profile. Profiles were traced from electron micrographs at either X 1000 (LP) OR X 3000 (HP) final magnification, and in some cases the same cell was traced at both magnifications. The magnification did not affect the volume calculations. Even when only every 30th profile was included, the error was less than ± 5%. For cell B, which had a total of 460 sections, this still represented 15 profiles when calculations were made using every 30th profile.

meter times section thickness would be an adequate estimate of the surface area of the cells using ultrathin sections (21). This fallacy is present in source material relating to surface measurements (22). For objects that do not change in shape along their length, such as a cylinder, this assumption is accurate, but not for the irregular complex shapes of vascular smooth muscle cells. Determination of an optimal surface using an algorithm that calculates areas of triangular tiles connecting the *x,y* coordinates of adjacent sections is required (23, 24). The perimeter times thickness method underestimates the surface area, with the discrepancy increasing with the steepness of the change between adjacent profiles (18). The more irregular a cell is, and the more it changes its cross-sectional area along its length, the greater the difference between the above two methods.

Since reconstructing the cell from digitized profiles is a minor extension, further information can be obtained directly from plotting the cell (5, 18, 21). The cell length can be measured. It is not number of sections times section thickness, because the individual cells are at varying angles in the vessels, and branches or projections may not be aligned with the long axis of the cell. The angle in the vessel wall is readily determined, since each cell is digitized as if it were viewed from a point directly opposite to it at the junction of the tunica media and adventitia. Orientation within the vessel wall is also obtained from the plots. The axis of the cell may veer toward the luminal or abluminal edges or perfectly follow the curvature of the vessel. The plot also shows overall clockwise or counterclockwise orientation (Fig. 5-3).

In any sampling method, the probability is that

larger cells will have a greater chance of being chosen (25, 26). This is particularly true if cells are infinitely large versus infinitely small. Our evidence, from random sampling of cells, suggests that within a given vessel there is an overall range within which most cells fall (5, 21). If, indeed, very small cells are being missed, they are not representative of the major population, and therefore are probably of little importance.

2.2. *Quantifying cell shape*

The question of how to define cell shape and changes in shape has still to be definitively resolved. Shape may well be a much more significant parameter than has been recognized previously. For example, it has been suggested in neurulation (27) that changes in cell shape may be an active causative factor in tissue shaping and not merely a passive response. Controversy still exists as to whether changes in cell shape beget higher blood pressures or whether they occur solely as a result of higher pressures. Changes in size and shape in vascular smooth muscle cells in the disease of hypertension certainly will affect fluid and electrolyte exchange or the plasma membrane available for receptor sites. In striated muscle, the size of the fiber was a critical factor in sodium fluxes (28). Some cells can be related to geometric shapes, that is, correlated with idealized cones, cylinders, spindles, etc. Also, these shapes all have a convex profile. Irregular shapes that do not resemble any standard geometric shape prove much more difficult to analyze, particularly when concave regions routinely occur. For example, some hypertrophic guinea pig intestinal smooth muscle cells had deep invaginations of the plasma membrane (6). Therefore, surface areas are often much larger than would be estimated from simple model shapes (22).

One method of giving a numerical value to a shape is to plot the distances from a central point to the periphery as a function of angle, and then carry out conventional Fourier analysis (22, 29). This analysis has limitations based on the possibility of the radius leaving and re-entering the profile as in smooth muscle where areas of concavity can occur. Another way of dealing with shapes is to use fractal dimensions (13, 22, 30, 31). This process was first described in relation to the configuration of the coast of England. If the total length (or perimeter or boundary) is determined, based on dividing the length into a series of fractions or strides, and each fraction is then halved, the perimeter will increase because more irregularities of the profile are defined. If this is continued with finer and finer steps, the slope of the plot of fraction versus perimeter is constant on a log plot. Mandlebrot (30) has carried the idea further so that with two-dimensional profiles, the fractal dimensions vary between values of one and two. Therefore, the more regular a profile is, the nearer to *one* it is, and the more irregular, the nearer to *two*. Fractals can also be carried into three dimensions when the limits would be between two and three, depending on the degree of irregularity. The strides or fractions have traditionally been mechanically measured, for example, using calipers, or by increasing the magnification and using any map-measuring device or determining line length using computer technology (32).

This type of analysis has been applied to the complex surfaces of naturally arising objects of interest to physicists and chemists (33), and to determine the surface ruggedness of pharmaceutical solids (29). In the latter case, the need for surface characterization is due to phenomena dependent on shape such as absorption, diffusion, and dissolution. Some of these, translated into biological terms, are directly applicable to smooth muscle. We have some preliminary results from vascular smooth muscle cells. Since we are defining the plasma membrane as the definitive boundary for the profiles, using x,y coordinates, the fractal dimensions start with all irregularities defined, and fraction or stride length then takes in multiples of the coordinates defining the perimeter. This allows a numerical value for shape, which is compatible with the type of unevenness occurring in smooth muscle, which can be qualitatively described from a common-sense interpretation of the shapes of the profiles.

3. Morphofunctional characteristics of smooth muscle

The information described in this section will emphasize more clearly the diversity of structure found among different types of smooth muscle, and how each type, being unique, is adapted for its particular function. In architectural terms, form follows function.

3.1. Cell size

Many reviews of smooth muscle group all smooth muscle together and give a range of sizes such as 100 to 500 μm in length and 2 to 5 μm in diameter (34), with the myometrial smooth muscle (35) being somewhat larger (300 to 600 μm by 5 to 10 μm). Even greater extremes in length from arteriolar (20 μm) to visceral (nearly 1 mm) smooth muscle have been reported (36). However, as Gabella (37) points out, cell length is a rather uncertain dimension, since the cells can relax and contract over a wide range and their measured length depends on physiological conditions as well as on fixation procedure.

In somes cases where the perfusion fixation pressure is critical, as in vascular tissue, some reports describe vessels fixed following experimentally induced maximum relaxation (38). However, it cannot be assumed that normotensive versus hypertensive would necessarily respond identically to induced relaxation. This method gives no indication as to the state of the vessels *in vivo*. Other investigators perfuse at the same pressure for normotensive versus hypertensive vessels (39), and similarly this does not preserve vessels at their functional dilation. In our studies on vascular tissue, we have come to the conclusion that perfusion at each animal's mean blood pressure is a reasonable compromise representing the physiological *in situ* situation (5).

A commonly used method to determine smooth muscle cell size or size changes is to determine the cross-sectional area of cells, either by direct measurement or by stereological morphometric methods (38, 39, 40, 41). For example, Osborne-Pellegrin (40) concluded that smooth muscle cells of the rat aorta and renal artery were the same size based on the area of nucleated profiles. In our studies on smooth muscle cells that were reconstructed using serial sections from rat vessels and perfusion-fixed at each animal's mean blood pressure (5), we found that the tail and femoral artery cells had the same length and same dimensions in the middle section. With only these parameters — and this is much more information than just mean areas from one (nucleated) region of the cell — it would be natural to assume that these cells were of similar size. However, when volumes were compared from the computer-assisted analysis of the serial sections, the tail artery cells (2505 ± 238 μm^3) were found to be nearly three times larger than smooth muscle cells of the femoral artery (919 ± 76 μm^3) in adult 16-week-old rats. This emphasizes the misinterpretations that can arise if only two-dimensional values are evaluated.

If all profiles in a section are assessed to estimate cell size, another problem can arise. One cannot make assumptions that each profile represents an individual cell, as Gabella (6) has so conclusively demonstrated in guinea pig hypertrophied small intestine smooth muscle. Many of the profiles in a single section in this tissue represent a number of processes from one cell, since each cell has many branched processes. He demonstrated the continuity by tracing the profiles through consecutive sections, and from these he also assessed dimensions and surface-area-to-volume proportions. We have also demonstrated that many of the profiles in a section can belong to one cell in vascular smooth muscle (5, 16, 18, 21), and examples are seen both in micrographs of a muscular artery (Fig. 5-1) and in the venous system (Fig. 5-9).

The same problems, namely what is a cell or what is part of a cell, arise when numbers of layers of smooth muscle cells in a tissue are evaluated. For example, if smooth muscle cells are likened to a shape such as a sphere, the possibility that they may branch is not taken into consideration. Spheres have been used to evaluate whether hyperplasia or hypertrophy would account for changes in overall dimensions of the vessel wall (38). As Baandrup and coworkers emphasize (42), it is often overlooked that stereological measurements are suited to tissues that are randomly oriented and have particles of similar size and shape, criteria that do not apply to most vascular smooth muscle. We have found that mesentery artery cells from young spontaneously hypertensive rats (16 weeks) actually have cells that are shorter but that in the center of the cell have the same dimensions as

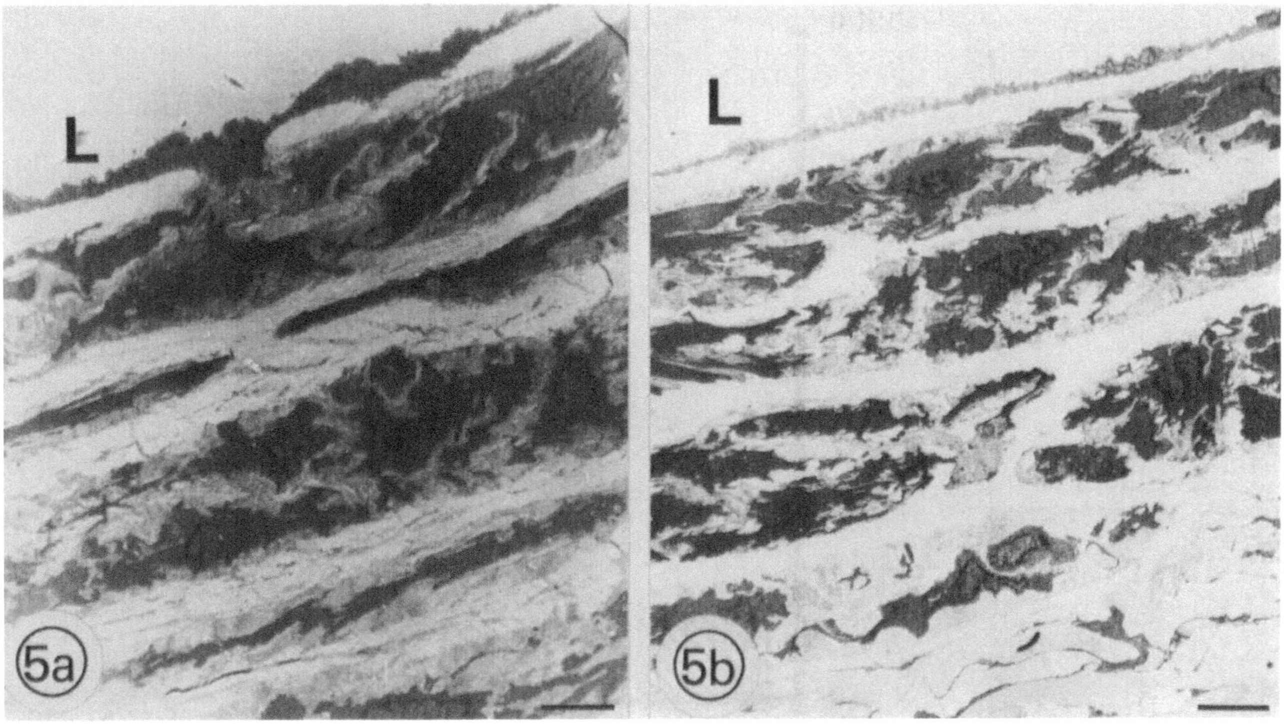

Figure 5-5. Electron micrographs of smooth muscle cells from a mesenteric artery from normotensive (a) and hypertensive (b) 16-week-old rats. The two vessels appear similar, and in fact the dimensions of the middle profile of traced cells (length and width averaged) are not different in the two groups (normotensive, 14 ± 1 μm; hypertensive, 18 ± 3 μm). However, the cells from the hypertensive animal are significantly shorter, 49 ± 3 μm versus 64 ± 4 μm ($p < 0.01$), and smaller in volume, 636 ± 68 μm^3 versus 918 ± 81 μm^3 ($p < 0.05$). These values were obtained from computer-assisted analyses from serial sets ($n = 16$ in each group). L: lumen. Bar = 5 μm.

control cells (Fig. 5-5). Therefore, indirect morphological measurement of any changes in the cell dimensions could miss this change in shape. For example, rat aortic cell size from hypertensive and normotensive strains was compared using the areas of nucleated profiles (43). In this same study, the cell size was estimated from number of profiles versus number of nuclei. Our results from serial sets would suggest that assumptions are being made that the available evidence does not substantiate: 1) that profiles with nuclei indicate cell size, and 2) that these cells have no forks or branches, and that therefore each profile represents a single cell.

Methods that use numbers of nuclei within a given volume of tissue would, however, reveal a mean decrease in cell size (42, 44, 45). The drawbacks of using nuclei to reveal the morphological characteristics of a particular smooth muscle is that only mean values can be derived. This method does not reveal any of the heterogeneity in cell size, shape, or orientation that may exist within a tissue. If cell dimensions are evaluated from nuclei, corrections can be made for angle if the cells are other than circumferential, but this may be difficult since cells in many blood vessel cells run in both clockwise and counterclockwise directions (5, 46). This method also will not identify whether or not there are differences within the layers, possibly a significant proportion of larger cells. With different surface-area-to-volume ratios, diffusion rates may be significantly influenced by cell size alone in a given tissue, as has been demonstrated in striated muscle (28).

The evidence from the smallest arterial vessels, using either serial sections or scanning electron microscopy, is that the cells are similar in size in arteriolar branches (3, 4, 47). In any one age group in growing rats, all arteriolar vessels, characterized by having a single smooth muscle cell layer forming the wall, have cells similar in

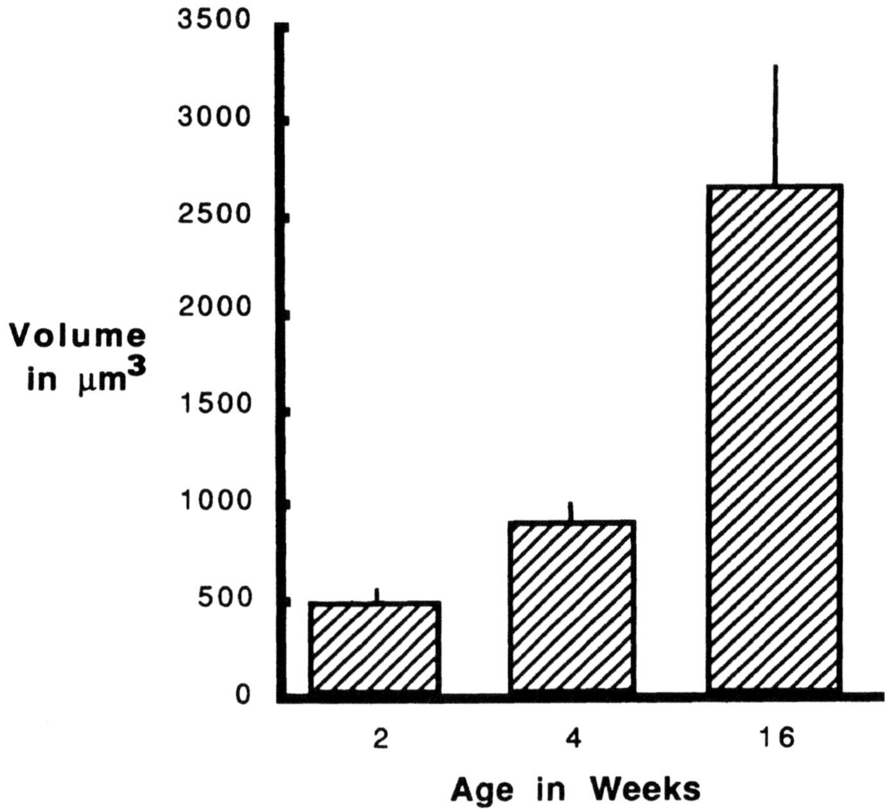

Figure 5-6. A comparison of mean cell volumes of smooth muscle cells from the tail artery in rats that were 2, 4, and 16 weeks old. Cells from electron micrographs of the proximal region only were compared. Each group is significantly different from the other two groups ($p < 0.01$). Standard error of the mean is indicated by vertical bars.

size, even though the vessels themselves vary in size by many diameters (47). We have found a decreased range of variation in cell size in a small muscular artery when compared with a muscular artery of larger size. Branches of the terminal mesenteric arcades of rat ileum were compared with the rat tail artery, with volumes derived from serial sections (21). Could this represent the beginnings of a pattern in the vascular system? As the muscular arteries get smaller, the cells decrease in size, and also have a smaller range of cell size. It cannot be postulated that a smaller vessel has smaller cells, since the cells in femoral and mesenteric arteries and in the aorta in the rat are much smaller in volume than those in a muscular artery of very much smaller diameter (5, 21). To test this hypothesis, we have carried out some preliminary studies on the first part of the puzzle: whether cells get smaller in a muscular artery with a decrease in diameter. An ultrastructural analysis of cells from the beginning of the first quarter (proximal) and beginning of the fourth quarter (distal) in the tail artery of two-week-old rats followed the apparent trend. The proximal cells had significantly larger cells volumes, $p < 0.01$ ($n = 6$, $494 \pm 74\ \mu m^3$), than distal cells ($n = 8$, $221 \pm 12\ \mu m^3$). The proximal tail artery cells are also significantly smaller in volume than cells at four weeks of age, and both two- and four-week cells are significantly smaller than cells in an adult (Figs. 5-6 and 5-7).

3.2. *Position of the smooth muscle nucleus*

In the classical spindle-shaped smooth muscle cell, the nucleus is assumed to be centrally located and in the thickest part of the cell (47, 48, 49). It certainly may be in the center in some smooth muscle, but our evidence from rat vascular smooth muscle (Figs. 5-3 and 5-7) indicates that the nucleus may be anywhere along the cell length, and it is most commonly off center (5,

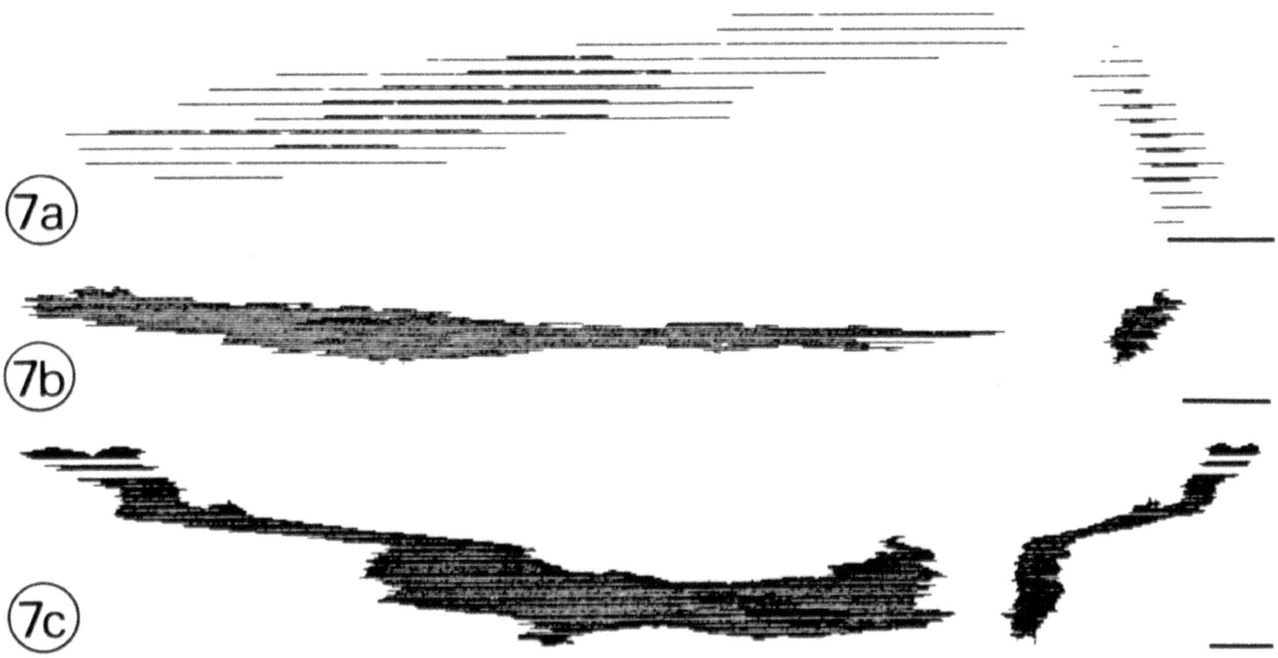

Figure 5-7. A comparison of plots of smooth muscle cells from electron micrographs of the tail artery. Micron bars are included to aid in indicating the differing sizes. Both $x = 90°$ and $y = 90°$ (see Fig. 5-3 for explanation) are shown for each cell. (a) A cell from the distal region, two-week-old animal. Every tenth profile is plotted. The nucleus is to the left in $x = 90°$, and the cell is oriented in a counterclockwise direction (6°) and veers toward the adventitia. Bar = 5 μm. (b) A cell from the proximal region, four-week-old animal. Every fifth profile is plotted. Circumferential orientation and veering toward the lumen. Bar = 2.5 μm. (c) A cell from the proximal region, 16-week-old animal. Every fifth profile is plotted. Clockwise orientation at an angle of 10°, and pronounced veering toward the lumen. The nucleus is toward the right. Bar = 2.5 μm.

21). The position of the nucleus is one structural parameter that,by itself, may not have functional importance unless the contraction abilities of the cell are more efficient with the nucleus eccentrically located. Does the contractile mechanism function better with a greater proportion toward one end, uninterrupted by a nucleus in these relatively small cellular units?

3.3. Smooth muscle cell orientation

The orientation of smooth muscle cells in vascular tissue has been thoroughly reviewed in all sizes of vessels and in both the arterial and venous sides by Rhodin (46). From Gabella's extensive studies and reviews, we have a very clear understanding of all layers of the intestinal wall, relaxed and contracted, and under conditions that induce hypertrophy, and also the arrangement in the urogenital system (7, 8, 17, 37).

Literally thousands of experiments have been reported concerning tension changes or forces developed by contracting (and relaxing) vascular smooth muscle cells from strips or rings cut from the vessel since such changes were first described by Furchgott and Bhadrakom (50). Herlihy (51) tested the force developed in aortic rings cut at various angles and found that the maximum force was developed with transversely cut strips, which would correspond to circumferential orientation. This was later confirmed by cutting the vessel at varying angles (43). More recently (52, 53, 54), similar studies carried out on the rat tail artery, using helical strips cut at varying angles, confirmed that the angle of the strip affected the result. From reconstructions of serial sets, we found that the tail artery cells in adult rats (16 weeks old) were oriented at a mean pitch or angle of 15 ± 2° in the vessel wall, which is in the same range as the approximately 20° angle found above. We have shown, however, that the cells are oriented in both clockwise and counterclockwise directions (5). Presumably, then, the helical strips could be cut in either direction, and as long as the axis was along that of the cells, the results would be comparable.

Many vessels in addition to the aorta have cells with circumferential orientation (46). We have found the cells of mesenteric and femoral arteries to have a lower pitch than in the tail artery (5). Others, using scanning electron microscopy, have reported that mesenteric arteriolar cells are circumferentially organized (47). In other arterial vessels, such as cerebral arteries (55), various sized arteries in the rabbit ear (45), and hamster cheek pouch arterioles (56), the orientation was found to be circumferential. The orientation in all of these was derived from nuclear orientation, and in the arteriolar vessels it was concluded that the greatest force developed was transmitted circumferentially (56).

Since smooth muscle is a dynamic tissue, responding to changing stimuli, one might postulate that the orientation can change just as cell size and shape have been shown to alter. When hypertension develops, does the orientation change in those vessels that react most dramatically to the higher blood pressure? This remains to be explored. We have evidence from developmental studies that the orientation of the cells in the muscular saphenous artery in the rat thigh increases from a low pitch (6 ± 1°) at three weeks of age to a pitch of 11 ± 1° at six weeks ($p < 0.01$). The cell volume also increases significantly in this period, $p < 0.01$ ($n = 24$ in each group, from 533 ± 45 to 1220 ± 70 μm^3). This certainly corresponds to the period when blood pressure is increasing. It is impossible to say without further investigation whether pressure is the prime stimulus, or whether the developing innervation (57,58) may play a role, or whether pressure and innervation interact. Trophic

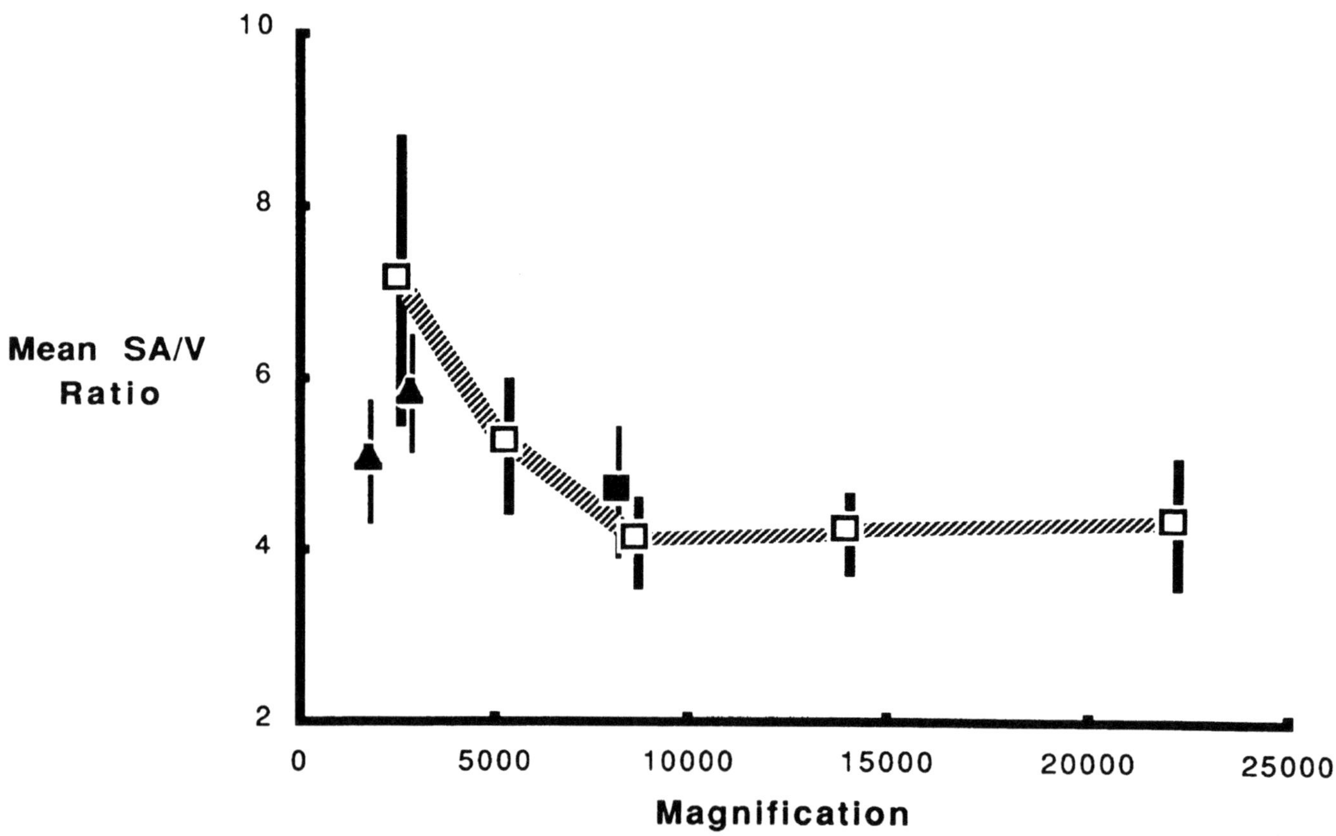

Figure 5-8. Three-week-old rat. Smooth muscle cells from the saphenous artery were analyzed. Surface-area-to-volume ratios from electron micrographs of portions of cells are indicated by open squares. The ratios were obtained from tracings of the same five cells through 31 serial sections at various magnifications. Another set (closed square), traced from 20 cells through 11 serial sets, suggests that combination is as suitable as fewer cells through more sections. The high values at the lower magnifications are due to the problem of lining up adjacent profiles in register, so that the surface is exaggerated. The triangles represent ratios obtained from whole cells ($n = 4$) using light microscopy. Since the values from whole cells fall within the expected curve, it suggests that ratios obtained from partial cells represent accurate estimations for whole cells. ± Standard error of the mean is indicated by vertical bars.

interactions between nerve and smooth muscle may be a factor. Evidence suggests that the vessel and neural tissue have strong trophic interactions, causing vasomotor nerves to grow directionally toward it (59).

3.4. Surface areas and shape

In determining structural parameters, surface areas of irregularly shaped objects pose the most problems. Where muscle cells are more regular in shape, as in the smooth muscle of the intestinal tract or vas deferens, surface areas of 5000 μm^2 per cell have been reported, giving surface-area-to-volume ratios of approximately 1.5 (60, 61). The ratio in myometrial muscle is approximately 1.1 based on an average volume of 21,000 μm^3 and surface area of 23,000 μm^2 (35). If cross-sectional area versus perimeter are compared, the smaller, more irregular cells of the sphincter pupillae smooth muscle have a higher surface-to-volume ratio of 2.7 (62), as do vascular aortic and renal cells (40).

Determinations of surface area depend strongly on the magnification, since the surface, in this case the plasma membrane or sarcolemma, must be visualized with all its projections and crenulations. The surface area, therefore, increases with magnification, unlike volume which can be accurately estimated at the light microscopic level, since the ins and outs cancel each other (13, 18). Our estimates of vascular smooth muscle surface areas using summated areas of triangular tiles connecting *x,y* coordinates of adjacent profiles (see Section 2.1) illustrated that surface areas initially do increase with an increase in magnification (Fig. 5-8). This was due to falsely high values because of the difficulty in getting each profile in precise register, as in the cell *in situ*, with the preceding and succeeding profiles. Some recent studies using an accurately defined laser-generated topographical reference that extends through the tissue and therefore can be lined up in adjacent sections may prove to be a method that solves this problem (63).

The falsely higher surface-area-to-volume values at lower microscopic magnifications is illustrated (Fig. 5-8). Light microscopic values represent complete cells and the values measured at the ultrastructural level reflect portions of cells only. Initially, ratios were estimated from five cells through 31 ultrathin serial sections. A second group, portions of 20 cells through 11 sections, gave similar values. Since the whole cells (n = 4) fit closely with the curve, it suggests that the values from partial cells, using sufficiently high magnifications, are indeed representative of the surface-area-to-volume ratios in the tissue. The results represent cells in developing animals (muscular saphenous artery, three weeks of age). We have also found that surface-area-to-volume ratios changed in hypertension in the portal vein smooth muscle, indicating that the cells have a greater proportion of plasma membrane per unit μm^3 of volume (16, 18).

Recently we have been exploring the possibilities of using fractal dimensions (see Section 2.2) to quantify cell shape. A mean fractal dimension was derived from 11 serial sections of ultrastructural profiles. Muscle cells in portal veins from hypertensive and normotensive 16-week-old rats had differences between the two groups. The mean value for the control profiles (n = 4, 1.097 ± 0.006), being nearer one, indicates a much more uniform profile than the value of 1.206 ± 0.038 (n = 7) found in cells from the hypertensive animal ($p < 0.05$). If micrographs or plots of cells from these two experimental groups are compared, then the differences are readily apparent (Fig. 5-9). Further investigation may reveal whether one can correlate these fractal dimensions with surface-area-to-volume proportions.

4. Conclusions

No attempt has been made here to give an exhaustive review of all previously described morphological characteristics of smooth muscle cells, since this area will be covered in other chapters of this volume. Rather, the attempt has been to emphasize how misconceptions can arise when interpreting from two dimensions, and how other methods such as those making use of serial sections can provide further information about these very heterogeneous populations of smooth muscle. Carrying out analyses from serial sets virtually necessitates computer assistance with sufficiently sophisticated software and sufficient storage to

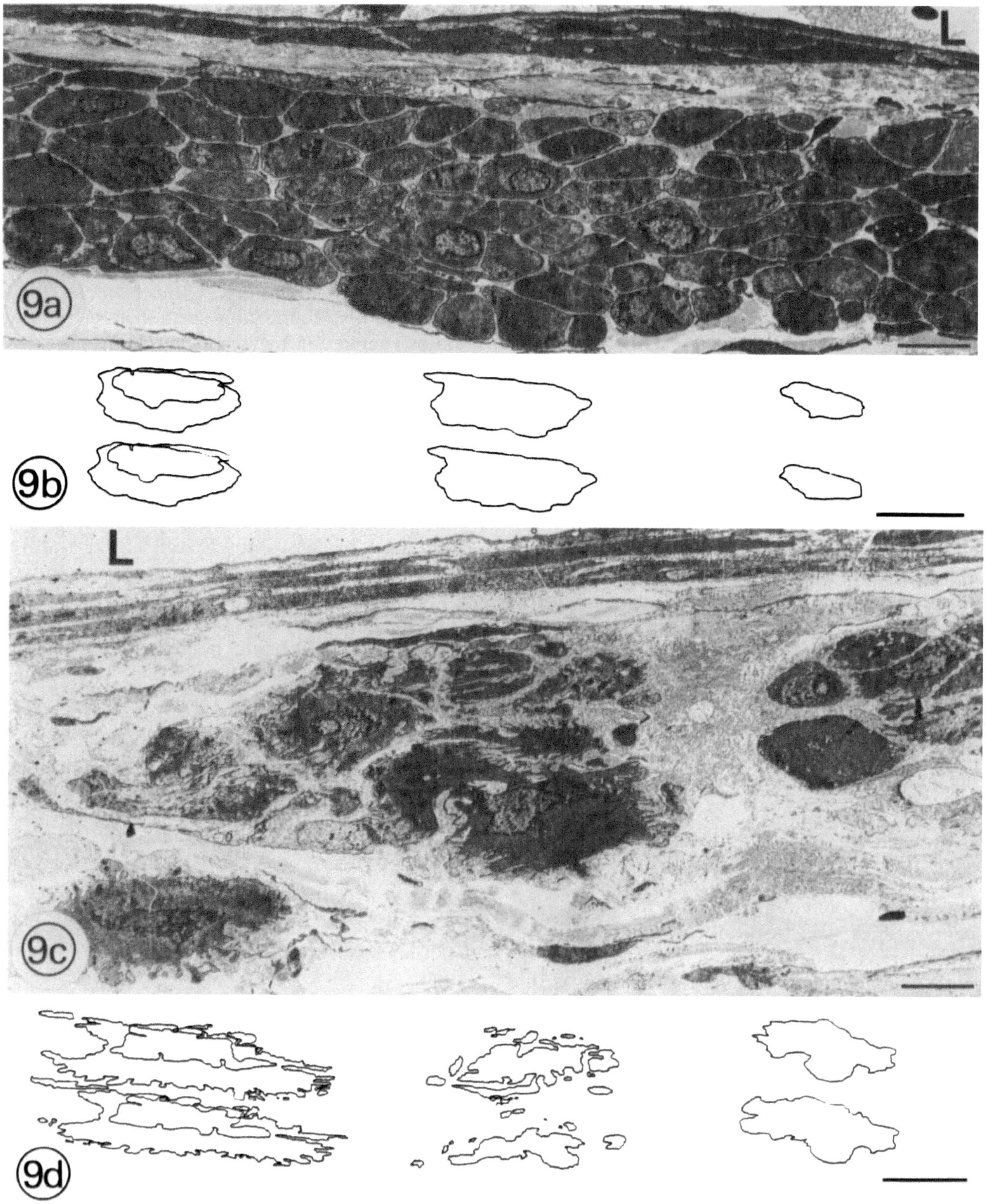

Figure 5-9. Electron micrographs of portal vein and plots of smooth muscle cells from the outer, longitudinal, layer. (a) Normotensive 16-week-old rat. The smooth muscle in the outer longitudinal layer shows a uniformity of profile shape. Bar = 5 μm. This is reflected in plots of typical profiles (b), with the nucleus present in the first pair only ($x = 60°$; see Fig. 5-3 for explanation). Each pair is represented by two plots ten consecutive sections apart. Bar = 2.5 μm. (c) Hypertensive 16-week-old rat. The longitudinal layer has smooth muscle cells with boundaries that are much more irregular in outline than in the normotensive animal, with many branches or projections. Bar = 5 μm. The irregularities are seen also in the plots of typical cells (d). Bar = 2.5 μm. The inner circular layer does not show any major changes. L: lumen.

cope with the millions of x,y coordinates that accumulate, particularly at the ultrastructural level. What also emerges is that the function of a particular group of smooth muscle cells is so unique that its members are specially adapted in size, shape, and orientation to perform at maximum efficiency. Therefore, at least at this stage, it is impossible to summarize briefly what constitutes smooth muscle in its overall dimensional parameters. Some questions have been posed that future research may answer, and some directions for further investigations have been suggested. A pattern must emerge, and more studies will reveal it, as long as we can overcome misconceptions that all smooth muscle is represented by spindle-shaped cells with a centrally located nucleus.

Acknowledgments

I gratefully acknowledge the British Columbia Heart Foundation and the Medical Research Council of Canada, which supported the research carried out in our laboratory. Appreciation is due Robert Wang for his skillful and painstaking efforts in translating our proposed biological investigations into workable computer programs. I am indebted to Brent Gowen and Fanny Chu for their innovative contributions toward developing techniques associated with studies involving serial sections. Cindy Gibson has been invaluable in the preparation of the manuscript. Judy Bysouth has again demonstrated her very high standards in the typing of the manuscript.

References

1. Stempak JG: Fixative effects on mitochondrial form in embryonic and neonatal rat liver cells. *Anat Rec* 148: 340 (abstr), 1964.
2. Stempak JG: Electron microscopic observations on serial sections of mitochondria from rat liver cells. *Anat Rec* 151: 420 (abstr), 1965.
3. Carlson EC, Burrows ME, Johnson PC: Electron microscopic studies of cat mesenteric arterioles: a structure–function analysis. *Microvasc Res* 24: 123–141, 1982.
4. Komuro T, Desaki J, Uehara Y: Three-dimensional organization of smooth muscle cells in blood vessels of laboratory rodents. *Cell Tissue Res* 227: 429–437, 1982.
5. Todd ME, Laye CG, Osborne DN: The dimensional characteristics of smooth muscle in rat blood vessels. A computer-assisted analysis. *Circ Res* 53: 319–331, 1983.
6. Gabella G: Hypertrophic smooth muscle. I. Size and shape of cells, occurrence of mitoses. *Cell Tissue Res* 201: 63–78, 1979.
7. Gabella G: Dynamic aspects of the morphology of the intestinal muscle coat. In: Cellular Physiology and Clinical Studies of Gastrointestinal Smooth Muscle. JH Szurszewski (ed), Amsterdam: Elsevier Science Publishers B.V., p 5–31, 1987.
8. Baluk P, Gabella G: Scanning electron microscopy of the muscle coat of the guinea-pig small intestine. *Cell Tissue Res* 250: 551–561, 1987.
9. Elias H: Identification of structure by the common sense approach. *J Microsc* 95: 59–68, 1972.
10. Williams MA: Introduction and stereological techniques. In: Practical Methods in Electron Microscopy. AM Glauert (ed), Amsterdam: North Holland Pub. Co., p 1–84, 1977.
11. Wootton GS, Goodford PJ: The ratio of smooth muscle cell volume to cell surface area measured by electron microscopy with corrections for shrinkage. *Cell Tissue Res* 162: 75–82, 1975.
12. Jones AW: Content and fluxes of electrolytes. In: Handbook of Physiology, Section 2, The Cardiovascular System. DF Bohr, AP Somlyo, HV Sparks (eds), Bethesda, MD: American Physiological Society, p 253–299, 1980.
13. Weibel ER: Stereological Methods. I. Practical Methods for Biological Morphometry. New York: Academic Press, 1979.
14. Gunderson HJG, Jensen EB: Stereological estimation of the volume-weighted mean volume of arbitrary particles observed on random sections. *J Microsc* 138: 127–142, 1985.
15. Miles RE: A comprehensive set of stereological formulae for embedded aggregates of not-necessarily-convex particles. *J Microsc* 138: 115–125, 1985.
16. Todd ME: Rat portal vein muscle cells change in shape, size and cytoplasmic organization in spontaneous hypertension. *Proc XXX Congress Int Un Physiol Sci*: 602 (abstr), 1986.
17. Gabella G: An introduction to the structural variety of smooth muscles. In: Vascular Neuroeffector Mechanisms. JA Bevan, M Fjuiwara, RA Maxwell, K Mohri, S Shibata, N Toda (eds), New York: Raven Press, 13–55, 1983.
18. Todd ME, Chu F, Gowen B: Vascular smooth muscle cell dimensional characteristics. In: Cells and Tissues: A Three Dimensional Approach by Modern Techniques in Microscopy. PM Motta (ed), New York: Alan R. Liss, p. 139–144, 1989.
19. Small JV: Measurements of section thickness. In: Proceedings of the 4th European Congress on Electron Microscopy Vol 1. DS Bocciarelli (ed), Rome: Tipografia Poliglotta Vaticanna, p 609, 1968.
20. Sakai T: Relation between thickness and interference colors of biological ultrathin section. *J Electron Microsc* 29: 369–375, 1980.
21. Todd ME: Vascular smooth muscle cell parameters from computer assisted reconstructions. In: Vascular Neuroeffector Mechanisms. JA Bevan, T Godfraind, RA Max-

well, JC Stoclet, M Worcel (eds), Amsterdan: Elsevier Science Publishers, p 265–269, 1985.

22. Russ JC: Practical Stereology. New York: Plenum Press, 1986.
23. Fuchs H, Kedem ZM, Uselton SP: Optimal surface reconstruction from planar contours. In: Graphics and Image Processing. J Foley (ed), *Comm ACM* 20: 693–702, 1977.
24. Shantz M: Surface definition for branching contour-defined objects. *Computer Graphics* 15: 242–270, 1981.
25. Cruz-Orive L-M: On the estimation of particle number. *J Microsc* 120: 15–27, 1980.
26. Sterio DC: The unbiased estimation of number and sizes of arbitrary particles using the dissector. *J Microsc* 134: 127–136, 1984.
27. Moore DCP, Stanisstreet M, Evans GE: Morphometric analyses of changes in cell shape in the neuroepithelium of mammalian embryos. *J Anat* 155: 87–99, 1987.
28. Menard MR: The "intermediate component" of the radiosodium efflux from frog skeletal muscle. *Can J Physiol Pharmacol* 62: 1492–1499, 1984.
29. Thibert R, Akbarieh M, Tawashi R: Application of fractal dimension to the study of the surface ruggedness of granular solids and excipients. *J Pharm Sci* 77: 724–726, 1988.
30. Mandelbrot BB: The Fractal Geometry of Nature. New York: Freeman, 1983.
31. West BJ, Goldberger AL: Physiology in fractal dimensions. *Am Sci* 75: 354–365, 1987.
32. Wright K, Karlsson B: Fractal analysis and stereological evaluation of microstructures. *J Microsc* 129: 185–200, 1983.
33. Stanley HE, Meakin P: Multifractal phenomena in physics and chemistry. *Nature* 335: 405–409, 1988.
34. Somlyo AP, Somlyo AV: Smooth muscle structure and function. In: The Heart and Cardiovascular System. HA Fozzard, E Haber, RB Jennings, AM Katz, HE Morgan (eds), p 845–864, New York: Raven Press, 1986.
35. Garfield RE, Somlyo AP: Structure of smooth muscle. In: Calcium and Contractility. AK Grover, EE Daniel (eds), Clifton NJ: Humana Press, p 1–36, 1985.
36. Burnstock G: Structure of smooth muscle and its innervation. In: Smooth Muscle. E Bülbring, AF Brading, AW Jones, T Tomita (eds), London: Edward Arnold, p 1–70, 1970.
37. Gabella G: Structure of smooth muscles. In: Smooth Muscle: An Assessment of Current Knowledge. E Bulbring, AF Brading, AW Jones, T Tomita (eds), London: Edward Arnold, p 1–46, 1981.
38. Lee RMKW, Forrest JB, Garfield RE, Daniel EE: Ultrastructural changes in mesenteric arteries from spontaneously hypertensive rats. *Blood Vessels* 20: 72–91, 1983.
39. Hadjiisky P, Peyri N, Grosgogeat Y: Tunica media changes in the spontaneously hypertensive rat (SHR). *Atherosclerosis* 65: 125–137, 1987.
40. Osborne-Pellegrin MJ: Some ultrastructural characteristics of the renal artery and abdominal aorta in the rat. *J Anat* 125: 641–652, 1978.
41. Lee RMKW, McKenzie R, Roy M: Ultrastructure and morphometric measurements of mesenteric arteries from newborn spontaneously hypertensive rats. *Blood Vessels* 25: 105–114, 1988.
42. Baandrup U, Gundersen HJG, Mulvany MJ: Is it possible to solve the problem: hypertrophy/hyperplasia of smooth muscle cells in the vessel wall of hypertensive subjects? *Prog Appl Microcirc* 8: 122–128, 1985.
43. Arner A, Uvelius B: Force–velocity characteristics and active tension in relation to content and orientation of smooth muscle cells in aortas from normotensive and spontaneously hypertensive rats. *Circ Res* 50: 812–821, 1982.
44. Olivetti G, Melissari M, Marchetti G, Anversa P: Quantitative structural changes of the rat thoracic aorta in early spontaneous hypertension. *Circ Res* 51: 19–26, 1982.
45. Walmsley JG, Owen MP, Bevan JA: Medial morphometry and mechanics of sequential rabbit ear arteries and myograph ring segments. *Am J Physiol* 245: H840–H848, 1983.
46. Rhodin JAG: Architecture of the vessel wall. In: Handbook of Physiology, Section 2, The Cardiovascular System. DF Bohr, AP Somlyo, HV Sparks (eds), Baltimore, MD: American Physiological Society, p 1–31, 1980.
47. Miller BG, Overhage JM, Bohlen HG, Evan AP: Hypertrophy of arteriolar smooth muscle cells in the rat small intestine during maturation. *Microvasc Res* 29: 56–69, 1985.
48. Friedman SM, Nakashima M, Mar MA: Morphological assessment of vasoconstriction and vascular hypertrophy in sustained hypertension in the rat. *Microvasc Res* 3: 416–425, 1971.
49. Walmsley JG, Canham PB: Orientation of nuclei as indicators of smooth muscle cell alignment in the cerebral artery. *Blood Vessels* 16: 43–51, 1979.
50. Furchgott RF, Bhadrakom S: Reactions of strips of rabbit aorta to epinephrine, isopropylarterenol, sodium nitrite and other drugs. *J Pharmacol Exp Ther* 108: 129–143, 1953.
51. Herlihy JT: Helically cut vascular strip preparation: geometrical considerations. *Am J Physiol* 238: H107–H109, 1980.
52. Packer CS, Stevens NL: Force–velocity relationships in hypertensive arterial smooth muscle. *Can J Physiol Pharmacol* 63: 669–674, 1985.
53. Packer CS, Stephens NL: Mechanics of caudal artery relaxation in control and hypertensive rats. *J Physiol Pharmacol* 63: 209–213, 1985.
54. Packer CS, Kagan ML, Stevens NL: Decreased velocity of shortening in arterial smooth muscle from older (28- to 31-week old) spontaneously hypertensive rats. *Can J Physiol Pharmacol* 64: 96–100, 1986.
55. Walmsley JG: Vascular smooth muscle orientation in straight portions of human cerebral arteries. *J Microsc* 131: 361–375, 1983.
56. Walmsley JG, Gore RW, Dacey RG, Jr, Damon DN, Duling BR: Quantitative morphology of arterioles from the hamster cheek pouch related to mechanical analysis. *Microvasc Res* 24: 249–271, 1982.
57. Todd ME: Development of adrenergic innervation in rat

peripheral vessels: a fluorescence microscopic study. *J Anat* 131: 121–133, 1980.
58. Todd ME, Tokito MK: An ultrastructural investigation of developing vasomotor innervation in rat peripheral vessels. *Am J Anat* 160: 195–212, 1981.
59. Todd ME: Trophic interactions between rat nerves and blood vessels in denervated peripheral arteries and in anterior eye chamber transplants. *Circ Res* 58: 641–652, 1986.
60. Merrillees NCR: The nervous environment of individual smooth muscle cells of the guinea pig vas deferens. *J Cell Biol* 37: 794–817, 1968.
61. Gabella G: Quantitative morphological study of smooth muscle cells of the guinea-pig taenia coli. *Cell Tissue Res* 170: 161–186, 1976.
62. Gabella G: The sphincter pupilae of the guinea-pig: structure of muscle cells, intracellular relations and density of innervation. *Proc R Soc Lond B* 186: 369–386, 1974.
63. Bron C, Gremillet P, Launay D, Jourlin M, Hatvani P, Gautschi HP, Bachi T, Schüpbach J: Three dimensional electron microscopy of entire cells (abstract). 4th Int Congress Cell Biol, p 201, 1988.

Author's address:
Dr. Mary E. Todd
Department of Anatomy
University of British Columbia
2177 Wesbrook Mall
Vancouver, B.C., V6T 1W5
Canada

CHAPTER 6

Morphology of smooth muscle and its diversity as studied with scanning electron microscopy

YASUO UEHARA, TAKASHI FUJIWARA, SATOSHI NAKASHIRO, & ZHOU DE SHAN

1. Introduction

Smooth muscles exhibit remarkable morphological diversity among different organs in their geometrical arrangement, shape, size, amount, and packing density of muscle fibers, as extensively reviewed by Burnstock (1) and Gabella (2, 3). These parameters have direct relevance to the overall behavior of individual organs and organ-specific physiological and mechanical properties of the muscles (4–8). The morphology of smooth muscles has been investigated on sections in a variety of organs, particularly and most intensively in the gastrointestinal tract by Gabella (9, 10). However, the parameters have not yet been fully scrutinized at the ultrastructural level in any given organ, primarily because of the intrinsic technical limitations of transmission electron microscopy (TEM). Reconstruction of ultrathin serial sections has been the only means for this sort of investigation, and has been occasionally adopted to assess the size and arrangement of smooth muscle fibers (11–15). Nevertheless, it involves considerable work and requires a skilled hand.

Recently a technique that selectively removes extracellular connective tissue components has been introduced to observe stromal surfaces of tissues and cells with scanning electron microscopy (SEM) (16, 17). With the improvement of the technique, it is now feasible to examine the overall morphology of normally hidden structures, such as nerves, blood vessels, and muscles, in much finer detail than hitherto achieved.

In an attempt to provide a structural basis for the better understanding of functional variability of smooth muscles, this chapter describes and compares the three-dimensional morphology of smooth muscles in some selected organs as evidenced with the SEM technique. The morphological diversity of smooth muscles is pronounced with respect to 1) the architecture, 2) the cell shape and size, 3) the fiber ending and intercellular relationships, and 4) the cell surface topography.

The overall morphology of ganglionated autonomic plexuses and of nerve terminals innervating smooth muscles has also been examined with SEM (18–22). The comparative aspect of the innervation pattern of smooth muscles will be reported elsewhere.

2. Methodological considerations

In classical histological studies, cells and tissues were isolated or macerated with various chemicals such as salicylic acid, sodium fluoride, osmic acid, hydrochloric acid, and potassium hydrochloride (for details, see 23). Likewise, isolation and maceration were frequently applied in early morphological studies of smooth muscles. With these techniques, Köelliker (24) noted, for the first time, the morphological diversity of smooth muscle fibers. Subsequently, McGill (25) demonstrated different types of interrelations between muscle fibers. Strong (26) also macerated blood vessels with hydrochloric acid and examined the arrangement of vascular smooth muscles. Until recently, tissue maceration with nitric acid or potassium hydroxide was commonly used for the quantitative analysis of smooth muscle cells (11, 27–30).

In early SEM studies of tissues and cells embedded within stromal connective tissue, specimens were either simply microdissected or enzymatically digested by various enzymes such as collagenase, hyaluronidase, amylase, pronase, and trypsin, either singly or in combination (31–35). Straight enzymatic digestion preserves the cell surface texture well, but often results in incomplete removal of connective tissue components. More recently, a more reliable method has been introduced, which is based on the classical acid maceration mentioned earlier. The method principally consists of the treatment of aldehyde-fixed tissues with concentrated hydrochloric acid, followed by collagenase digestion (26). Potassium hydroxide can be substituted for hydrochloric acid (36). With this method, connective tissue can be almost completely removed, and cells and tissues are preserved apparently unaffected. However, prolonged acid or alkaline treatment often causes serious tissue distortion, pittings, and ruptures of the cell membrane.

The procedure routinely used in our laboratory is a combination of enzymatic digestion and acid hydrolysis (18). With this method, the time required for acid hydrolysis can be minimized to reduce artifacts with thorough removal of connective tissue components. Nevertheless, we must admit some degree of tissue and cell shrinkage due to the drastic acid treatment.

The practical processing may be outlined as followed. Unfixed fresh specimens are treated with trypsin solution (DIFCO 1:250, 2.5 mg/ml in phosphate buffered saline) for 10 to 35 minutes at 37° C followed by fixation with 2%–3% glutar-

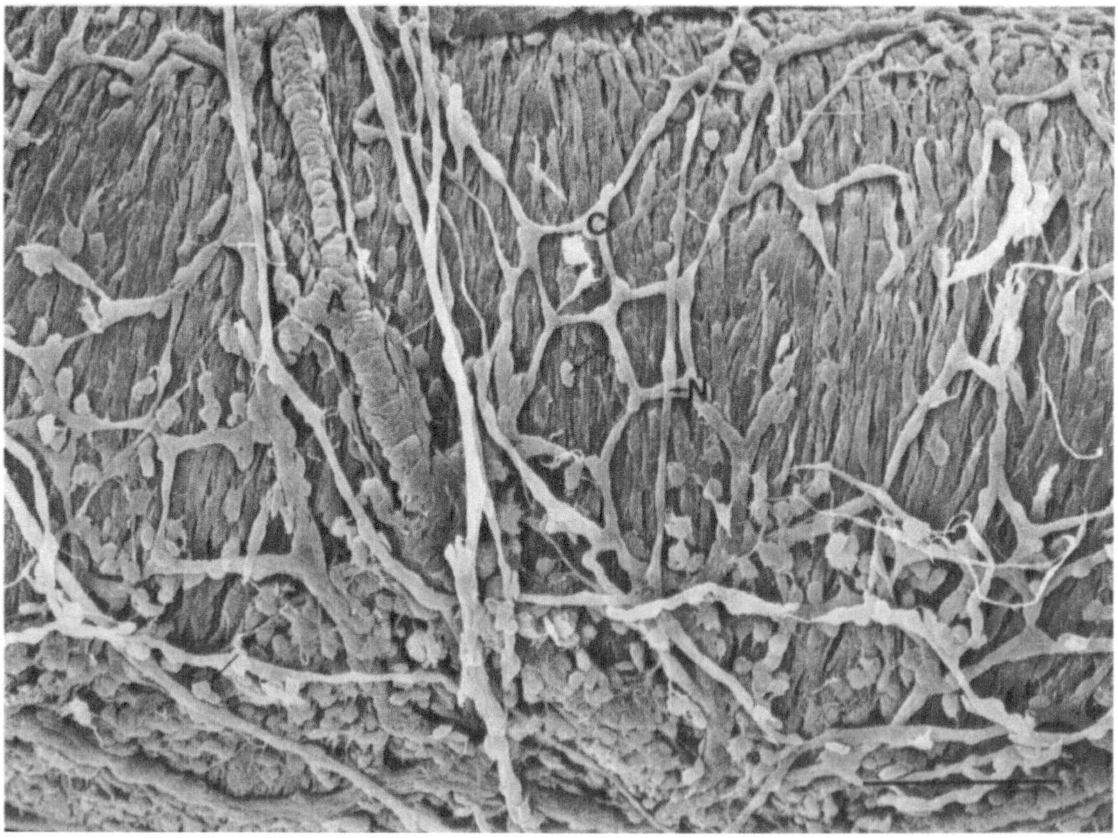

Figure 6-1. Overall SEM image of the adventitial aspect of the guinea pig oviduct. The muscular coat consists of a parallel array of circularly disposed smooth muscle fibers. Blood vessels (A: arteriole; C: capillary) and autonomic nerve fibers (N) are identified on the surface of the muscular coat. Scattered corpuscles (arrows) represent round-out fibroblasts. Bar: 50 μm.

aldehyde in 0.1 M phosphate buffer solution at pH 7.3. The specimens are then washed in the buffered saline and are treated with 8N hydrochloric acid for 10–30 minutes at 60° C. After thorough washing with distilled water, the specimens are dehydrated through a graded series of ethanol, immersed in isoamyl acetate, and critical-point dried. Platinum-coated specimens are examined in a Hitachi S-500A SEM.

3. Architecture of smooth muscles

In the specimens in which adventitial and intramural connective tissue components have been almost completely removed, the overall wall cytoarchitecture of organs is readily viewed with SEM. As an example of our preparations, Figure 6-1 shows the entire SEM image of the guinea pig oviduct. Smooth muscle can be identified as consisting of fusiform cells that are tightly packed together in a continuous layer. Blood vessels and autonomic nerves are also seen on the adventitial surface of the muscular coat. All the structural components of the organ wall are preserved apparently as normal without detectable artifacts. A number of spherical bodies about 5 μm in diameter are scattered over the muscle; these represent round-out fibroblasts with their intercellular contacts dissociated during the specimen preparation. In the small intestine, the cells appear stellate and form a continuous cellular network. Komuro (21, 22) suggested that these stellate cells correspond to the interstitial cells of Cajal. Figure 6-6 also shows the general muscular architecture in the guinea pig ureters and associated nerve fibers.

Smooth muscles of the outer muscle layer are directly viewed in all preparations. Those in the deeper muscle layer can be exposed when the outer muscles are removed by microdissection or by simply rolling a dried specimen onto double

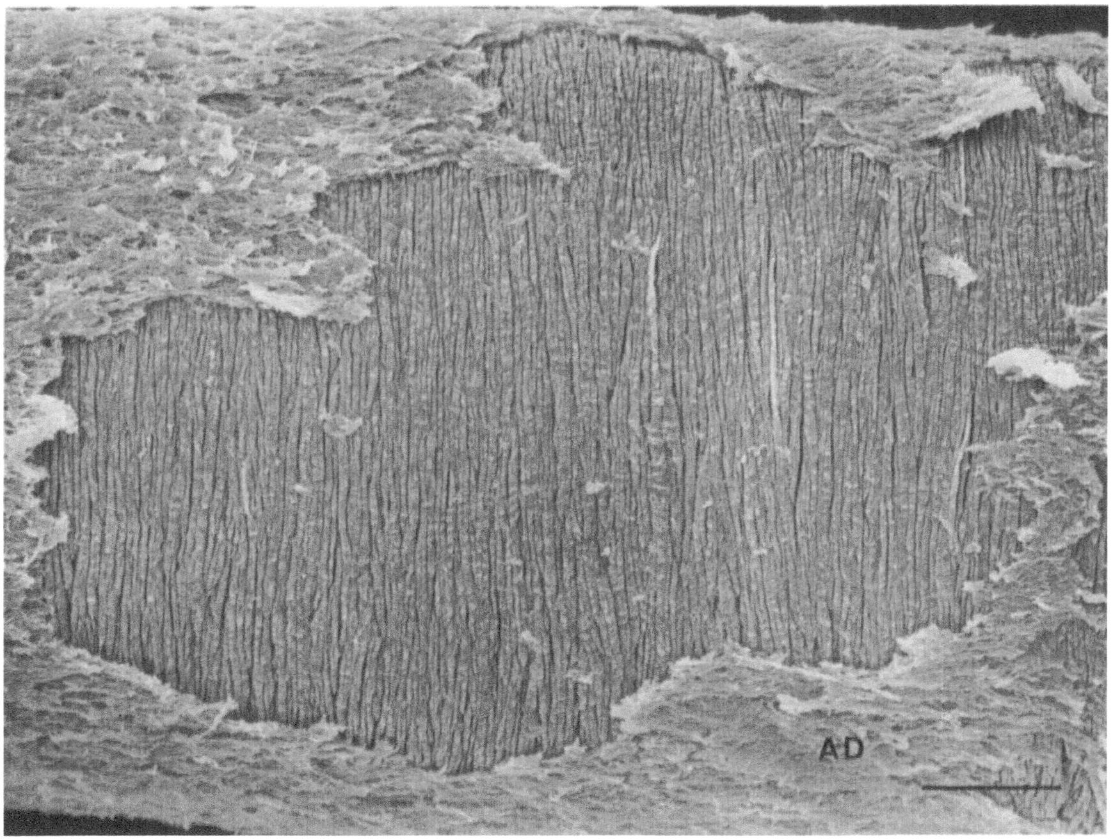

Figure 6-2. The medial architecture of a small mesenteric artery about 300 μm in diameter. Smooth muscle fibers run parallel to each other, forming a compact circular layer. The adventitial connective tissue (AD) is partially removed. Bar: 50 μm.

sticky tape adhered to the specimen holder. When the endothelium or epithelium has been exfoliated, the innermost muscles can also be examined (37). Smooth muscles thus exposed vary strikingly in their three-dimensional architecture among different organs.

The most ordered circular arrangement can be found in small arteries. As shown in Figure 6-2, the monkey mesenteric artery, about 300 μm in diameter, has a muscular coat consisting of tightly packed muscle fibers that are arranged parallel to each other and are oriented almost transversely with respect to the long axis of the vessel. Muscle fibers in the deeper media are also arranged in a regular circular fashion (37). The findings confirm the light microscopic observations by Staubesand (38) and Halpern et al. (39) but conflict with the reports that suggested a helical or diagonal arrangement (26,40). Contrary to previous light microscopical observations (41,42), the circular disposition remains unaltered during vasoconstriction (43). A detailed description of vascular smooth muscle cells will be reported in a separate chapter of this book. The muscular coat, which consists mainly of circular muscles, has been demonstrated with SEM in the guinea pig trachea (44) and in the rat thoracic duct (45). The guinea pig oviduct also has well-developed circular muscles in the outer muscular coat (Fig. 6-1), but has additional longitudinal muscles in the submucous layer, as demonstrated in the rabbit, monkey, and human (46–48). The muscular architecture of the bird oviduct has been reported to differ entirely from that of the mammals; in the hen, the muscular coat consists of the outer longitudinal and inner circular layers (49), and in the quail, outer muscles are also oriented longitudinally with a spiral bias and become circular towards the center of the organ (50). The bird oviduct is subject to extensive stretching and release during the transport of ova that are much larger than those of the mammal.

Highly developed longitudinal outer muscles are best known to occur in the taenia coli and also

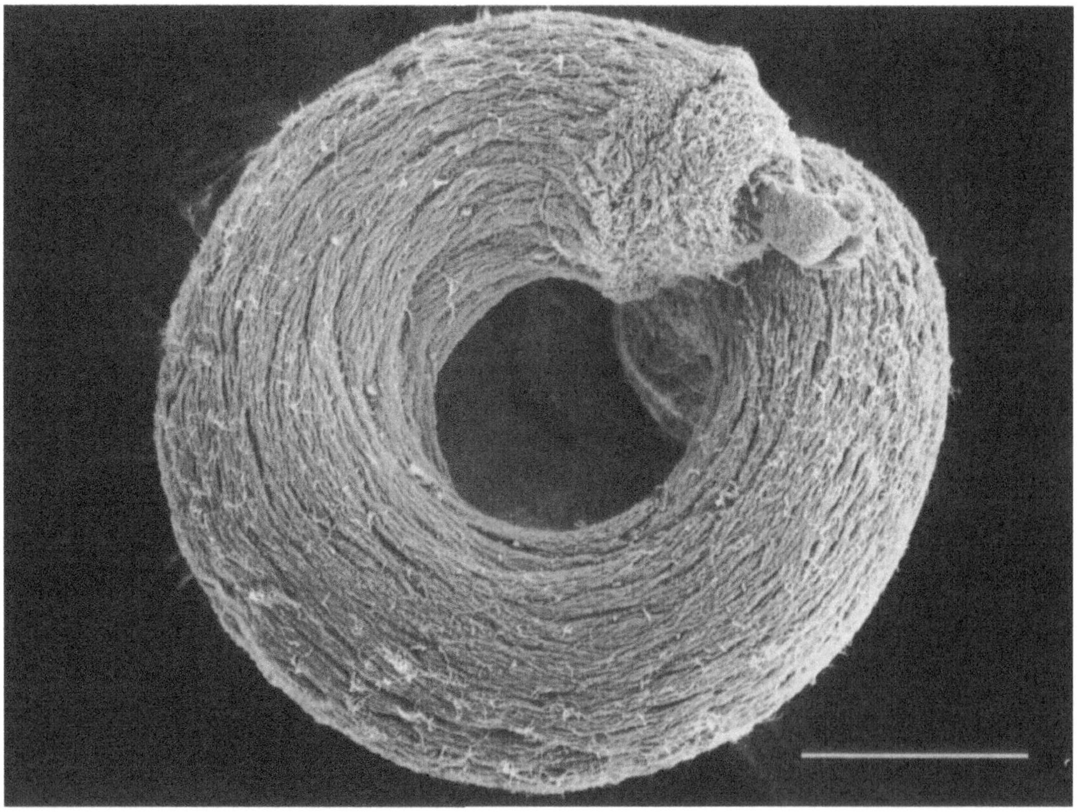

Figure 6-3. Low-power SEM picture of the guinea pig ductus deferens. Muscle fibers in the outer muscle layer are organized into longitudinal bundles. Circularly or diagonally arranged deeper muscle can be seen at the cutting end of the ductus. Bar: 500 μm.

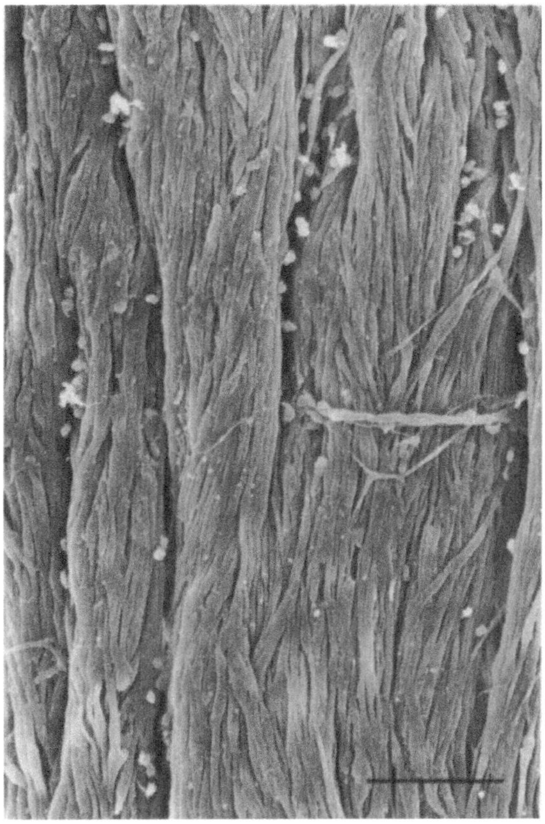

Figure 6-4. Interconnecting muscle bundles in the outer muscle layer of the guinea pig ductus deferens. Muscle fibers within a bundle are disposed slightly obliquely with respect to the long axis of the bundle, assuming a braided appearance. Bar: 50 μm.

occur in the guinea pig ductus deferens which has, in addition, circular or oblique muscles in the inner muscle layer (Fig. 6-3). In the ductus deferens, longitudinal muscles form indistinct bundles (Fig. 6-4).

The most regular two-layered organization of smooth muscles is generally known to occur in the small intestine, where the outer longitudinal layer and the inner circular layer are arranged almost at right angles to each other. The feature can be best seen in a superimposed image that is occasionally obtainable in the perinatal animals, where muscle fibers are still poorly developed and form a thin, discontinuous layer (Fig. 6-5). The orthogonal disposition of smooth muscles is related to coordinating peristaltic movements in an antagonistic manner.

A less regular and more intricate musculature is found in most of the urogenital system, though many histology textbooks describe the musculature as consisting of the inner longitudinal, middle circular, and outer longitudinal layers with indistinct boundaries. The muscular architecture of the system varies considerably in different organs and even in different portions of the same organ. Tachibana et al. (51) reported that muscle fibers in the middle guinea pig ureter were organized into interconnecting bundles that ran longitudinally or obliquely and were intermingled with underlying, more or less circularly oriented smooth muscle bundles (Fig. 6-6). In the upper ureter, bundle formation was less evident and muscle fibers were arranged predominantly circularly. In the lower ureter, outer muscles were predominantly longitudinal and were again intermingled with the underlying circular muscle bundles. The findings conflict with the earlier light microscopic observations, which suggested

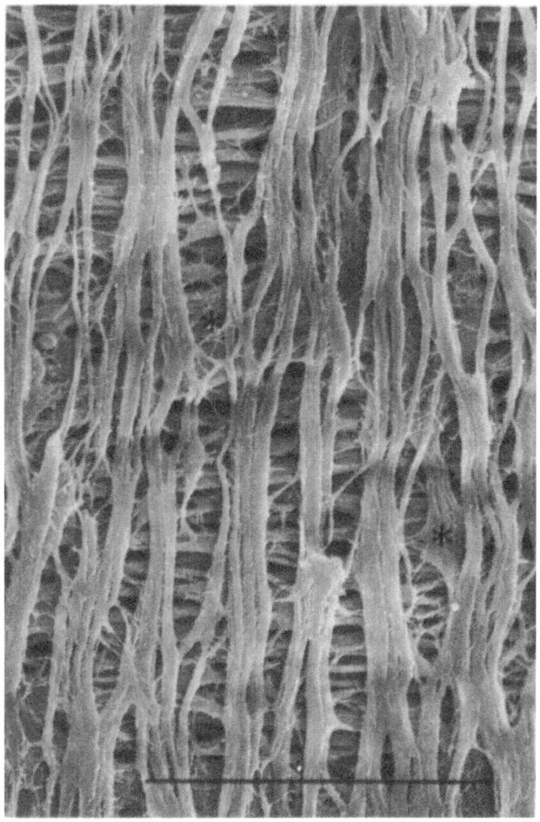

Figure 6-5. A regular orthogonal arrangement of outer longitudinal and inner circular muscle layers in the small intestine of neonatal rat. Muscle fibers, sparsely distributed, and the two layers can be seen in a superimposed image; sandwiched between the two layers is the myenteric plexus (asterisks). Bar: 50 μm.

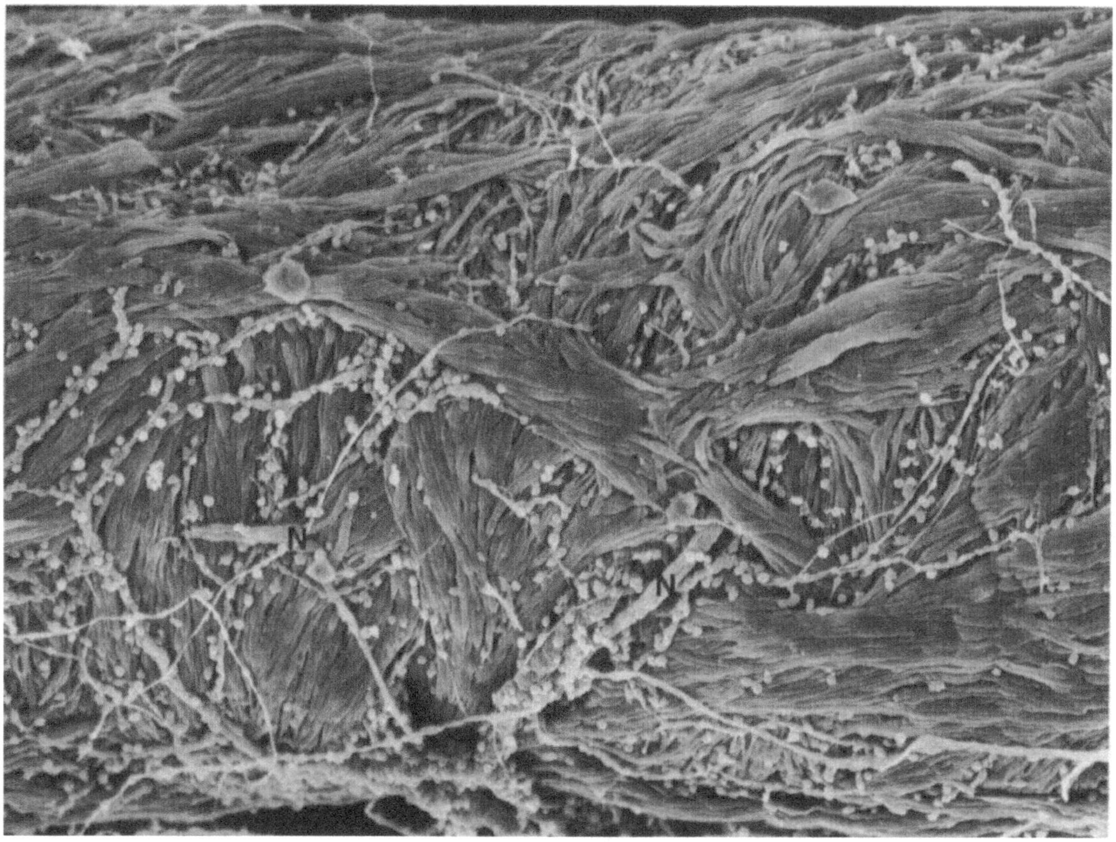

Figure 6-6. Disordered architecture of the muscular coat of the middle portion of the guinea pig ureter. Muscle fiber bundles are irregularly disposed with respect to each other and to the long axis of the ureter, being in contact with and overlapping to each other. N: nerve fibers and fiber bundles. Bar: 50 μm.

that muscle bundles were arranged in an irregular helix throughout the length of the ureter in the rabbit and human (52–54).

A number of light microscopic and ultrastructural studies have indicated that the structure of the muscular coat of the urinary bladder is highly irregular and varies considerably in different areas. Most previous studies indicate that muscle fiber bundles in individual layers are interconnected in a complex manner. When examined with SEM, there occur, in the dome, longitudinal bundles in the outermost muscular layer that radiate from the apex and partly cover deeper circular bundles (Fig. 6-7). In the ventromedial and lateral areas, muscle bundles run in all directions to form an interlacing network, assuming a knitting-ball aspect as a whole (Fig. 6-8). The musculature of the trigone and the structural relationship of the detrusor muscles to the ureteric and urethral muscles await a further elucidation with SEM.

An intricate arrangement of muscle bundles has also been demonstrated for the gall bladder in the guinea pig by histochemical staining for NADH-diaphorase in the whole mount preparation (55) and with SEM in the dogs by MacPherson et al. (56). They suggest that the three-dimensional meshwork of muscle bundles produce radial contractile forces directed toward the lumen. There are striking changes in the thickness of the musculature and the dimensions of muscle fibers during distension and constriction of the urinary bladder (29, 57). We are currently examining the changes in the morphology of the muscles in different states of filling of these spherical organs.

The male genital tract of the rat, for the most part, has a poorly developed muscular coat. In

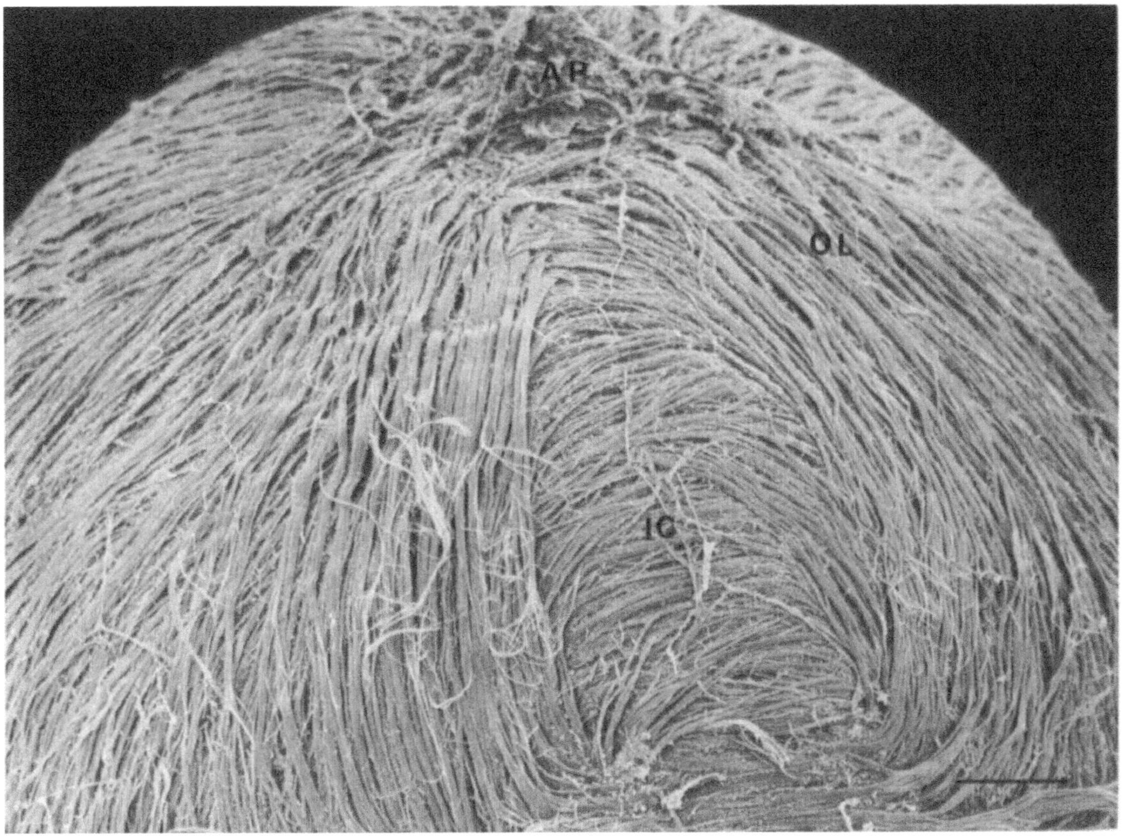

Figure 6-7. Superiomedial aspect of the muscular coat in the dome of the guinea pig urinary bladder. The outer longitudinal muscle bundles (OL) radiate from the apex (AP) and partly cover the inner circular muscle bundles (IC). Bar: 500 μm.

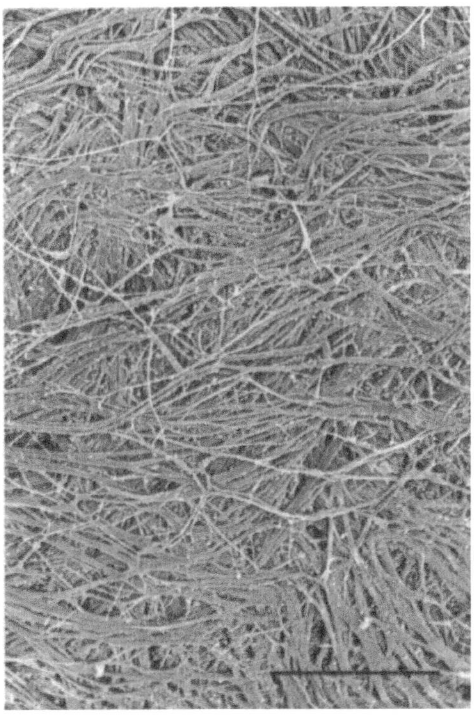

Figure 6-8. Interlacing muscle bundles in the ventrolateral portion of the guinea pig urinary bladder. The lateral portions also exhibit a similarly disordered muscle architecture. Bar: 500 μm.

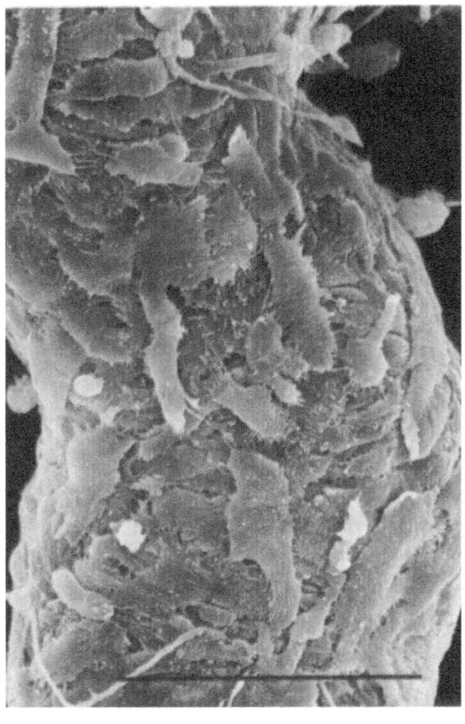

Figure 6-9. Muscle cells of the rat ductulus efferentis are small and polygonal, or short and rectangular, and appear to be flattened against the radial direction of the organ, forming a thin layer. Bar: 50 μm.

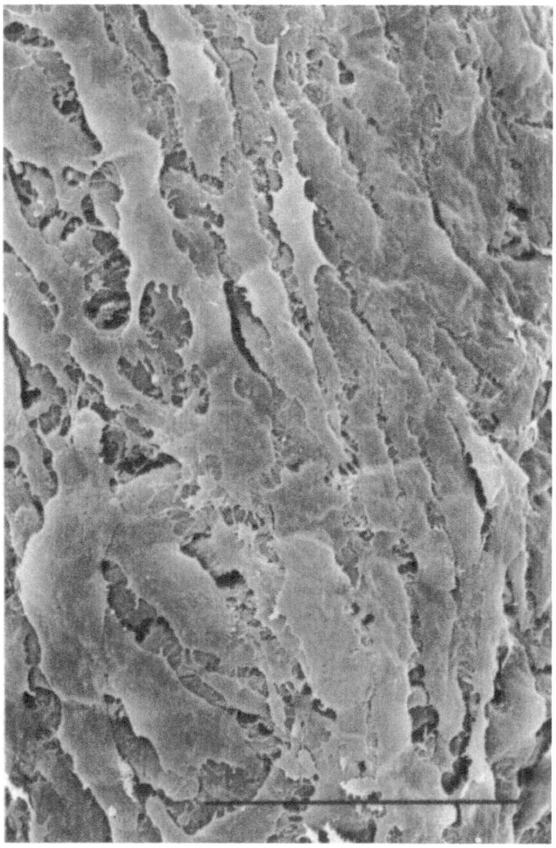

Figure 6-10. The corpus of the rat epididymis has a muscular coat consisting of flattened irregular ribbonlike muscle cells with branches and small lateral projections, being arranged longitudinally or diagonally. Circularly arranged muscle cells can be seen in the deeper layer. Bar: 50 μm.

the ductulus efferentis, the muscular coat consists only of one or two thin polygonal or rectangular muscle cells, while muscle cells of the outer layer are disposed longitudinally or diagonally and those of the inner layer are more or less circularly oriented (Fig. 6-9). In the caput and corpus of the epididymis, muscle cells of the outer layer are elongated and tapelike, forming a continuous longitudinal sheet that spreads over the circular muscles (Fig. 6-10). Towards the cauda, the outer longitudinal layer becomes thicker, and eventually forms the outer muscle of the ductus deferens. Our findings are consistent with the previous light microscopic studies on the rabbit and human (58, 59). In contrast to the rat, the epididymis of the guinea pig has a thicker muscular coat consisting of anastomosing fiber bundles that are oriented longitudinally or obliquely (Fig. 6-11). Individual muscle fibers are not flattened but appear to be fusiform. There may be underlying circular muscles.

4. Bundle formation of muscle fibers

In such organs as the monkey artery and the rat oviduct mentioned earlier, muscle fibers are arranged in more or less continuous layers or sheets. However, in many other organs, they are organized into bundles that vary in size, arrangement, and interrelationship in different muscles. So far in our examinations, the most distinct bundles have been found in the inner circular layer of the small intestine of the chicken (Fig. 6-12). Individual bundles are about 30 to 50 μm in diameter and are sharply bounded by an interstice 20 to 25 μm wide. In the guinea pig ductus deferens, muscle bundles are 40 to 60 μm in diameter and frequently split and anastomose each

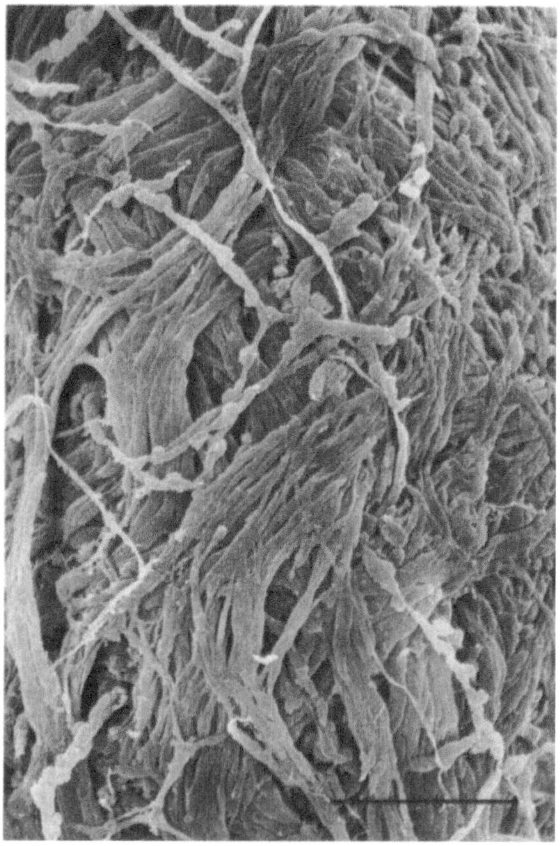

Figure 6-11. The muscular cost of the guinea pig epididymis consists of interconnecting loose muscle bundles that run in various directions. Unlike in the rat epididymis, individual muscle cells are not flattened. Bar: 50 μm.

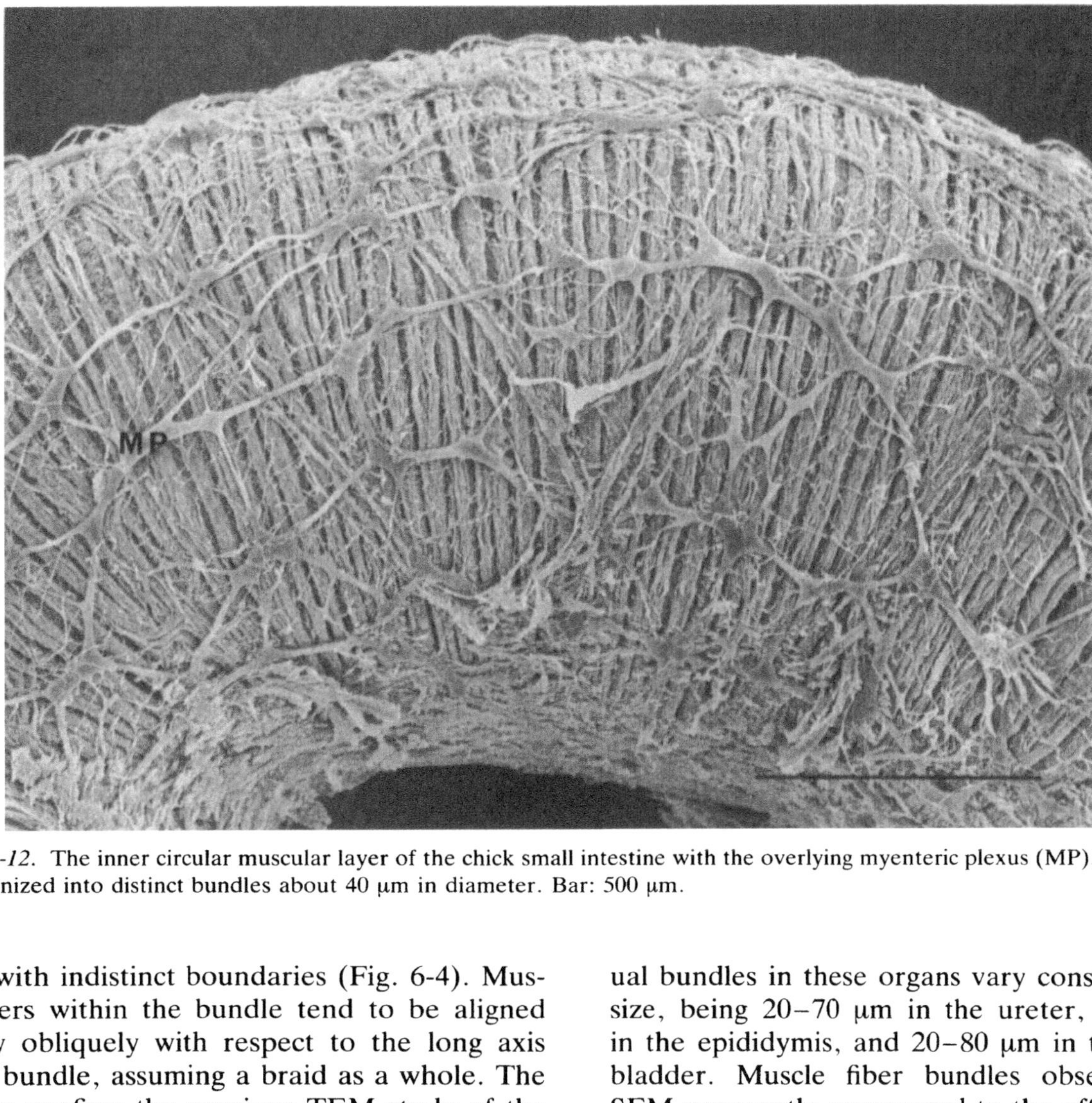

Figure 6-12. The inner circular muscular layer of the chick small intestine with the overlying myenteric plexus (MP). Muscle fibers are organized into distinct bundles about 40 μm in diameter. Bar: 500 μm.

other with indistinct boundaries (Fig. 6-4). Muscle fibers within the bundle tend to be aligned slightly obliquely with respect to the long axis of the bundle, assuming a braid as a whole. The findings confirm the previous TEM study of the same muscle by Merrillees (13). He examined serial ultrathin sections and found that a muscle bundle quickly lost its identity and was anastomosed with neighboring bundles. Relative positions of neighboring muscle fibers changed because of losses and gains of fibers within the group.

In such organs as the ureter and urinary bladder of the guinea pig and the epididymis of the rat, muscle bundles are frequently branched and intermingled with each other in a complex fashion, though the complexity differs in various organs (Figs. 6-6, 6-8, 6-11). Muscle bundles of adjacent layers are also frequently overlapped and/or interconnected to form a more or less continuous three-dimensional network. Individual bundles in these organs vary considerably in size, being 20–70 μm in the ureter, 10–50 μm in the epididymis, and 20–80 μm in the urinary bladder. Muscle fiber bundles observed with SEM apparently correspond to the effector units of electrophysiologists, i.e., the smallest muscle strip from which a propagated action potential can be initiated (60–63).

5. Cellular morphology

5.1. Cellular size and shape

The SEM procedure enables us to measure the size of smooth muscle fibers with a certain accuracy. However, the size — the length in particular — is largely subject to the state of muscle contraction and also to the preparative methods applied. The length and diameter reported in this chapter are measured in moderately distended organs. The results are summarized in Table 6-1 with the published data of the comparable muscles. So far in our examinations, flattened polygonal muscle cells found in the rat ductulus efferentis are the smallest, being about 15 μm long and 5 μm wide. Arteriolar smooth muscle cells are also small being 30–40 μm long and 4–5 μm wide. Muscle fibers in the guinea pig urinary bladder are highly elongated, and may reach 1000 μm.

The overall shape of smooth muscle fibers varies considerably in different muscles (Table 6-1). Muscle cells in many organs are fusiform with tapered ends, as can be typically seen in the monkey mesenteric arteries, in the guinea pig ureter and ductus deferens, the rat small intestine, and the chicken gizzard.

Smooth muscle cells possessing a few branches are found in the guinea pig urinary bladder and ureter (Fig. 6-13). Branched smooth muscle cells

Table 6-1. Shape and size of smooth muscle cells

Tissue	Animal	Shape	Length × Width (μm) (μm)	Method	Reference
Artery					
Mesenteric	Monkey	Sicklelike	(65–85 × 6.5)	SEM	(37)
Mesenteric	Rat	—	(61)	CAA	(81)
Mesenteric	Rat	Fusiform	(65 × 4)	NIM	(82)
Femoral	Mouse	—	(60 × 1.5–2.5)	TEM	(83)
Arteriole					
Brain	Dog	Fusiform	(40–50 × 3–4)	SEM	(64)
Fascia	Rabbit	Fusiform	(30–40 × 5)	TEM	(14)
Ileum	Guinea pig	Fusiform	(47 × 4.2)	LM	(84)
Intestine					
	Rat	Fusiform	60–120 × 2–3	SEM	PS
	Mouse	—	(400)	TEM	(11)
	Cat	—	(120 × 6)	NAM	(27)
Gizzard	Finch	Fusiform	150–250 × 2–3	SEM	PS
Urinary bladder					
	Guinea pig	Fusiform with a few branches	250–1000 × 3–5	SEM	PS
	Guinea pig	—	(160–580)	NAM	(57)
	Rabbit	—	(200–700)	NAM	(57)
Ureter	Guinea pig	Fusiform with a few branches	(100–150 × 5)	SEM	(20)
Ductus deferens					
	Guinea pig	Fusiform	60–80 × 4–5	SEM	PS
	Guinea pig	Ribbon- or rodlike	(380–450)	TEM	(13)
	Rat	Irregular with a few branches	100–150 × 8–10	SEM	PS
Epididymis					
	Rat	Tapelike	60–100 × 5–15	SEM	PS
Ductulus efferentis					
	Rat	Rectangular or polygonal	15–40 × 3–10	SEM	PS
Oviduct					
	Guinea pig	Fusiform	60–100 × 3–5	SEM	PS

NIM: Normarski's interference microscopy; CAA: computer-assisted analysis; LM: light microscopy; TEM: transmission electron microscopy; NAM: nitric acid maceration; PS: present study.

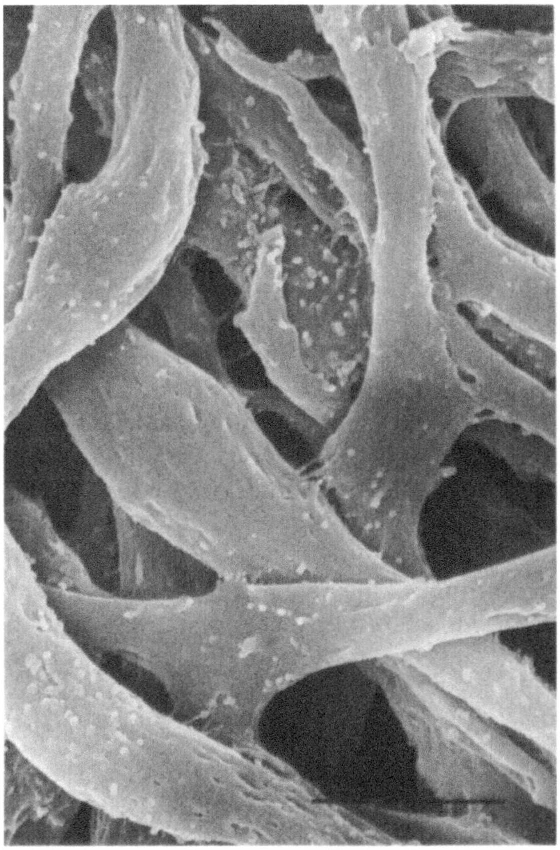

Figure 6-13. Smooth muscle cells in the guinea pig ureter with uneven thickness along the cell length. They often have a few side branches. Bar: 5 μm.

also occur in many of the rat genital organs. Figure 6-14 shows a typical example of branched muscle cells found in the guinea pig epididymis, where branches are connected to the neighboring cells in an end-to-side fashion. Highly branched smooth muscle cells are also present in the medio-adventitial border of some brain arteries, which are closely attached to the underlying circular muscle (64).

Muscle cells with a number of ramifying branches are best known to occur in the terminal portions of some exocrine glands. Because of their direct association with the epithelial cells and their possible epithelial origin, they are called myoepithelial cells. Figure 6-15 shows the SEM image of the myoepithelial cells in the lactating mammary gland. The shape of the cells and the number and width of the branches varies considerably in different glands, possibly reflecting the different viscosity of the secretory products to be expelled from the terminal portion to the duct (65). Flattened smooth muscle cells are found in various organs. They are compressed against the surface of the organs to form thin layers. Flattened cells in the small mesenteric veins of the monkey are irregular and ribbonlike, with several processes ranging from 40 μm to 100 μm in length, the largest having a width of 8 μm. They are randomly oriented and overlap each other in a squamous fashion (66). The muscle cells in the muscular venules are also ribbonlike, but they are much more attenuated, being less than 5 μm wide and more than 100 μm long. They run parallel to each other and are oriented almost circularly. A number of thin projections arise from the lateral cell border to connect adjacent muscle cells (19). Flattened muscle cells also occur widely in the rat genital organs. In the epididymis and distal portion of the ductus deferens, they are either rectangular

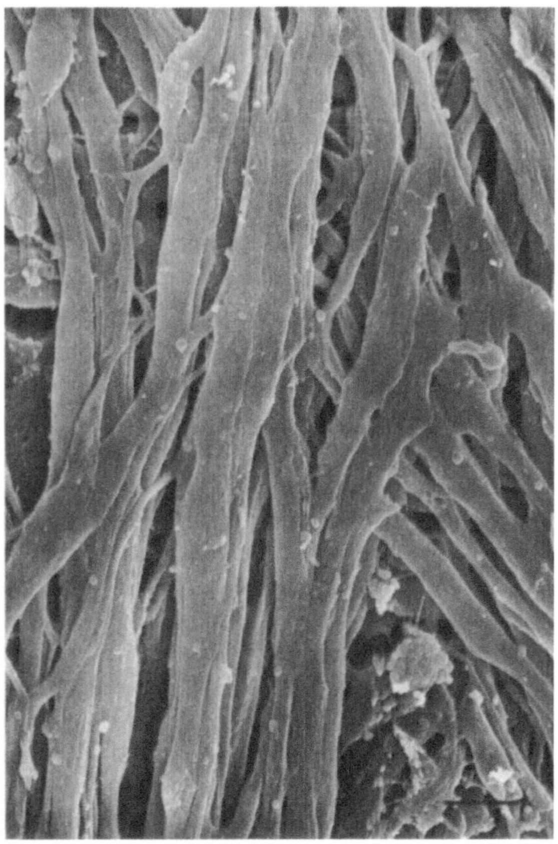

Figure 6-14. Branched muscle cells of the guinea pig epididymis. Adjacent cells contact and overlap each other in a end-to-side or side-to-side fashion. Bar: 5 μm.

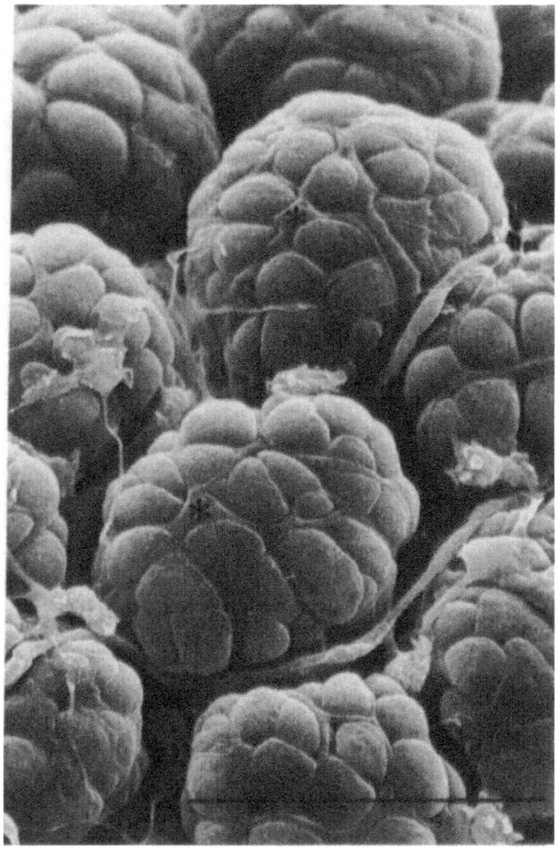

Figure 6-15. Stellate myoepithelial cells (asterisks) associated with terminal portions of the rat lactating mammary gland. Bar: 50 μm.

or thin and tapelike, about 10 μm wide and 60 μm to 100 μm long with occasional branches. Those in the ductulus efferentis are somewhat similarly shaped but much smaller in size, being less than 10 μm wide and 40 μm long (Fig. 6-16). SEM has demonstrated flattened smooth muscle cells around the seminiferous tubules of the monkey and rat. Their structure resembles a tile roof or stone pavement (67, 68). In ultrathin sections, the lamellar processes of these cells in the human seminiferous tubules are reported to be less than 0.5 μm in thickness (69). It is likely that the flattened muscle cells observed in the ductulus efferentis and epididymis are continuous with those of the seminiferous tubules. According to Suvanto and Kormano (70), the muscle contraction of the rat seminiferous tubule gives rise to a local indentation rather than to circular peristaltic waves.

5.2. Fiber endings and interrelationships

Smooth muscle fiber ends attach to collagenous fibrils via the basal lamina and microfibrils to form an anchoring device that transmits the force generated within the cell to the connective tissue framework of the muscles. When examined with SEM, fusiform and branched muscle fibers usually terminate with simply tapered, or occasionally bifurcated, fiber ends, which are tightly associated with the neighboring fiber in an end-to-side fashion (Fig. 6-17). Highly elaborate fiber ends are found in the central tendinous portion of the finch gizzard (Fig. 6-18). They are either conical or obtuse, possessing a number of longitudinal fingerlike projections 0.5 μm to 1.0 μm thick and 1.0 μm to 10.0 μm long with fingerlike or slitlike invaginations. This feature closely resemble the skeletal muscle fiber ends observed with SEM (71). Sectional profiles of this sort of elaborate

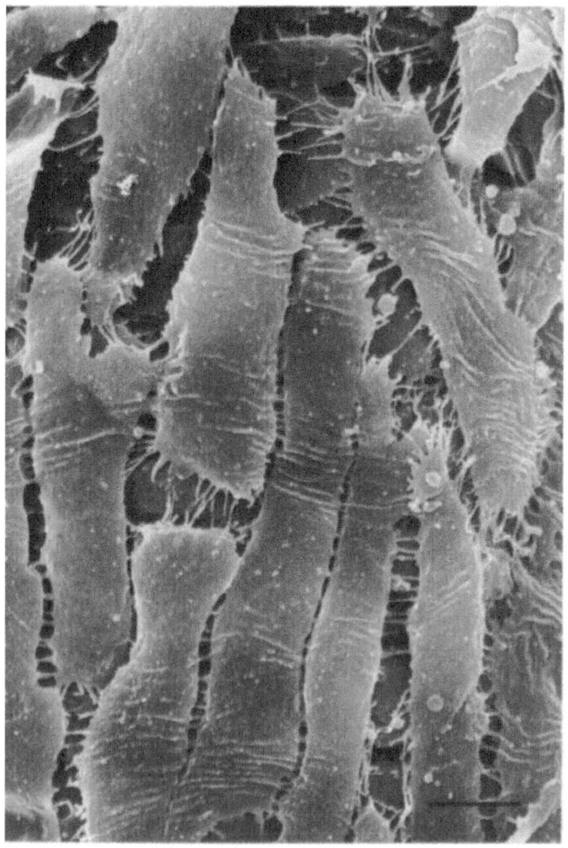

Figure 6-16. Rectangular muscle cells in the rat ductulus efferentis with numerous thin lateral projections bridging adjacent cells. There are faint folds on the cell membrane that suggest that the cells are under slight contraction. Bar: 5 μm.

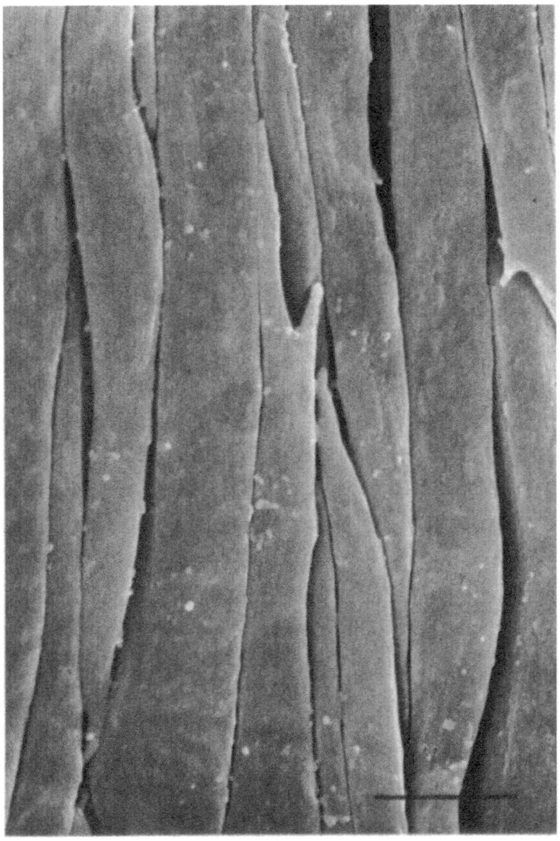

Figure 6-17. Smooth muscle fiber ends shown in the finch gizzard. At the junction between smooth muscle and submucosal and subserosal connective tissue, the muscle fiber ends exhibit elaborate structural specialization with a number of fingerlike projections and invaginations. This feature resembles the skeletal muscle fiber ends at myotendinous junctions. Bar: 5 μm.

cell ends have been demonstrated in the guinea pig ureter, ductus deferens (13, 72), taenia coli (73), and also the rabbit portal vein (74).

Various types of intercellular junctions have been described in smooth muscles. They are interdigitations with fingerlike projections, nexuses or gap junctions, intermediate junctions (see reviews by Henderson (75), Uehara et al. (72), and Gabella (2)). Side-by-side connections with interdigitations are evidenced with SEM in such organs as the guinea pig ureter (Fig. 6-13) and epididymis (Fig. 6-14), where muscle fibers are irregularly arranged with respect to each other. Gap junctions and intermediate junctions cannot be properly identified in our SEM preparations. As we have reported previously, adjacent muscle fibers are interconnected either by cylindrical, spiny, or squamous lateral projections in the monkey mesenteric vein (66), in arterioles and venules in the mammary gland (19), and in the guinea pig ureter (51). In these organs, cylindrical projections 0.1 μm to 0.5 μm in diameter are frequently encountered (Fig. 6-19). In the ureter, muscle fibers are known to be organized into effector bundles with highly developed intercellular couplings. The cylindrical projections are comparable in overall diameter to gap junctions as viewed in freeze-fracture preparations (2). It is therefore likely that the junctions with cylindrical projections represent gap junctions. If this is indeed the case, the SEM method will be helpful for a morphometrical analysis of the distribution of gap junctions in various smooth muscles.

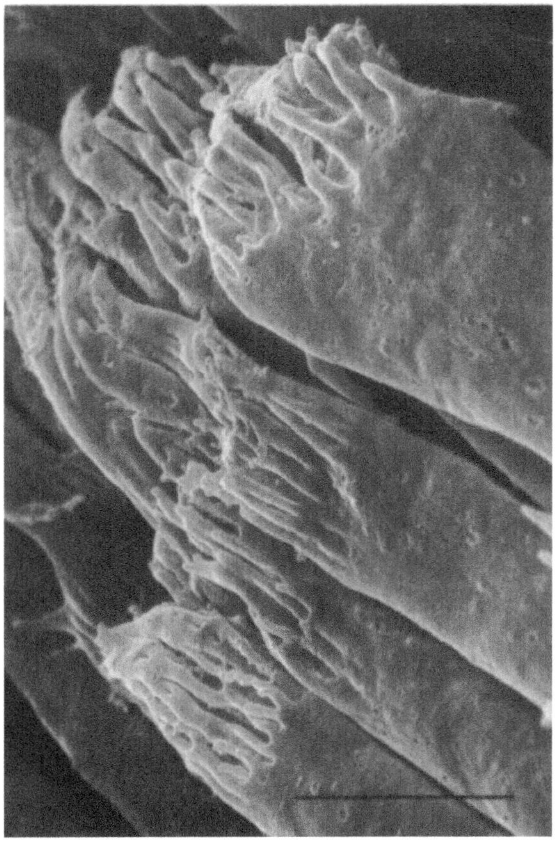

Figure 6-18. Smooth muscle fiber ends, shown within a parallel muscle bundle of the finch gizzard. The fiber ends often bifurcate and are simply tapered to contact the adjacent cells. Bar: 5 μm.

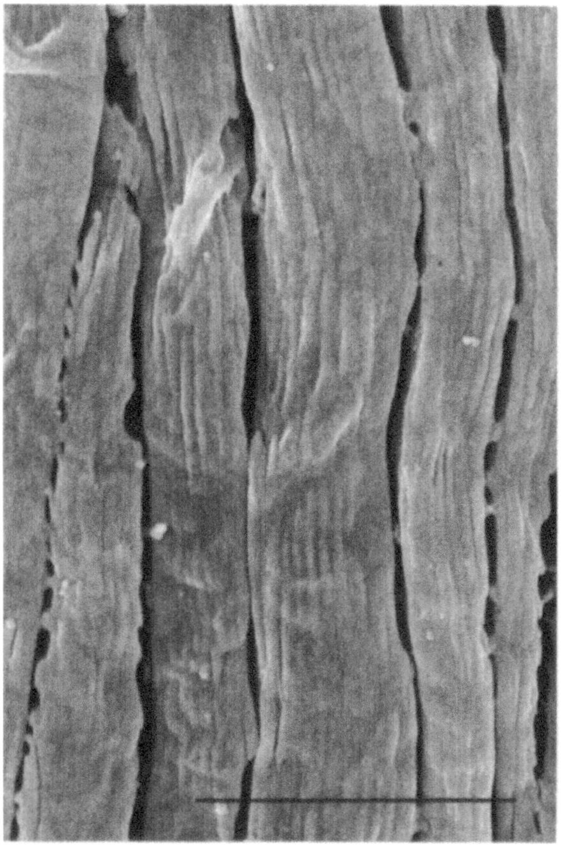

Figure 6-19. Smooth muscle fibers of the small mesenteric artery of the rat. A number of small cylindrical projections (0.1 to 0.5 μm in diameter) bridge adjacent fibers, which may represent gap junctions. Fine longitudinal striations seen on the cell surface correspond to the dense areas of attachment sites of actin filaments. Bar: 5 μm.

5.3. Surface topography

When examined with SEM, the surface of smooth muscle cells is usually smooth in distended organs. Surface caveolae that decorate the cell membrane cannot be detected, due to the insufficient resolving power of our scanning electron microscope. In some preparations, fine parallel striations occur along the longitudinal cell axis (Fig. 6-19), which may correspond to the attachment sites of actin filaments, known as dense bands. Their longitudinal orientation with alternative areas of surface caveolae has been demonstrated (2).

Some smooth muscle cells in the pelvic portion of the guinea pig ureter are characterized by a highly rugged surface with many projections and depressions (Fig. 6-20; see also 51); the feature entirely differs from that of contracted muscle cells. They may represent pacemaker cells that were identified as such by Gosling and Dixon (76, 77) in the renal part of the pelvis and in the pelviureteric junction in the rat and guinea pig (see also chapter 8 in this volume). The pacemaker cells were specialized in that they had extremely irregular outlines with numerous outpouchings of their cell membrane. Nakamura and Yamamoto (45), with the SEM procedure, reported the presence of large sarcoplasmic invaginations on the surface of smooth muscle cells of the rat thoracic duct. The invaginations were 200 nm to 500 nm wide and 150 nm to 200 nm deep, arranged in regular rows disposed parallel to the longitudinal cell axis. The authors suggested that such invagination may enlarge the surface area of the muscle cells.

The muscle cells in distended arteries often

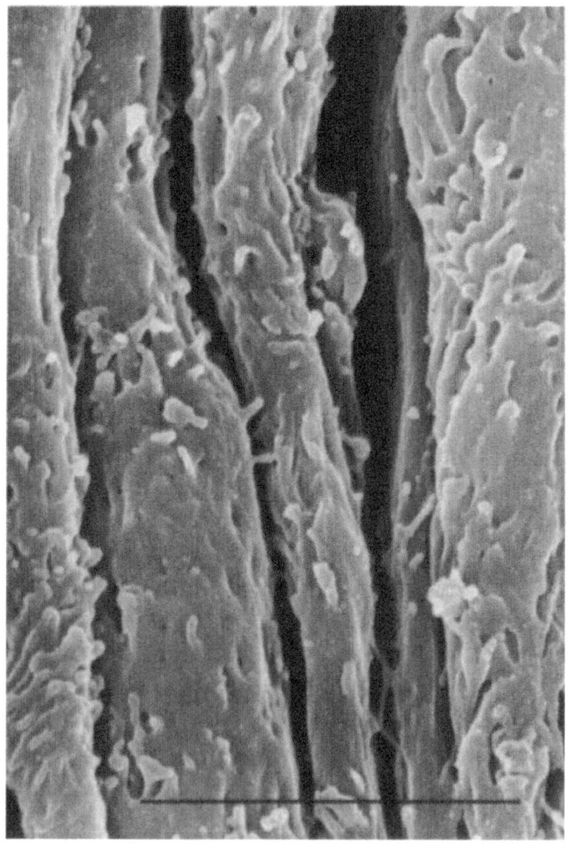

Figure 6-20. A unique surface texture of smooth muscle fibers found in the pelvic portion of the guinea pig ureter, which is characterized by a number of projections and indentations. Bar: 5 μm.

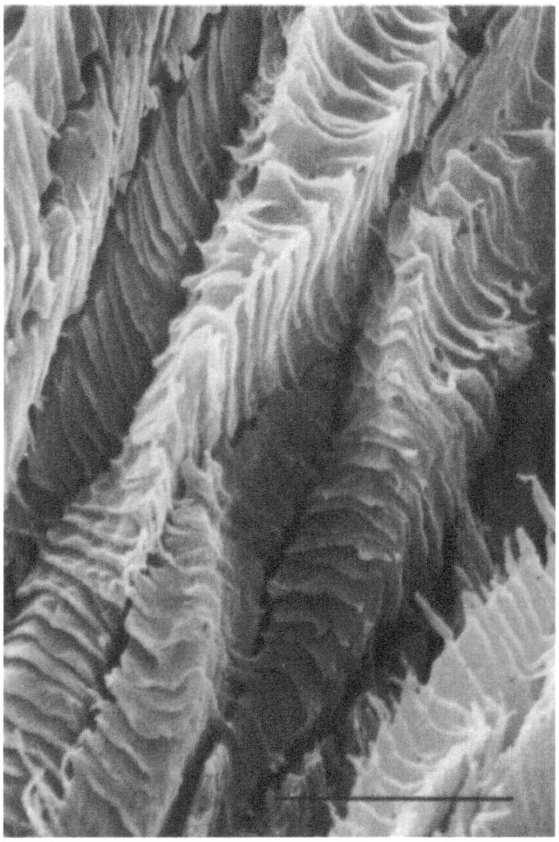

Figure 6-21. Contracted smooth muscle cells in the chicken gizzard give rise to numerous transverse lamellar folds on the cell surface. Bar: 5 μm. (Courtesy of Dr. S. Matsuda.)

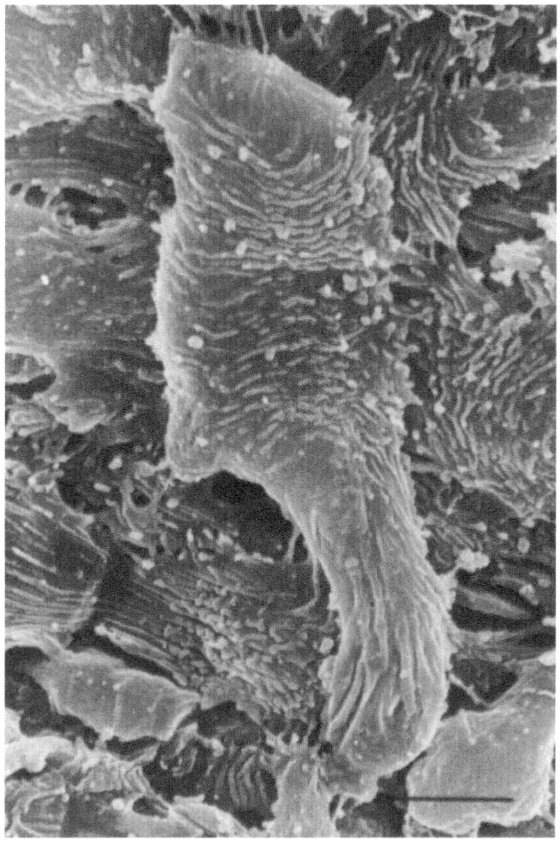

Figure 6-22. Contracted flattened muscle cells in the rat ductulus efferentis have many lamellar folds and short ridges that vary in their arrangement in the same cell. Bar: 5 μm.

have nodular projections on their adventitial surface (37). These protrusions may represent the attachment sites of the muscle cell membranes to elastic components as shown with TEM (2).

The surface texture undergoes drastic changes during shortening; the cell membrane is thrown into myriads of folds and processes (78–80). Similar changes have been demonstrated with SEM in the mesenteric arteries of the monkey, where the muscle cells give rise to numerous transverse ridges and bulbous protrusions during chemically and mechanically induced vasoconstriction (43). Smooth muscle cells of the chicken gizzard that have been fixed in slices immediately after excision so as to produce contraction exhibit prominent transverse or diagonal folds (Fig. 6-21). In some sites, folds of adjacent cells are interdigitated; this feature has been recognized with TEM (80). Similar but less prominent folds also occasionally occur on the surface of flattened muscle cells in the rat ductulus efferentis (Fig. 6-22). Folds are arranged longitudinally or transversely in different areas of the same cell. The arrangement of folds is related to the attachment of myofilaments to the cell membrane and also possibly to connections between the cell membrane and collagen fibrils (2).

References

1. Burnstock G: Structure of smooth muscle and its innervation. In: Smooth Muscle. E Bülbring, AF Brading, AW Jones, T Tomita (eds), London: Edward Arnold, p 1–70, 1970.
2. Gabella G: Structure of smooth muscle. In: Smooth Muscle: An Assessment of Current Knowledge. E Bülbring, AF Brading, AW Jones, T Tomita (eds), London: Edward Arnold, p 1–46, 1981.
3. Gabella G: An introduction to the structural variety of smooth muscles. In: Vascular Neuroeffector Mech-

anisms: 4th International Symposium. JA Bevan et al. (eds), New York: Raven Press, p 13–35, 1983.
4. Brading AF: Ionic distribution and mechanisms of transmembrane ion movements in smooth muscle. In: Smooth Muscle: An Assessment of Current Knowledge. E Bülbring, AF Brading, AW Jones, T Tomita (eds), London: Edward Arnold, p 65–92, 1981.
5. Casteels R: Membrane potential in smooth muscle cells. In: Smooth Muscle: An Assessment of Current Knowledge. E Bülbring, AF Brading, AW Jones, T Tomita (eds), London: Edward Arnold, p 105–126, 1981.
6. Kuriyama H: Excitation–contraction coupling in various visceral smooth muscles. In: Smooth Muscle: An Assessment of Current Knowledge. E Bülbring, AF Brading, AW Jones, T Tomita (eds), London: Edward Arnold, p 171–198, 1981.
7. Tomita T: Electrical activity (spikes and slow waves) in gastro intestinal smooth muscles. In: Smooth Muscle: An Assessment of Current Knowledge. E Bülbring, AF Brading, AW Jones, T Tomita (eds), London: Edward Arnold, p 171–198, 1981.
8. Creed KE: Functional diversity of smooth muscle. *Br Med Bull* 35: 243–247, 1979.
9. Gabella G: Quantitative morphological study of smooth muscle cells in the guinea-pig taenia coli. *Cell Tissue Res* 170: 161–186, 1976.
10. Gabella G: On the musculture of the gastro-intestinal tract of the guinea-pig. *Anat Embryol* 163: 135–156, 1981.
11. Taxi J: Contribution a l'etude des connexions des neurones moteurs du systeme nerveux autonome. *Ann Sci Nat (Zool)* 7: 413–674, 1965.
12. Bennett MR, Rogers DC: A study of the innervation of the taenia coli. *J Cell Biol* 33: 573–596, 1967.
13. Merrillees NCR: The nervous environment of individual smooth muscle cells of the guinea-pig vas deferens. *J Cell Biol* 37: 794–817, 1968.
14. Rhodin JAG: The ultrastructure of mammalian arterioles and precapillary sphincters. *J Ultrastruct Res* 18: 181–223, 1967.
15. Komuro T, Desaki J, Uehara Y: Three-dimensional organization of smooth muscle cells in blood vessels of laboratory rodents. *Cell Tissue Res* 227: 429–437, 1982.
16. Evan AP, Dail WG, Dammrose D, Palmer C: Scanning electron microscopy of cell surfaces following removal of extracellular material. *Anat Rec* 185: 433–446, 1976.
17. Uehara Y, Suyama K: Visualization of the adventitial aspect of the vascular smooth muscle cells under the scanning electron microscope. *J Electron Microsc* 27: 157–159, 1978.
18. Fujiwara T, Uehara Y: Scanning electron microscopy of myenteric plexus: A preliminary communication. *J Electron Microsc* 29: 397–400, 1980.
19. Fujiwara T, Uehara Y: The cytoarchitecture of the wall and the innervation pattern of the microvessels in the rat mammary gland: A scanning electron microscopic observation. *Am J Anat* 170: 39–54, 1984.
20. Tachibana S, Takeuchi M, Fujiwara T: Visualization of autonomic varicose terminal axons by scanning electron microscopy. *J Electron Microsc* 34: 136–138, 1985.
21. Komuro T: Three-dimensional visualization of the intraganglionic structures of the rat myenteric plexus: scanning electron microscopy with the connective tissue digestion method. *Neurosci Lett* 72: 49–53, 1986.
22. Komuro T: Three-dimensional observation of the fibroblast-like cells associated with the rat myenteric plexus, with special reference to the interstitial cells of Cajal. *Cell Tissue Res*, 255: 343–351, 1989.
23. Romeis B: Mikroskopische Technik. München: Oldenburg, 1968.
24. Kölliker VA: Beiträge zur Kenntnis der glatten Muskeln. *Z wiss Zoll* 1: 48–87, 1849.
25. McGill C: The structure of smooth muscle in the resting and in the contracted condition. *Am J Anat* 9: 493–545, 1909.
26. Strong KC: A study of the structure of the media of the distributing arteries by the method of microdissection. *Anat Rec* 72: 151–168, 1938.
27. Prosser CL, Burnstock G, Kahn J: Conduction in smooth muscle: Comparative structural properties. *Am J Physiol* 199: 545–552, 1960.
28. Cooke PH, Fay FS: Correlation between fiber length, ultrastructure, and the length–tension relationship of mammalian smooth muscle. *J Cell Biol* 52: 105–116, 1972.
29. Uvelius B: Isometric and isotonic length–tension relations and variations in cell length in longitudinal smooth muscle from rabbit urinary bladder. *Acta Physiol Scand* 97: 1–12, 1976.
30. Driska SP, Murphy RA: Estimate of cellular force generation in an arterial smooth muscle with a high actin: myosin ratio. *Blood Vessels* 15: 26–32, 1978.
31. Boyde A, Williams JC: Surface morphology of frog striated muscle as prepared for and examined in the scanning electron microscope. *J Physiol (London)* 197: 10P–11P, 1968.
32. Finlay JB, Hunter JA, Steven FS: Preparation for human skin for high-resolution scanning electron microscopy using phosphate buffered crude bacterial alpha-amylase. *J Microsc* 93: 73–76, 1971.
33. Papa CM, Farber B: Direct scanning electron microscopy of human skin. *Arch Dermatol* 104: 262–270, 1971.
34. Sommerlad BC, Creasey JM: A technique for preparing human dermal and scar specimens for scanning electron microscopy. *J Microsc* 103: 369–376, 1975.
35. Sawada H: Scanning electron microscopy of guinea pig taenia coli. *Biomed Res* 2 (Suppl): 153–158, 1981.
36. Miller BG, Woods RI, Bohlen HG, Evan AP: A new morphological procedure for viewing microvessels: A scanning electron microscopic study of the vasculature of small intestine. *Anat Rec* 203: 493–503, 1982.
37. Fujiwara T, Uehara Y: Scanning electron microscopical study of vascular smooth muscle cells in the mesenteric vessels of the monkey: Arterial smooth muscle cells. *Biomed Res* 3: 649–658, 1982.
38. Staubesand J: Anatomie der Blutgefässe. I. Funktionelle Morphologie der Arterien, venen und arterio-venösen Anastomosen. In: Angiologie. M Ratchow (ed), Stuttgart., p 23–82, 1959.
39. Halpern W, Mulvany MJ, Warshaw DM: Mechanical

properties of smooth muscle cells in the walls of arterial resistance vessels. *J Physiol* 275: 85–101, 1978.
40. Fischer H: Über die funktionelle Bedeutung des Spiralverlaufes der Muskulatur in der Arterienwand. *Gegenbaurs Morphol Jahrbuch* 91: 394–445, 1951.
41. von Hayek H: Uber die Kontraktionsfahigkeit der kleinsten Lungenarterien. *Z Anat Entwickl Gesch* 116: 373–376, 1952.
42. Lang J: Mikroskopische Anatomie der Arterien. *Angiologica* 2: 225–284, 1965.
43. Uehara Y, Fujiwara T: The morphological changes of arterial smooth muscle cells upon vasodilation and vasoconstriction. In: Progress in Microcirculation Research II. FC Courtice, DG Garlick, MA Perry (eds), Kensington: CPME, The University of New South Wales, p 405–410, 1984.
44. Baluk P, Fujiwara T, Matsuda S: The fine structure of the ganglia of the guinea-pig trachea. *Cell Tissue Res* 239: 51–60, 1985.
45. Nakamura K, Yamamoto T: Morphology of smooth muscle cells in the rat thoracic duct. A scanning and transmission electron-microscope study. *Cell Tissue Res* 251: 243–248, 1988.
46. David A, Czernobilsky B: A comparative histologic study of the uterotubal junction in the rabbit, rhesus monkey, and human female. *Am J Obstet Gynecol* 101: 417, 1968.
47. Woodruff JD, Pauerstein CJ: The Fallopian Tube. Baltimore: Williams & Wilkins, 1969.
48. Pauerstein CJ, Alexander FRW, Mobley JA, Fremming BD: Comparative anatomy of the inner longitudinal muscle layer of the oviductal isthmus. *Obstet Gynecol* 35: 504–512, 1970.
49. Hodges RD: The Histology of the Fowl. London: Academic Press, 1974.
50. Arjamaa O, Talo A: Description of the structural control systems of ovum transport in the quail oviduct. *Acta Physiol Scand* 117: 405–410, 1983.
51. Tachibana S, Takeuchi M, Uehara Y: The architecture of the musculature of the guinea-pig ureter as examined by scanning electron microscopy. *J Urol* 134: 582–586, 1985.
52. Murnaghan GF: Mechanisms of congenital hydronephrosis with reference to factors influencing surgical treatment. *Ann Roy Coll Surg Engl* 23: 25, 1958.
53. Tanagho EA: Ureteral embryology, developmental anatomy, and myology. In: Urodynamics: Hydrodynamics of the Ureter and Renal Pelvis. S Boyarski, GW Gottshalk, EA Tanagho, PD Zimskind (eds), New York: Academic Press, p 3–27, 1971.
54. Tanagho EA, Miller ER: Abnormal voiding and urinary tract infection. *Urol Nephrol* 4: 165–173, 1972.
55. Cai C, Gabella G: The musculature of the gall bladder and biliary pathways in the guinea pig. *J Anat* 136: 237–250, 1983.
56. MacPherson BR, Yiu V, Lee W, Scott GW: A scanning electron-microscopic study of the muscle layer of the canine gallbladder. *Acta Anat* 127: 59–64, 1986.
57. Uvelius B, Gabella G: Relation between cell length and force production in urinary bladder smooth muscle. *Acta Physiol Scand* 110: 357–365, 1980.
58. Holstein AF: Muskulatur und Motilität des Nebenhodens beim Kaninchen. *Z Zellforsch* 76: 498–510, 1967.
59. Baumgarten HG, Holstein AF, Rosengren E: Arrangement ultrastructure, and adrenergic innervation of smooth musculature of the ductuli efferentes, ductus epididymidis and ductus deferens of man.*Z Zellforsch* 120: 37–79, 1971.
60. Burnstock G, Prosser CL: Conduction in smooth muscles: comparative electrical properties. *Am J Physiol* 199: 553–559, 1960.
61. Nagai T, Prosser CL: Pattern of conduction in smooth muscle. *Am J Physiol* 204: 910–914, 1963.
62. Tomita T: Electrical responses of smooth muscle to external stimulation in hypertonic solution. *J Physiol* 183: 450–468, 1966.
63. Bennett MR: Autonomic neuromuscular transmission. In: Monographs of the Physiological Society, No. 30, Cambridge, 1972.
64. Shiraishi T, Sakaki S, Uehara Y: Architecture of the media of the arterial vessels in the dog brain: A scanning electron-microscopic study. *Cell Tissue Res* 243: 329–335, 1986.
65. Nagato T, Yoshida H, Yoshida A, Uehara Y: A scanning electron microscope study of myoepithelial cells in exocrine glands. *Cell Tissue Res* 209: 1–10, 1980.
66. Fujiwara T, Ikeuchi M, Uehara Y: Scanning electron microscope study of smooth muscle cells in the mesenteric veins of the monkey. *Biomed Res* 4: 225–230, 1983.
67. Hamasaki M, Murakami M: SEM observation of the contractile cells of Japanese monkey seminiferous tubules treated with HCl-collagenase. *J Electron Microsc* 28: 154–158, 1979.
68. Murakami M, Hamasaki M, Okita S, Abe J: SEM surface morphology of the contractile cells in the rat seminiferous tubules. Experientia 35: 1099–1101, 1979.
69. Böck P, Breitenecker G, Lunglmayr G: Peroxysomen im Ovar der Maus. *Z Zellforsch Mikrosk Anat* 133: 519–527, 1972.
70. Suvanto O, Kormano M: The relation between in vitro contractions of the rat seminiferous tubules and the cyclic stage of the seminiferous epithelium. *J Reprod Fertil* 21: 227–232, 1970.
71. Ishikawa H, Sawada H, Yamada E: Surface and internal morphology of skeletal muscle. In: Handbook of Physiology, Section 10, Skeletal Muscle. LD Peachey, RH Adrian, SR Geiger (eds), Bethesda, MD: American Physiological Society, p 1–21, 1983.
72. Uehara Y, Campbell GR, Burnstock G: Muscle and its Innervation: An Atlas of Fine Structure. London: Edward Arnold, 1976.
73. Gabella G: Arrangement of smooth muscle cells and intramuscular septa in the taenia coli. *Cell Tissue Res* 184: 195–212, 1977.
74. Komuro T, Burnstock G: The fine structure of smooth muscle cells and their relationship to connective tissue in the rabbit portal vein. *Cell Tissue Res* 210: 257–267, 1980.
75. Henderson RM: Cell-to-cell contacts. In: Methods in Pharmacology, Vol 3, Smooth Muscle. EE Daniel, DM Paton (eds), New York: Plenum Press, p 47–77, 1975.
76. Gosling JA, Dixon JS: Structural evidence in support of an urinary tract pacemaker. *Br J Urol* 44: 550–560, 1972.

77. Gosling JA, Dixon JS: Species variation in the location of upper urinary tract pacemaker cells. *Invest Urol* 11: 418–423, 1974.
78. Richardson KC: The fine structure of autonomic nerve endings in smooth muscle with special reference to the vas deferens. *Acta Neuroveg (Wien)* 26: 373–376, 1964.
79. Lane BP: Alterations in the cytologic detail of intestinal smooth muscle cells in various stages of contraction. J Cell Biol 27: 199–213, 1965.
80. Gabella G: Structural changes in smooth muscle cells during isotonic contraction. *Cell Tissue Res* 170: 187–201, 1976.
81. Todd ME, Laye CG, Osborne DN: The dimensional characteristics of smooth muscle in rat vessels. *Circ Res* 53: 319–331, 1983.
82. Mulvany MJ, Halpern W: Mechanical properties of vascular smooth muscle cells in situ. *Nature* 260: 617–619, 1976.
83. Rhodin JAG: Fine structure of vascular walls in mammals. *Physiol Rev* 42 (Suppl) 5: 48–81, 1962.
84. Hua C, Cragg B: Measurements of smooth muscle cells in arterioles of guinea-pig ileum. *Acta Anat* 107: 224–230, 1980.

Author's address:
Prof. Yasuo Uehara
Department of Anatomy
Ehime University
School of Medicine
Shigenobu
Ehime 791–02
Japan

CHAPTER 7

Smooth muscle in the gut and airways

GIORGIO GABELLA

1. Architecture of the intestinal musculature

The main muscle component of the gastrointestinal tract of vertebrates is a layer of smooth muscle known as the muscularis externa or muscle coat (Fig. 7-1). Additional musculature is found in the muscularis mucosae, in the core of intestinal villi, in the media of blood vessels, and as individual muscle cells in the core of villi. The muscle coat varies greatly in thickness in different regions of the gut and in different animal species. In the ileum of man it measures, at rest, over one millimeter, while in a mouse it is less than 50 micrometers. In a given animal, the thickness of the muscle coat in the jejunum and ileum is uniform around the circumference and along the length of the organ. In the initial part of the duodenum, the muscle is almost twice as thick as in the rest of the small intestine. In the large intestine the musculature is more abundant than in the small intestine. In any part of the gut, upon full contraction the thickness of the muscle coat can treble. The muscle coat is made of a longitudinal (outer) layer and a circular (inner) layer (see the next paragraph for a few exceptions). In each layer the muscle cells are oriented parallel to one another, and in the two layers they run orthogonal to each other. The two layers have well-defined boundaries and are distinct and separate, although it is common to find bundles of musculature that turn around and pass from one layer to the other (Fig.7-2). In both layers all muscle cells lie parallel to the plane of the serosa. Generally speaking, the arrangement of the musculature in the gut is more geometrical and more regular than in any other visceral muscle (Fig. 7-3).

The ratio in thickness or volume of circular to longitudinal musculature varies over a wide range. In both the large and small intestine of mammals the circular musculature predominates. A longitudinal muscle is virtually absent in some places, for example, over most parts of the stomach of amphibia and birds or in the intestine of reptiles such as the turtle. There are no examples of a clear predominance of the longitudinal musculature, except in the muscularis mucosae. In mammals, the longitudinal musculature of the caecum and parts of the proximal colon (depending on the species) are gathered into thick cords or taeniae that run uninterruptedly for many centimeters. Between the taeniae, the wall bulges out into regular pouchlike evaginations, or haustrations, where the longitudinal muscle is extremely thin and the muscle coat is made almost exclusively of circular muscle. Accordingly, the myenteric plexus of these regions lies very close to the serosa. In the mammalian stomach, the arrangement of the musculature is more complicated, and often additional layers or bundles of musculature are found. As in the intestine, however, the musculature forms discrete layers, quite regular in thickness and in the arrangement of muscle cells, and these run orthogonal to each other in adjacent layers. The overall thickness of the muscle exceeds that in the small intestine. In the esophagus, where the musculature is smooth only over part of the length (depending on the

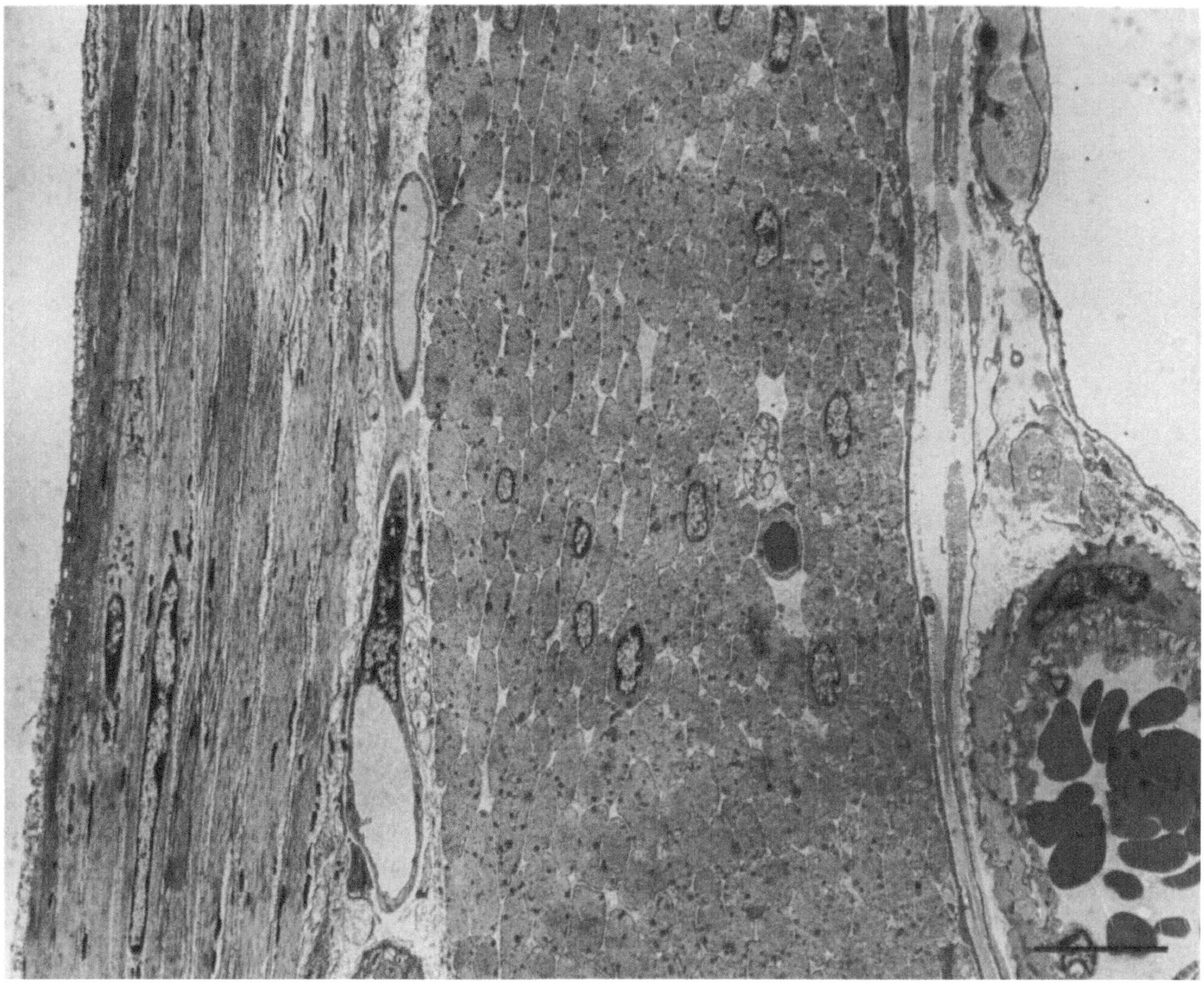

Figure 7-1. Transverse–longitudinal section of part of the wall of a guinea pig's small intestine as seen in the electron microscope. To the right is the submucosa with an arteriole (with a one-cell-thick media and containing red blood cells), a lymphatic vessel (empty-looking), and bundles of collagen fibrils. To the left is the serosa and the longitudinal muscle. The circular muscle is in transverse section; it shows a special layer of small and dark cells in its innermost part, and it is separated from the longitudinal muscle by blood capillaries and small nerve trunks. Calibration bar: 10 μm.

species), the boundary between smooth and striated musculature is blurred and the two types of muscle mix or lie side by side. Continuity between smooth and striate musculature is also found at the anal canal.

Within the muscle coats of the gut there are many vessels. In the regions adjacent to the insertion of the peritoneum, large blood vessels pierce the muscle coat very obliquely to reach the submucosa. Other blood vessels are not in transit but supply the muscle itself, the tissue generally being well vascularized; the oxygen consumption of the muscle is one fourth to one third that of the mucosa (1). Muscle contractions affect blood flow through the intestinal wall (2). The truly intramuscular blood vessels, as opposed to those running within septa, are mainly capillary, and these are nonfenestrated. Large lymphatic vessels pass through the muscularies externa to reach the subserosal space; before reaching the serosa they course for some distance between circular and longitudinal muscle (Figs. 7-3B, C). Within the muscularis externa, in the interstice between circular and longitudinal muscle layers, also lies

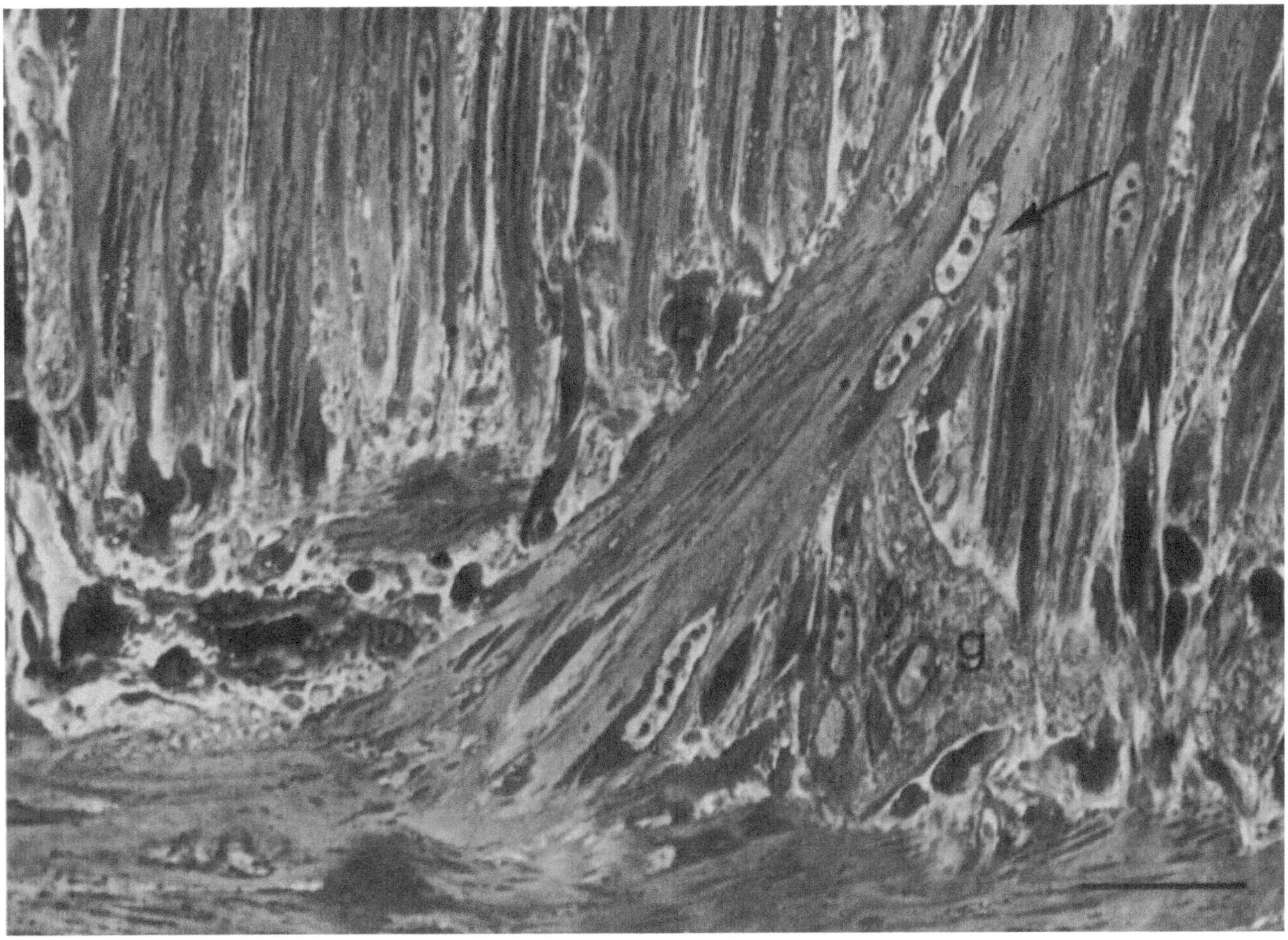

Figure 7-2. Muscle coat of the ileum of a mouse, in a section nearly parallel to the serosa. A bundle of muscle passes from the longitudinal layer (bottom) to the circular layer (top). The arrow points to a binucleate muscle cell. g: a ganglion of the myenteric plexus. Calibration bar: 2.5 μm.

the myenteric plexus, with its ganglia and connecting strands and several cells that accompany them; these include fibroblasts, macrophages, and interstitial cells (3, 4).

2. Special small and dark muscle cells

The innermost portion of the circular musculature, nearest to the submuscosa, is made of a thin layer of special muscle cells that differ in appearance from those of the bulk of the circular layer (5) (Fig. 7-3A). They are smaller in diameter (but approximately of the same length) and denser both in light and electron microscopy than the principal circular muscle cells. These special small and dark (s.a.d.) cells usually form a layer one or two cells thick that extends for the full length of the small intestine, but is not found in the large intestine or the stomach. This special muscle layer is found, with some modifications, in the small intestine of all vertebrates. In some species, such as the sheep, the special circular muscle spreads over intramuscular septa, and some of its bundles approach the longitudinal muscle layer; in other species it forms discrete bundles rather than a continuous layer. Because of their small size, these special muscle cells have a higher surface-to-volume ratio than ordinary visceral muscle cells. They are packed with thin filaments and a few organelles (mitochondria, caveolae). They are surrounded by connective tissue that is more abundant and qualitatively different from that in the rest of the circular layer;

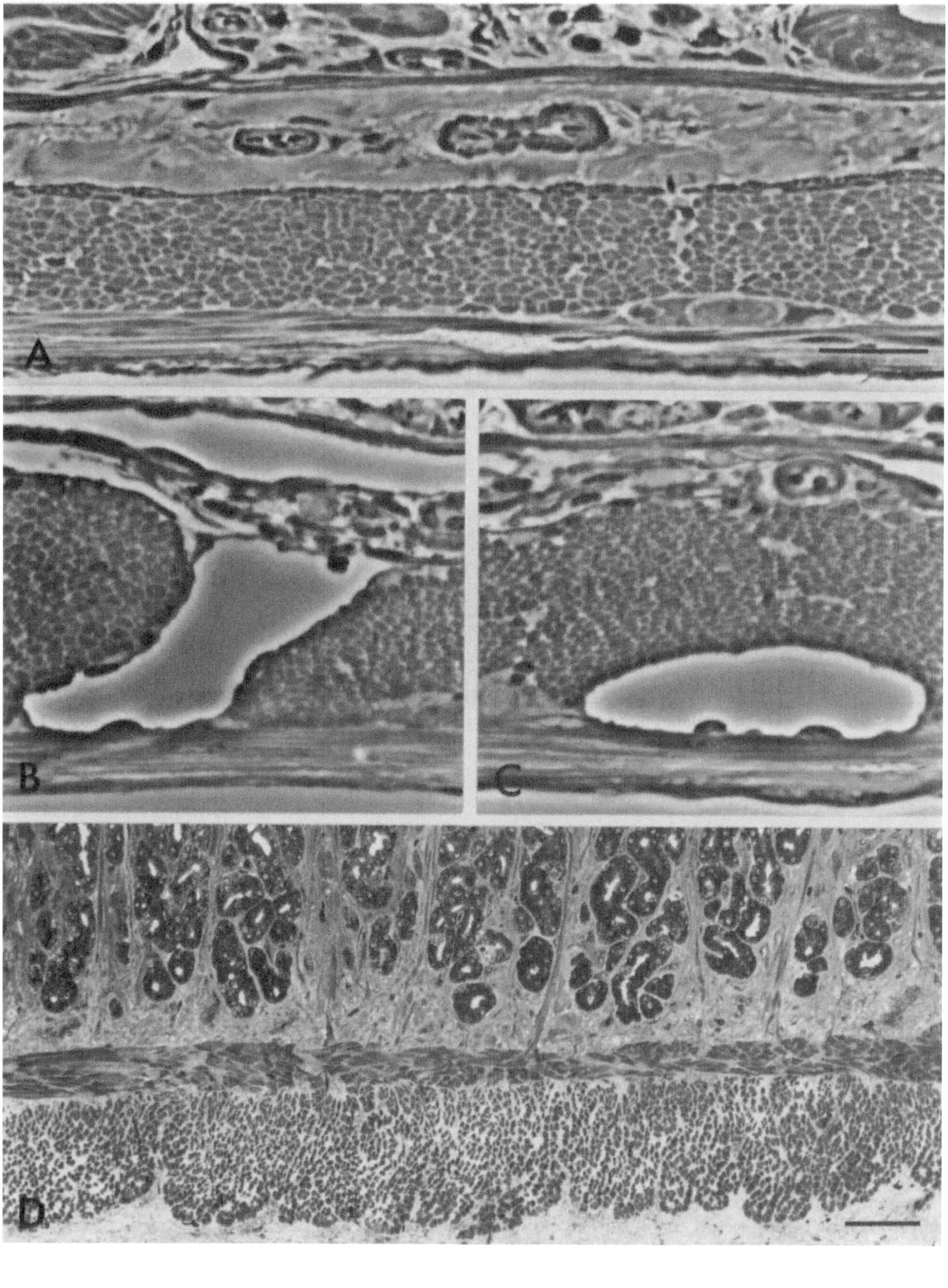
A
B
C
D

it contains many small elastic fibers and collagen fibrils of heterogeneous size. Between the layer of small and dark muscle cells and the bulk of the circular layer lie many interstitial cells and many nerve bundles. The great majority of intramuscular nerve fibers are concentrated in this particular region of the wall.

3. Muscularis mucosae

The muscularis mucosae forms the boundary between mucosa and submucosa and it is much thinner than the muscle coat (Fig. 7-3A). It is only 2–4 cells thick in the small intestine of a guinea pig, but about 100 micrometers in the ileum of a horse. A muscularis mucosae is absent over Peyer's patches and often shows other, smaller discontinuities; it is pierced by many lymph and blood vessels. It is formed by an outer component of longitudinally arranged muscle cells, and an inner component of circular cells; the latter is the thinner of the two and can be absent. The muscularis mucosae is thicker in the esophagus and in the terminal part of the large intestine than in the rest of the gut, and in these two sites it is made entirely of bundles of longitudinal musculature. In the stomach of amphibia, the muscularis mucosae is well developed and its cells are embedded in an abundant stroma (Fig. 7-3D, 7-4). Isolated muscle cells are found along the axis of intestinal villi. Special arrangements of the musculature exist at the junction between esophagus and stomach (cardia), between stomach and duodenum (pylorus), between bile duct and duodenum (ampulla), and between ileum and colon. Finally, there are some conspicuous cordlike smooth muscles anchoring the gut to the posterior abdominal wall near the midline (muscle suspensor duodeni, muscle anococcygeus, and recto coccygeus).

4. Stroma of intestinal muscles

Connective tissue is well in evidence in intestinal muscles in the form of septa separating groups or bundles of muscle cells. Septa, which are best recognized when the muscle is transversely sectioned, have an extent and distribution that vary characteristically in different muscles. The largest intramuscular septa of the mammalian intestine are radially arranged and are anchored to the collagen of the submucosa. Septa often occupy the full thickness of the muscle, but they extend only a short distance along the length of the muscle. Therefore, the bundles of musculature outlined by the septa are not consistent structures in that they merge which each other or split into two, and the lateral continuity of the musculature is not completely interrupted. Although when looking at a transverse section of a muscle one has a strong impression of the muscle being subdivided into discrete units, or bundles, this impression is not confirmed when the three-dimensional architecture of the muscle is examined and one sees the continuity of the muscle bundles with each other. In the gut of amphibia and reptiles, especially where the longitudinal musculature is absent, intramuscular septa in the circular layer often lie parallel to the serosal surface. An intriguing trellislike pattern of conspicuous intramuscular septa is found in the gizzard (muscular stomach) of birds (6).

The intramuscular septa are made of collagen, and they also contain fibroblasts and vessels, and a relatively small number of elastic fibers. The collagen merges without a clear boundary with the collagen fibrils around the individual muscle cells (Fig. 7-5). Each muscle cells is thus surrounded by a more or less abundant amount of collagen and this is linked with larger aggregates of fibrils as are found in the septa. This pattern is of paramount importance in the transmittal of

←

Figure 7-3. (A) Transverse–longitudinal section through part of the wall of a guinea pig's small intestine as seen in a phase contrast microscope. Calibration bar: 25 μm. (B) Similar preparation as in (A), showing a lymphatic vessel located between bundles of circular musculature. Another lymphatic vessels is visible in the submucosa. Magnification as in (A). (C) Similar preparation as in A, showing a lymphatic vessel located between circular and longitudinal muscle layers. Magnification as in A. (D) Transverse–circumferential section of part of the wall of a toad's stomach, showing a thick muscularis mucosae and glands of the mucosa. The muscularis mucosae in made of a thicker outer longitudinal layer (in transverse section) and a thinner inner circular layer; from the latter, small bundles of muscle cells penetrate between the glands. Calibration bar: 100 μm.

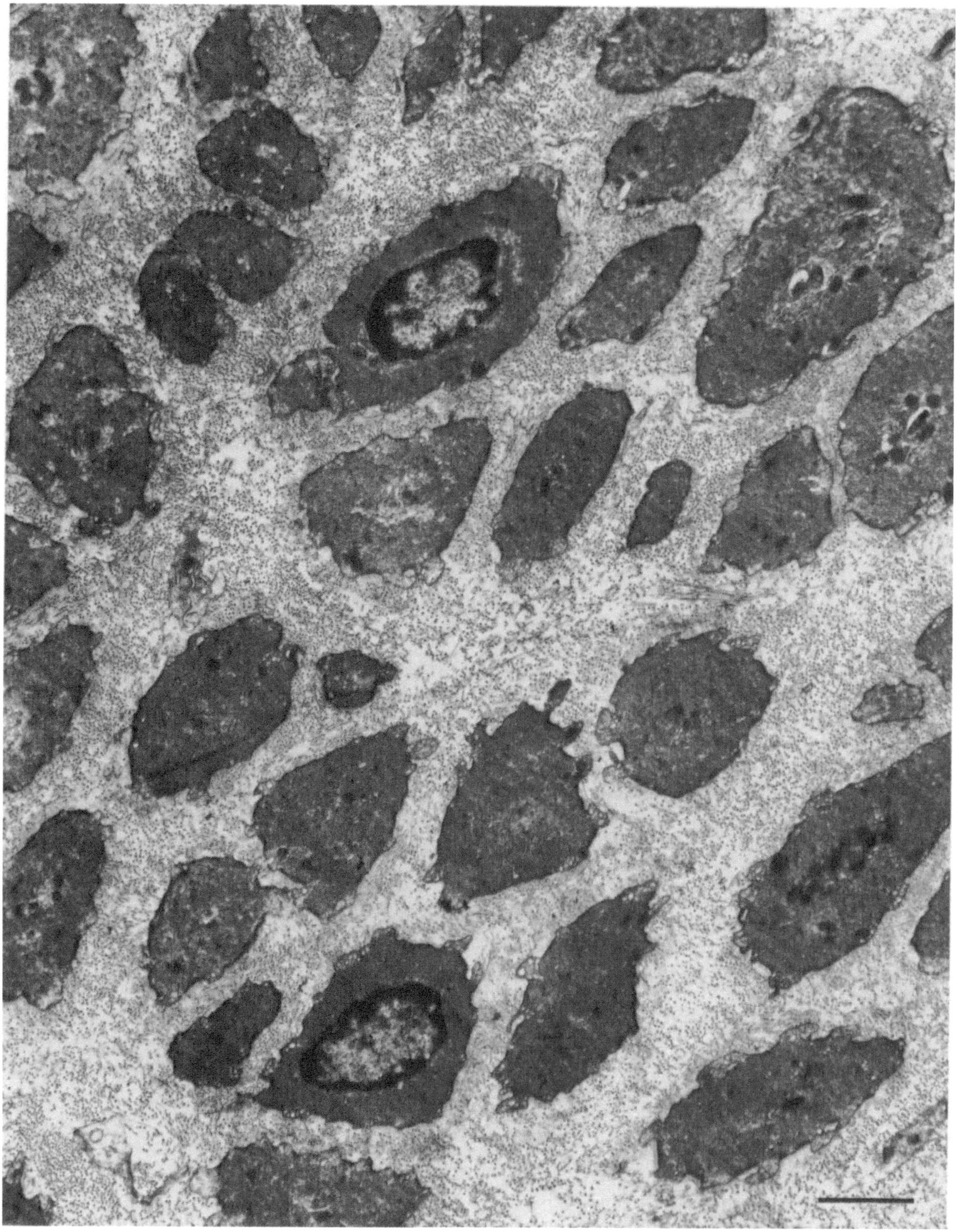

Figure 7-4. Electron micrograph of the muscularis mucosae of a bullfrog's stomach. The muscle cells are in transverse section and two of them show the nucleus. Note the large amount of connective tissue, and the considerable separation between the cells. Calibration bar: 2 μm.

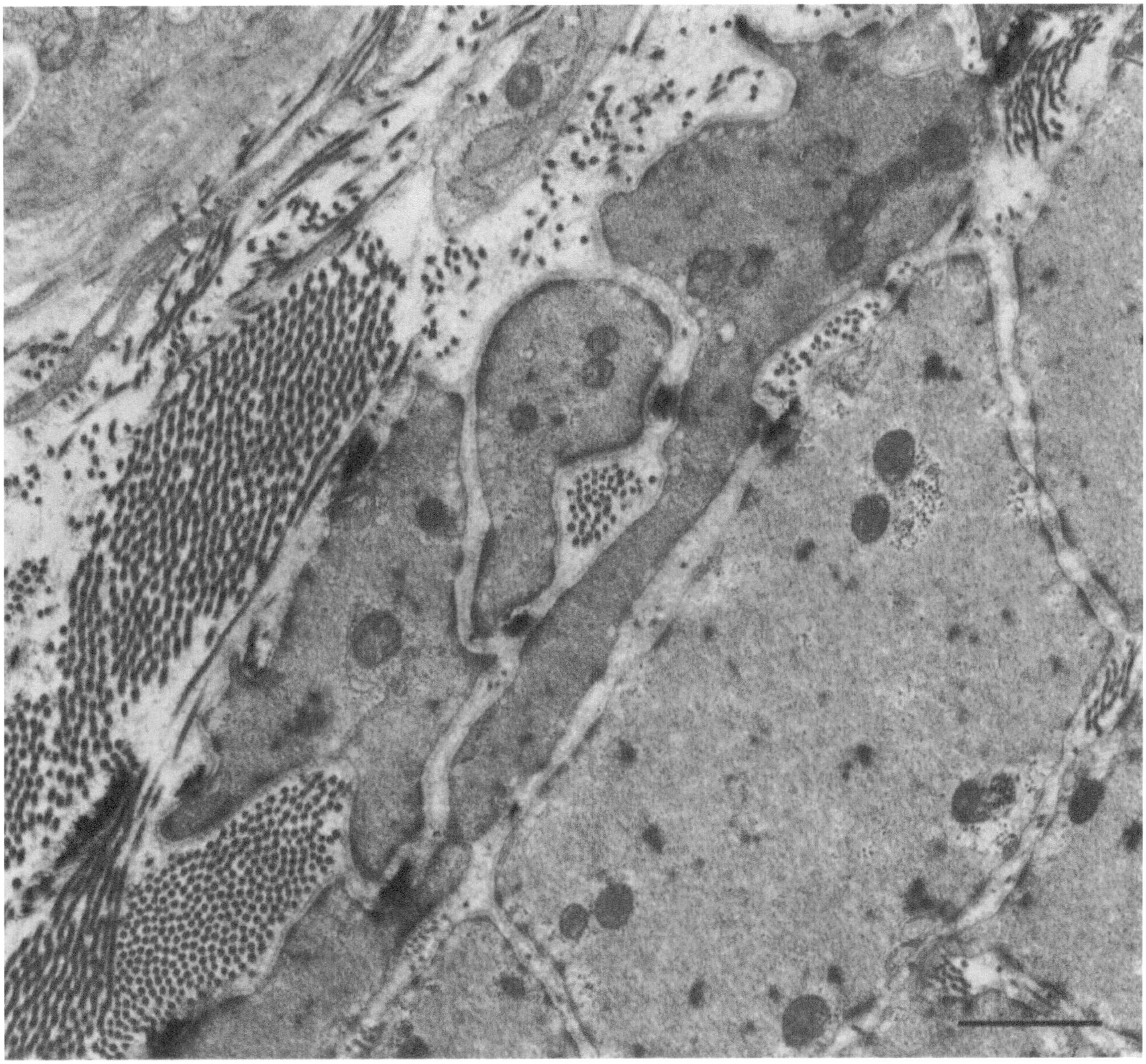

Figure 7-5. Innermost portion of the circular layer of the guinea pig ileum, showing ordinary muscle cells (bottom right) and a layer of small and dark special muscle cells. The latter are surrounded by abundant collagen fibrils and elastic fibers. At the top right is part of a ganglion of the submucosal plexus. Calibration bar: 1 μm.

force and shortening over the gut wall. The contraction of the individual muscle cells is transmitted from cell to cell over a short distance and is then discharged onto the pericellular collagen fibrils and then onto intramuscular septa. The septa in their turn are anchored to the submucosa where an elaborate apparatus of collagen fibers constitutes a kind of skeletal element of the gut wall, and onto it the contraction of the muscle cells is eventually discharged. Collagen is by far the largest component of the submucosa. The collagen fibrils are gathered into large fibers, a few microns in diameter, that form two parallel but intertwined systems. One runs as clockwise helices the other as anticlockwise helices, each set of helices being the mirror image of the other (7, 8). The helical pattern of the collagen fibers of the submucosa is not rigid but changes with the movement of the intestinal wall. Changes in length or diameter of the intestine are reflected in precise changes of the angle between the two sets of helices. The cross-ply arrangement of the collagen fibres of the submucosa allows the intestine to undergo reversible changes in length and diameter, and to maintain its structural integrity while offering a remarkable resistance to excessive distension.

5. Contraction of intestinal muscles

The structure of smooth muscles in contraction has been described in Chapter 1. Many of the studies discussed there were carried out on intestinal muscles. Isotonic contractions, by altering the shape and the dimensions of the muscle, bring about changes in the length or circumference of portions of the gut, and hence displacement of their contents. The change in the shape of a segment of intestine, for example in peristalsis, is ultimately due to an active change in shape of some of the constituent muscle cells. The chief mechanical effect of (smooth) muscle contraction can be described as the *shortening* of the muscle (*lengthwise pull*); equally correctly, however, the contraction could be regarded as the

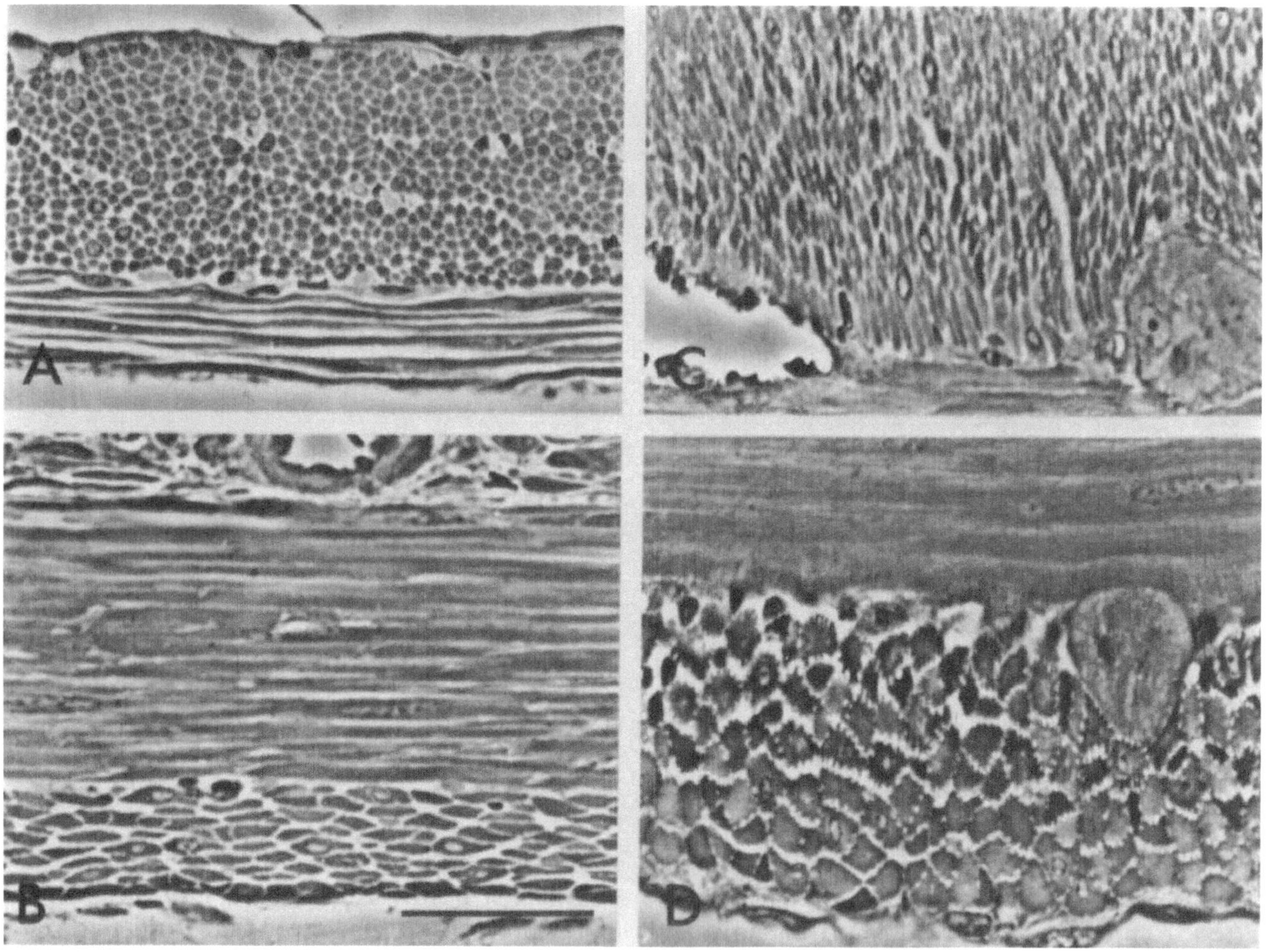

Figure 7-6. Guinea pig ileum. (A and B) The intestine is at rest and moderately distended by injection of fluid into the lumen. Muscle cells of the circular layer have approximately circular profiles (A), whereas muscle cells of the longitudinal layer have circumferentially flattened profiles (B). (C and D) An adjacent segment of the intestine was stimulated to contract with carbachol. Both muscle layers have thickened. Muscle cells of the longitudinal layer have profiles that are large, have a corrugated surface, and are roughly isodiametric (D), the characteristic appearance of isotonically contracted muscle cells. Cells of the circular layer in the same segment of intestine are not contracted, and their profiles are not circular but flattened radially (C), a passive change in shape due to contraction of the longitudinal muscle. Calibration bar: 100 μm. (From G Gabella: Handbook of Physiology, 1989, see note on page 150)

increase in girth of *fattening* of the muscle (*sideways push*). The sideways push is particularly extensive in smooth muscles and mechanically important in tubular organs with circular musculature, such as the gut. Contraction of the circular musculature of the small intestine, for example, shortens the muscle and reduces the circumference of that segment of gut; however, there is also a considerable lateral expansion of the muscle, and this produces an increase in *thickness* of the circular layer (hence a further reduction of the size of the lumen) and an increase in *width* of the muscle along the length of the intestine (hence an elongation of the intestine). The extent of this elongation of the intestine depends on the arrangement of the connective tissue septa and on whether or not there is a simultaneous contraction of the longitudinal musculature.

There is a complex mechanical interaction between longitudinal and circular muscle layers, and contraction in one layer induces passive changes in structure in the adjacent layer (Fig. 7-6). Moreover, muscle contraction compresses and alters the shape of intramural ganglia; intramuscular nerve bundles and capillaries acquire a wavy course.

6. Fine structure of muscle cells

The structural features of intestinal muscle cells are similar to those of other viscera and correspond to the description in Chapter 1. Within each layer the cells are rather uniform in appearance. The main features of the cell surface membrane are the rows of caveolae, which are regular and alternate with areas of the membrane bearing dense bands. Cell-to-cell junctions are common and can be grouped into three types (Fig. 7-7). The ability of the muscles to produce an effective contraction depends on the existence of junctions that allow the excitation, arising either from nerve or from pacemaker cells, to spread to all

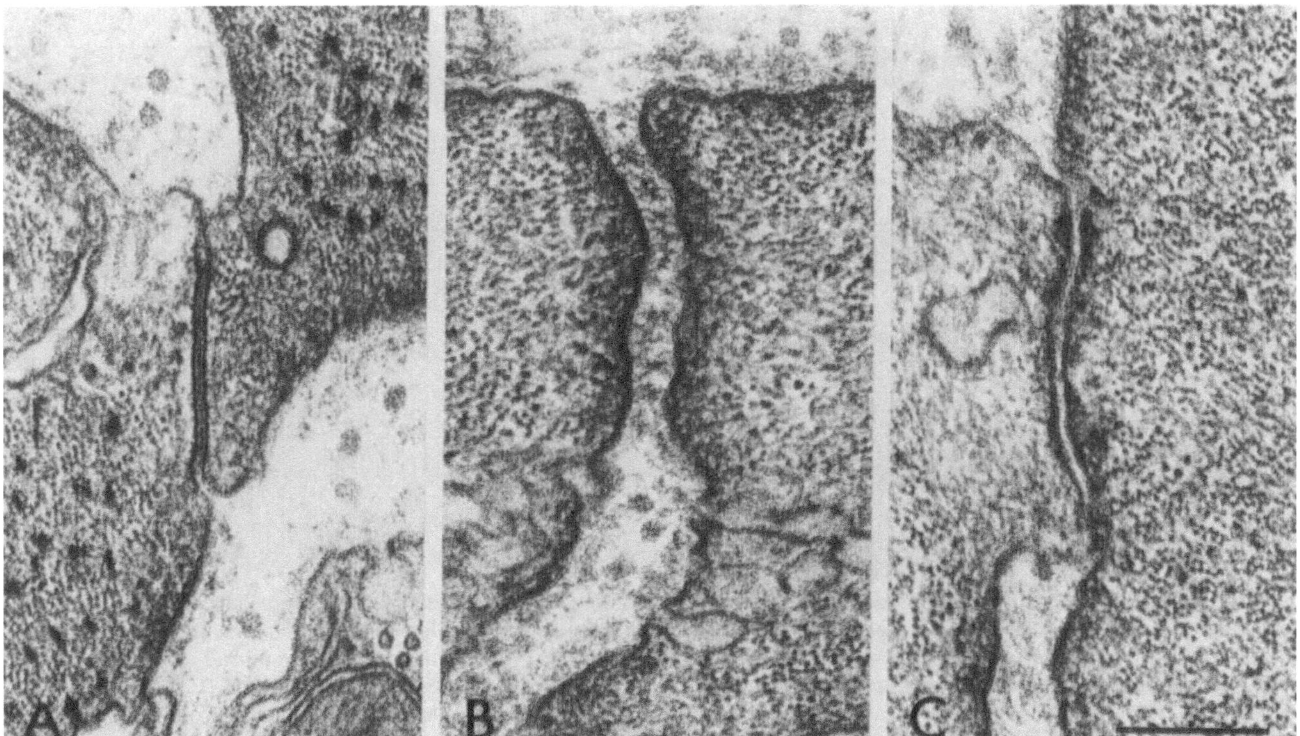

Figure 7-7. Electron micrographs of guinea pig intestinal muscle showing three different cell-to-cell junctions at the same magnification. (A) Gap junction (macula communicans). (B) Intermediate junction (macula, or probably fascia adherens). (C) Third type of junction, probably of adherens type, with 20 nm intercellular cleft and less obvious association with intracellular filaments. Calibration bar: 0.2 μm. (From, G Gabella, Handbook of Physiology, 1989, see note on page 150)

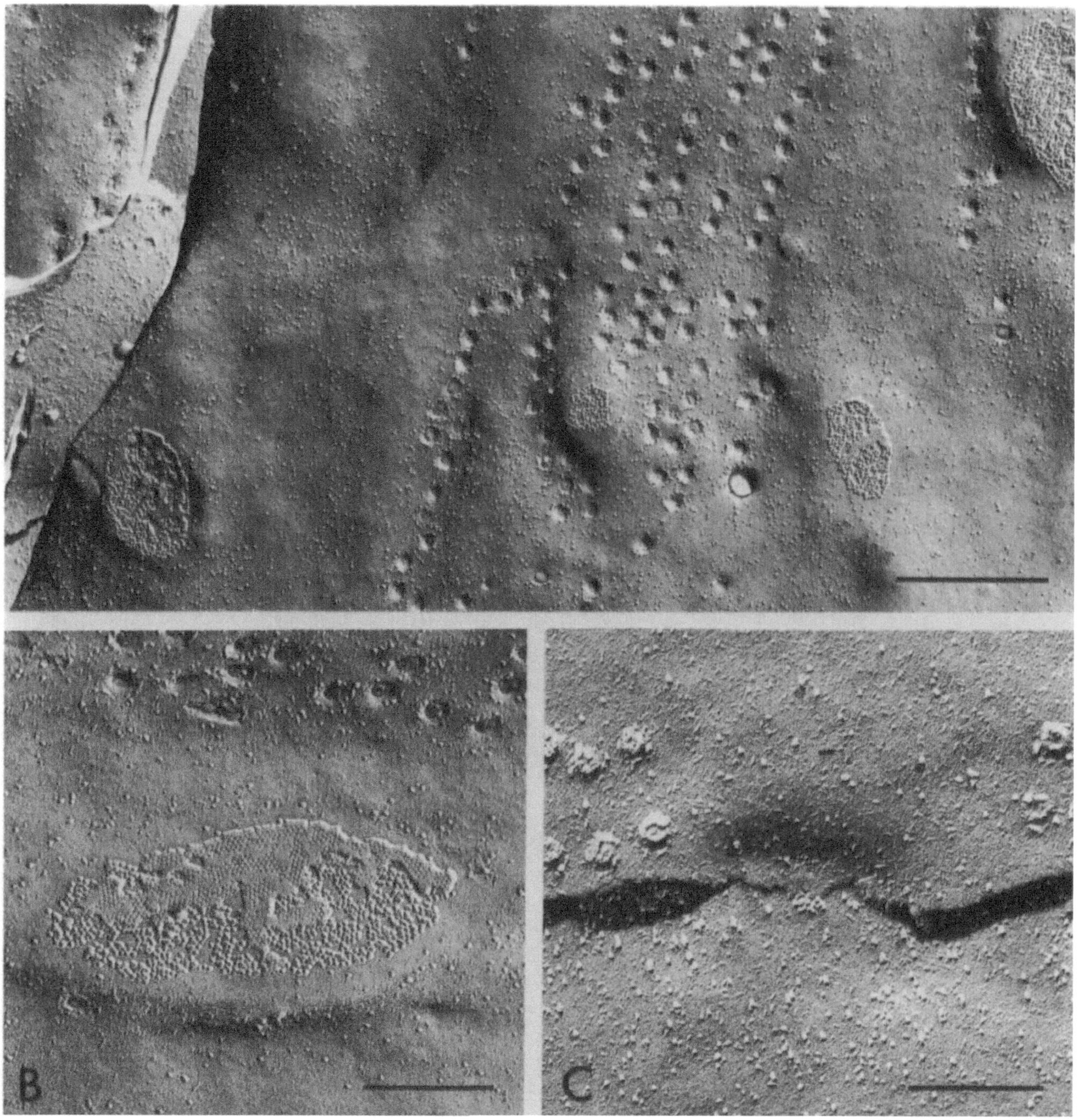

Figure 7-8. Freeze-fracture preparations of the sheep small intestine. (A) Muscle cell of the circular layer showing the plasma membrane on its P-face pitted with several caveolae. There are four gap junctions. Calibration bar: 0.5 μm. (B) Gap junction on a muscle cell of the circular layer seen partly as an aggregate of particles on the P-face of the cell membrane and partly as an aggregate of pits located on the E-face of a patch of membrane of the adjacent muscle cells. Calibration bar: 0.25 μm. (C) Small gap junction between two muscle cells of the longitudinal layer of the same specimen as (B). Calibration bar: 0.25 μm. (From G Gabella, Handbook of Physiology, 1989, see note on page 150)

muscle cells, and on the existence of junctions that allow the contraction of each cell to be added to that of its neighbors. Additional forms of junctions are those between muscle cell membrane and stroma.

Gap junctions or nexuses (Fig. 7-7A; see also page 7 in Chapter 1) are recognized by a close apposition of the membranes of the two cells; there are no structural specializations on the cytoplasmic site of these patches of membrane. By freeze-fracture, the connections forming the junction are recognized as intramembrane particles on the P-face of each membrane (and the corresponding intramembrane pits when the E-face is exposed) (Fig. 7-8). There can be from a few to many hundreds of connexons grouped into one junction, but even where they are best developed the gap junctions of intestinal muscle cells never reach the size found in other tissues, for example, the rat liver, where a junction can be up to a square micron in area. The distribution and number of gap junctions vary in different

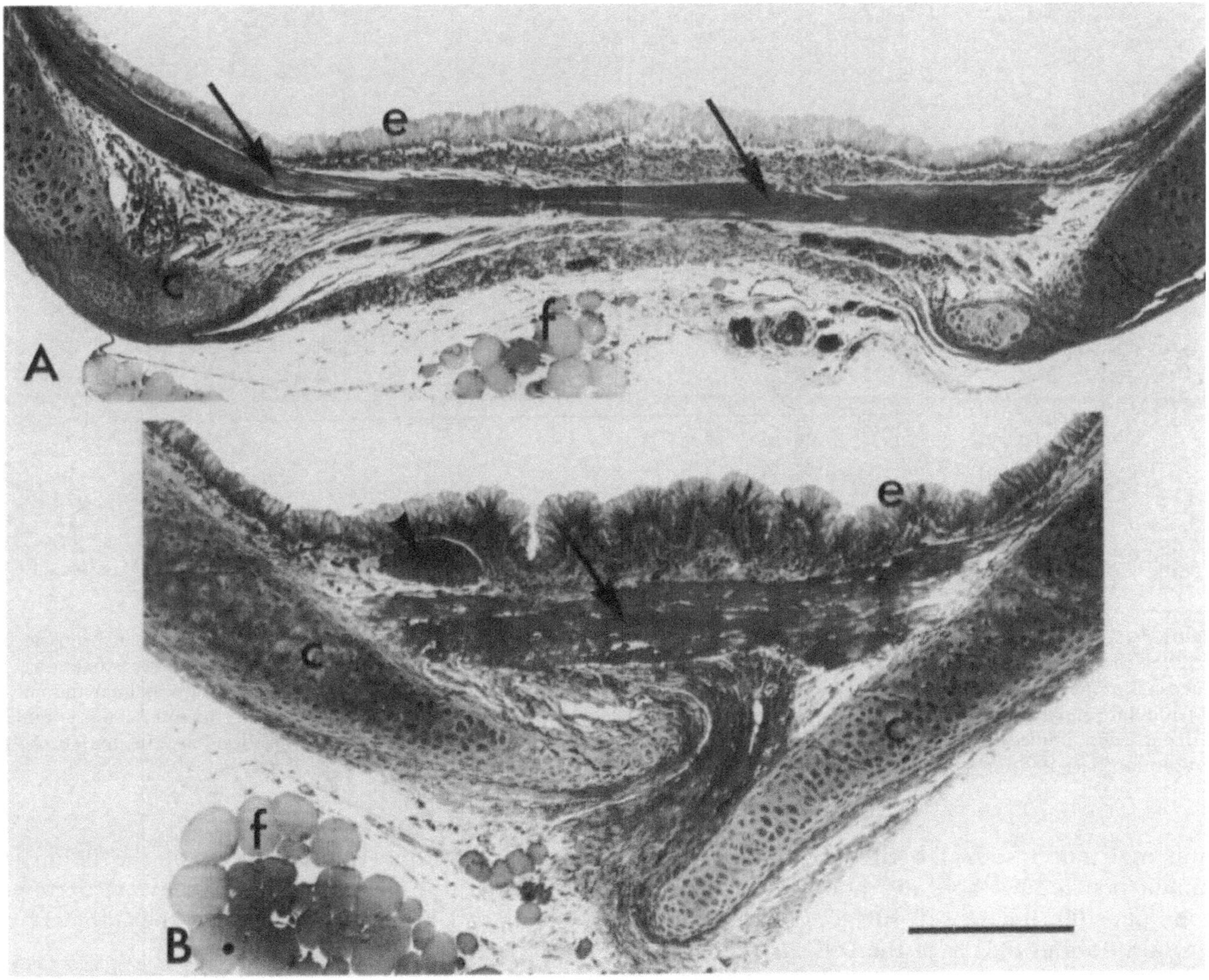

Figure 7-9. (A) Transverse section of a guinea pig's trachea, stained with toluidine blue. The muscle (arrows), which is in longitudinal section, was made to relax by incubating the trachea in calcium-free solution immediately before fixation. e: epithelial lining of the trachea; c: cartilage; f: fat tissue. The arrowhead points to a bundle of longitudinal musculature. (B) Similar preparation to (A), except that the muscle was made to contract isotonically with carbachol immediately before fixation. The muscle is markedly shortened, and its insertions to the cartilage are visible. The mucosa is thrown into longitudinal folds and is pushed ventrally. The tips of the cartilage are brought together and partly overlap. Calibration bar: 250 μm. (From 10.)

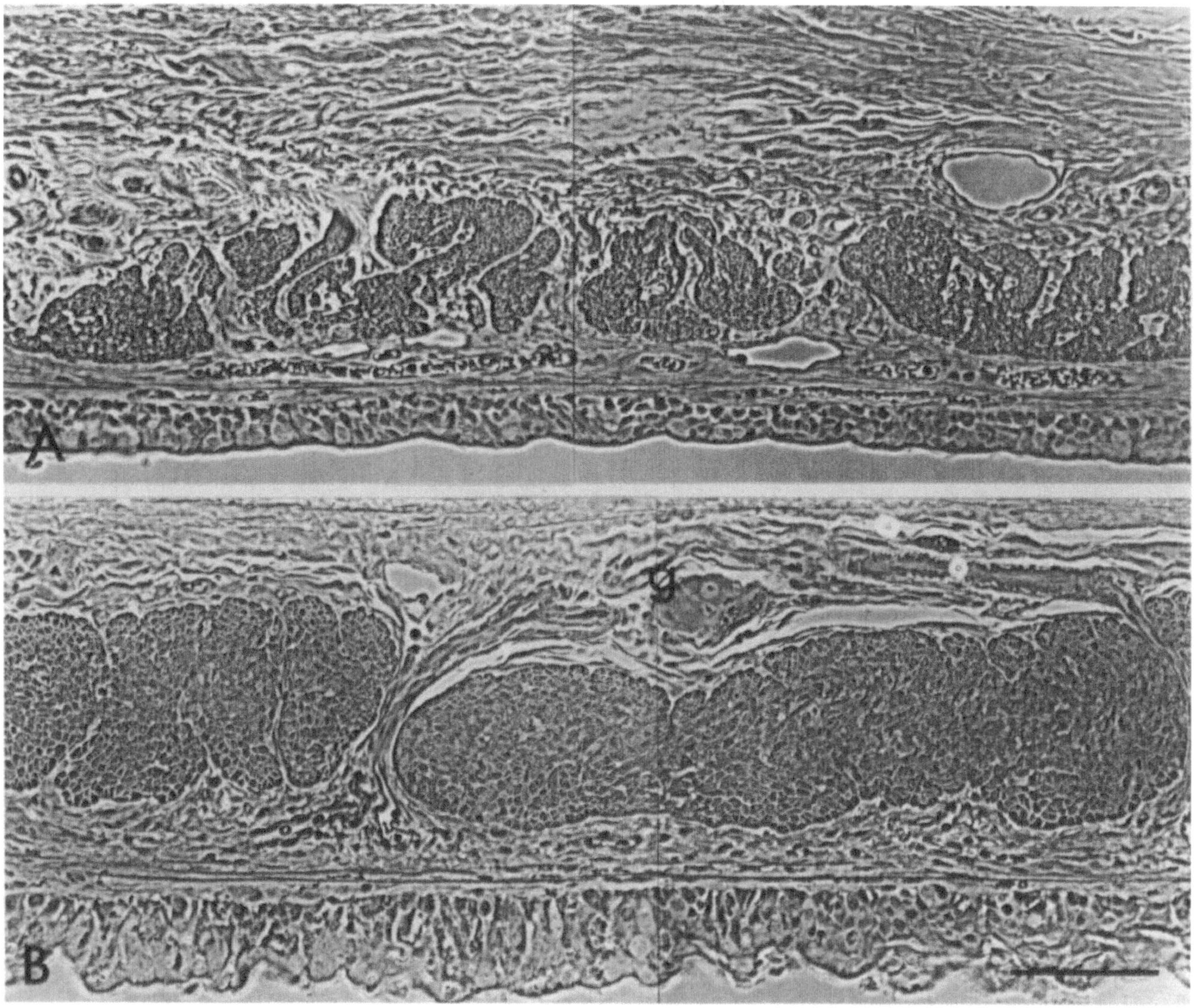

Figure 7-10. (A) Longitudinal section of the trachea through the middle of the membranous portion. The tracheal muscle is in transverse section and is in relaxed condition (the trachea was incubated in calcium-free solution immediately prior to fixation). The mucosa is at the bottom, and many blood vessels and many elastic fibers running longitudinally lie between epithelium and muscle. (B) Similar preparation as in (A), except that the trachea muscle is in isotonically contracted condition (the muscle was stimulated with carbachol immediately before fixation). A ganglion of the tracheal plexus is visible (g). Calibration bar: 100 μm. (From 10.) Calibration bar: 100 μm = 19.5 mm.

intestinal muscles. In the circular muscle of the guinea pig ileum, there are about 48 gap junctions per 100 μm^2 of cell surface, amounting to a total of about 0.21% of the cell surface. In the duodenum of the same species they are twice as abundant. Interestingly, however, in the circular muscle of the same organ, gap junctions are very few or absent. The same situation has been found in the small intestine of other mammalian species. Even in species where gap junctions do occur in the longitudinal muscle layer of the ileum, for example, the sheep (Fig. 7-8), they are extremely small and much fewer than in the adjacent circular layer.

Other junctions (Fig. 7-7B) are of the fascia adherens type and are associated with intermediate filaments and bundles of thin filaments; the intercellular gap is 40–60 nm wide and is occupied by a layer of dense material with period densities, which is in continuity with the basal laminae of the two cells. These junctions contribute to the mechanical coupling between muscle cells. The third type of junction (Fig. 7-7C) displays dense material on the cytoplasmic side of the membrane but not a clear association with filaments; the intercellular gap is electron-lucent and measures 20 nm or less. The functional significance of these junctions is still obscure.

Other cytological characteristics of intestinal muscle cells are described in Chapter 1.

7. Smooth muscle in the airways

Smooth muscle in the airways of mammals is found in the trachea and in the main extraparenchymal and intraparenchymal bronchi. (Smooth muscle is absent or poorly represented in the trachea of nonmammalian species.) The tracheal muscle is a narrow and thin band of smooth muscle running transversely within the dorsal, or membranous, wall of the trachea (Fig. 7-9). Thin septa of connective tissue, carrying blood vessels and nerves, divide the muscle into bundles (Fig. 7-10). These septa, like those found in the intestinal muscles, are of short length, and the muscle bundles split and merge repeatedly so that the lateral continuity of the muscle is maintained over the full length of the trachea. The muscle is inserted onto the C-shaped tracheal cartilages (Fig. 7-9); in some species (ferret) the insertion is on the outer surface of the cartilage,

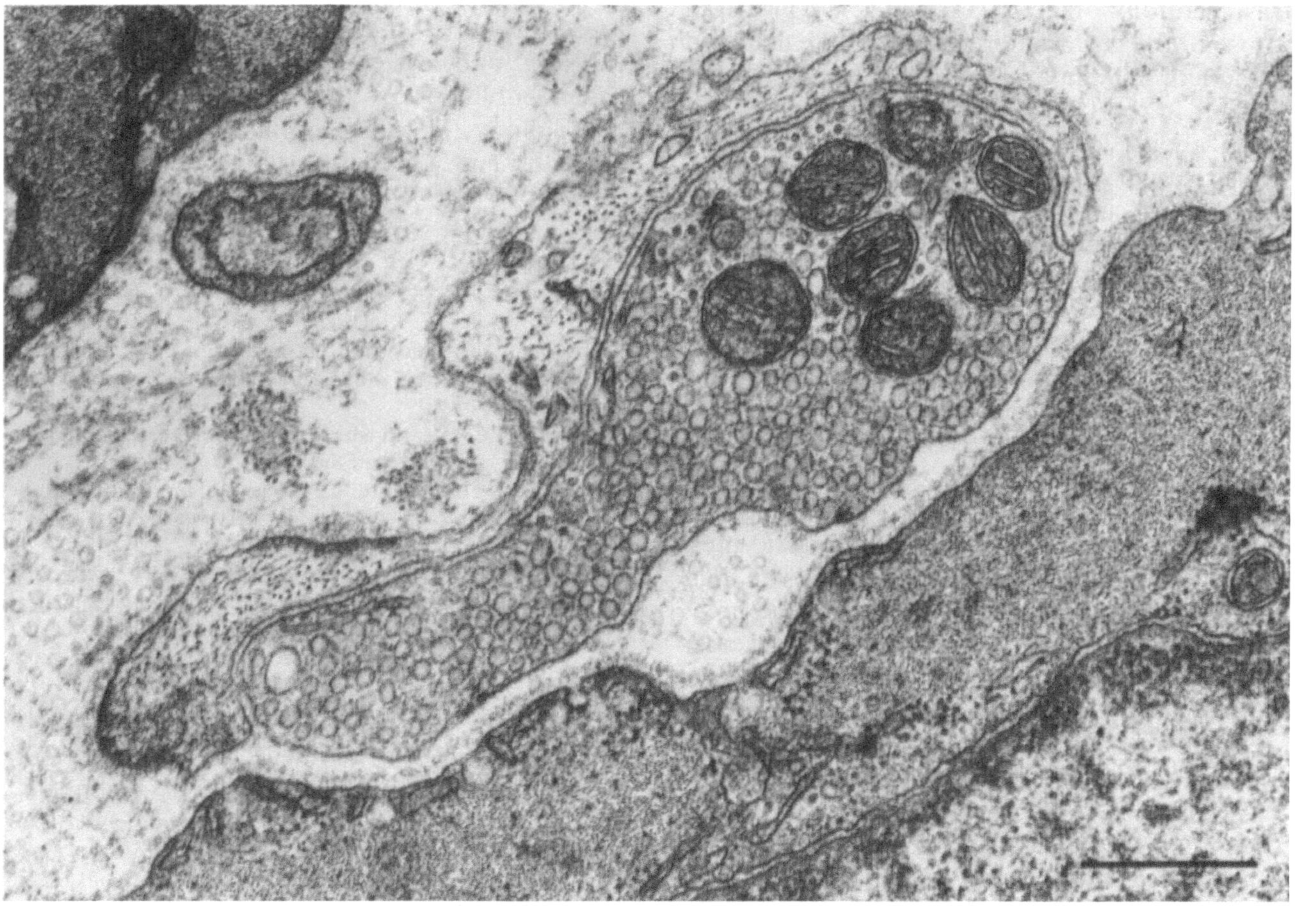

Figure 7-11. Transverse section of the tracheal muscle of a rat. The electron micrograph shows a nerve ending packed with agranular vesicles, mitochondria, endoplasmic reticulum, and microtubules. The nerve ending is partly covered by the slender process of a Schwann cell containing gliofilaments and membrane-bound densities. A few dense projections are attached to the prejunctional membrane. The muscle cell profile at the bottom right corner shows part of its nucleus, caveolae, smooth sarcoplasmic reticulum, and actin and myosin filaments. Calibration bar: 0.5 μm.

in others (rat) it is on the tips of the cartilage, and in others (guinea pig, sheep) it is on the inner surface of the cartilage. Therefore, the length of the muscle can be considerably greather than the distance between the tips of the cartilage. Bundles of longitudinal musculature are occasionally found in some species such as rat and human (9). Upon contraction, the tracheal muscle shortens and thickens and the ends of the cartilage are brought close together, the curvature of the cartilage is increased, and the lumen of the trachea is reduced (10).

In bronchi and bronchioles, the musculature is a system of muscle bundles arranged as geodesic lines within the wall and close to the cartilagenous plaques and an abundant amount of elastic fibers (11).

Smooth muscle cells of the airways resemble ultrastructurally other visceral muscle cells, such as those of the gut. Cameron et al. (12) calculated a cell length of 0.8 mm and a cell volume of about 3000 μm^3 in the bovine trachea. With a cell surface of about 7400 μm^2, the surface-to-volume ratio is relatively high, 2.5 μm^2 of cell surface for every μm^3 of cell volume, a value much higher than that found in intestinal muscles. A similar situation is found in the tracheal muscle cells of other species because of the irregular contours of the muscle cells and the large number of cell processes and invaginations. The cell membrane displays many caveolae, which are arranged in rows between dense bands. Gap junctions are consistently found, often at the end of slender cell processes. There is, however, great variation in frequency of gap junction in the tracheal muscle of different animal species. The muscle cells are coated by a basal lamina, except in the areas forming gap junctions. The basal lamina increases with the age of the animal and is particularly prominent in human bronchial musculature. Between the muscle cells there are abundant collagen and elastic fibers and also elaunin-oxytalan fibers (13).

Few blood vessels run in the connective tissue septa between muscle bundles, and none are truly intramuscular. There are no interstitial cells comparable to those of the intestine and only few intramuscular fibroblasts. However, there are numerous mast cells that often lie close to muscle cells and to nerve endings. There are many nerve endings (Fig. 7-11), the afferent ones originating mainly from the nodose ganglion, and the efferent ones originating from tracheal ganglia and from the stellate ganglion.

The connective tissue ventral to the tracheal muscle, or tunica propria of the tracheal mucosa, is rich in elastic fibers running longitudinally; these fibers are under tension in the trachea in situ. On the dorsal side of the tracheal muscle there is a thicker layer of connective tissue made mainly of collagen bundles running transversely or with a crisscross pattern. A more complex arrangement of musculature, cartilages, and connective tissue is found in the bronchi.

Note

An expanded version of this chapter with a fuller description of the fine structure of intestinal muscles and an extensive list of references has been published by this author in Handbook of Physiology, The Gastrointestinal System, Vol. 1, Motility and Circulation, ed. by J.D. Wood, pp. 103–139 (1989).

References

1. Walus KM, Jacobson ED: Relationship between small intestinal motility and circulation. *Am J Physiol* 241: G1–G15, 1981.
2. Chou CC: Relationship between intestinal blood flow and motility. *Annu Rev Physiol* 44: 29–42, 1982.
3. Taxi J: Contribution à l'étude des connexions des neurones moteurs du système nerveux autonome. (1983) *Ann Sci Nat Zool* 7: 413–674, 1983.
4. Mikkelsen HB, Thuneberg L, Wittrup IH: Selective double staining of interestitial cells of Cajal and macrophage-like cells in small intestine by an improved supravital methylene blue technique combined with FITC-dextran uptake. *Anat Embryol* 178: 191–195, 1988.
5. Li P-L: Neue Beobachtungen über die Struktur der Zirkulärmuskels im Dünndarm bei Wirbeltieren. *Z Anat Entwicklungsgesch* 107: 212–222, 1937.
6. Bennett T, Cobb JLS: Studies on the avian gizzard: morphology and innervation of the smooth muscle. *Z Zellforsch* 96: 183–195, 1969.
7. Gabella G: The cross-ply arrangement of collagen fibres in the submucosa of the mammalian small intestine. *Cell Tissue Res* 248: 491–497, 1987.
8. Komuro T: The lattice arrangement of the collagen fibres in the submucosa of the rat small intestine: scanning electron microscopy, *Cell Tissue Res* 251: 117–121, 1988.
9. Ferner H, Müller I: Mikroskopische Anatomie und Archi-

tektonik der membranösen Trachealwand des Menschen. *Z Mikrosk Anat Forsch* 67: 571–591.
10. Amiri MH, Gabella G: Structure of the guinea-pig trachea at rest and in contraction. *Anat Embryol* 178: 389–397, 1988.
11. Macklin CC: The musculature of the bronchi and lungs. *Physiol Rev* 9: 1–60, 1929.
12. Cameron AR, Bullock CG, Kirkpatrick CT: The ultrastructure of bovine tracheal smooth muscle. *J Ultrastruct Res* 81: 290–305, 1982.
13. Böck P, Stockinger L: Light and electron microscopic identification of elastic, elaunin and oxytalan fibers in human tracheal and bronchial mucosa. *Anat Embryol* 170: 145–153, 1984.

Author's address:
Prof. Giorgio Gabella
Department of Anatomy and Developmental Biology
University College London
Gower Street
London WC1E 6BT
England

CHAPTER 8

Ultrastructure of smooth muscle cells in the urinary system

JOHN S. DIXON & JOHN A. GOSLING

1. Introduction

This chapter provides a review of current knowledge on the ultrastructure of smooth muscle and its innervation in the urinary system including the ureter, renal calices and pelvis, and the urinary bladder. Emphasis is placed on the human urinary tract, since this has been a major field of study by the authors over the last several years. Tissue for examination in the electron microscope has been obtained either at operation or by biopsy with the cooperation of numerous local urological surgeons whose help is gratefully acknowledged.

The detailed fine structure of smooth muscle cells in the wall of the urinary tract is similar in all mammalian species so far examined. However, species variation occurs in the muscular architecture of the renal calices and pelvis, since some species have a unicaliceal system whereas others are multicaliceal. In addition, species variation occurs in the density and distribution of autonomic nerve fibers that supply different regions of the urinary tract. These variations are referred to in the text where appropriate.

2. The ureter

The muscle coat of the ureter gradually increases in thickness in a proximodistal direction and in the human varies in width from about 600 μm in the upper ureter to around 900 μm in the lower ureter (1). The ureteric muscularis is composed of muscle bundles separated from one another by large amounts of connective tissue (2). However, the individual muscle cells that form each bundle are closely packed together with very little intervening connective tissue. The muscle bundles frequently branch and unite with one another so that separate layers of muscle are not readily discernable. Nevertheless, in the upper ureter, the innermost muscle bundles tend to lie longitudinally or obliquely while those on the outer aspect have a generally circular orientation. In the middle and lower thirds of the ureter, additional outer longitudinally orientated muscle bundles are present (3, 4). Near the ureterovesicle junction, the muscle coat consists almost entirely of obliquely or longitudinally orientated muscle bundles (1).

2.1. Fine structure of ureteric smooth muscle cells

Ureteric muscle bundles are composed of closely packed, elongated smooth muscle cells that are fusiform in shape with tapering ends. Within a bundle, the cells are arranged approximately parallel to one another and appear circular or oval in transverse section. The cell surface becomes highly folded in the contracted state such that adjacent cells frequently interdigitate with their neighbors. Ureteric smooth muscle cells are approximately 300–400 μm in length, although this is a rather uncertain parameter since the cells can shorten and lengthen over a wide range. Generally each cell measures between 4 μm and 7 μm at its widest part (Fig. 8-1).

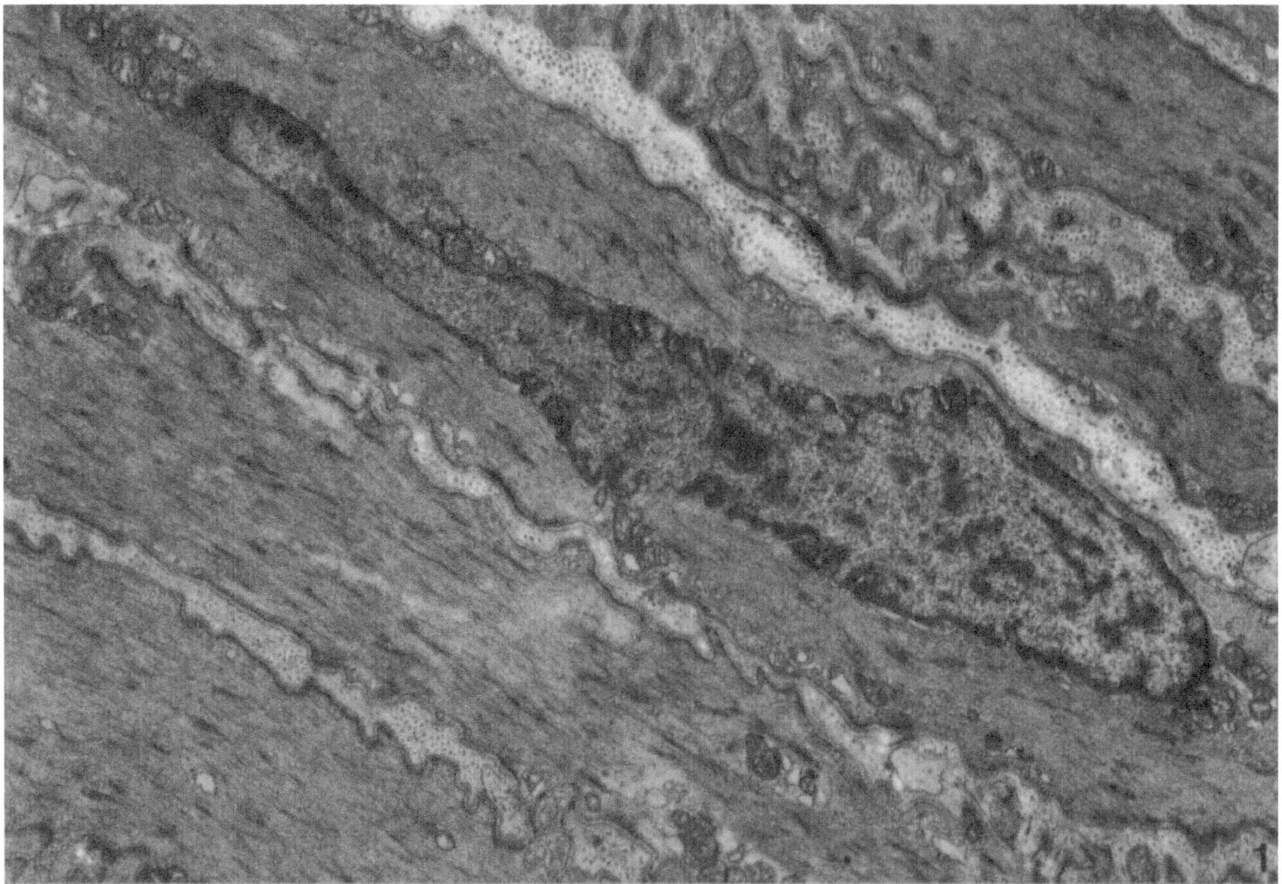
1

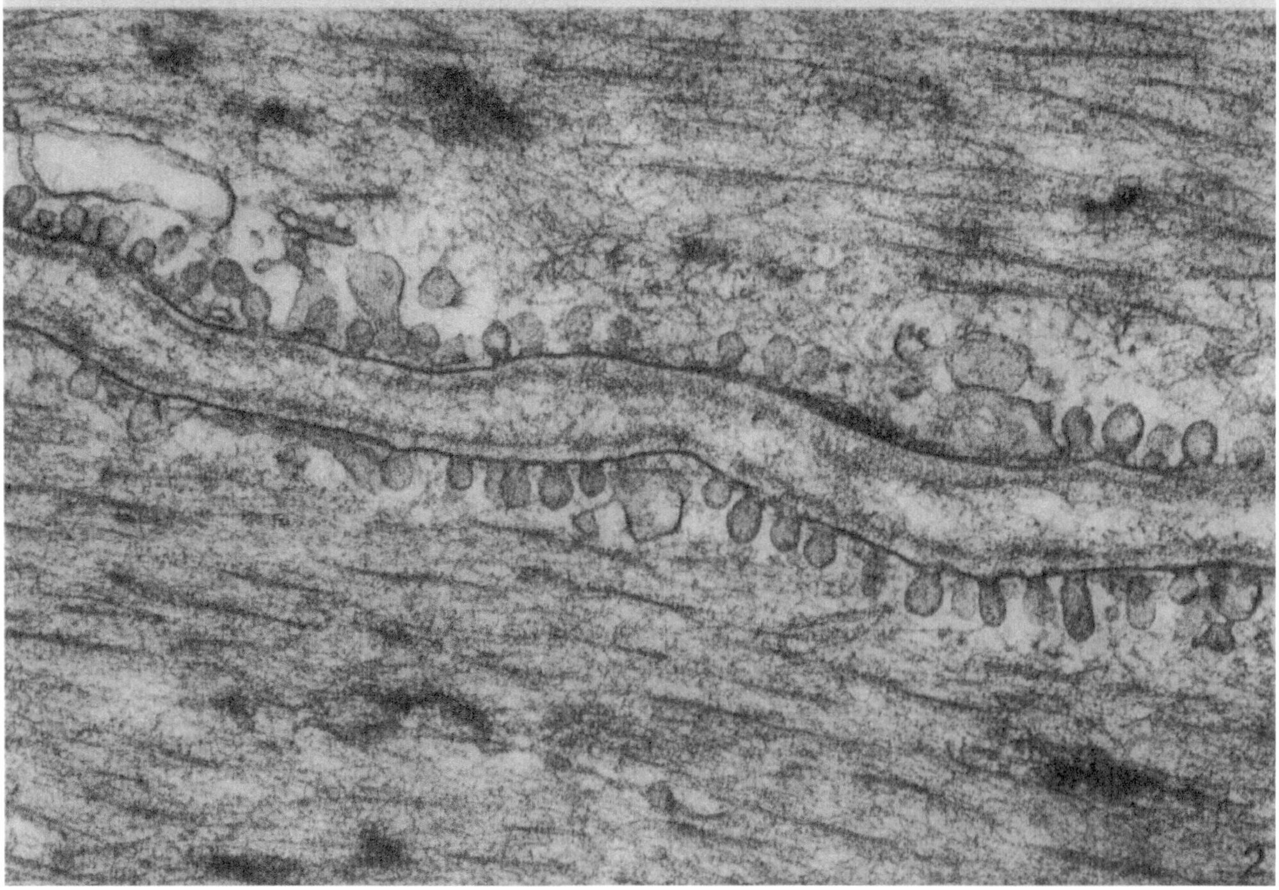
2

Each smooth muscle cell is surrounded by a trilaminar plasma membrane (the sarcolemma) on the outer aspect of which is a layer of amorphous electron-dense material, the basal lamina (Fig. 8-2). The basal lamina is approximately 40 nm in thickness and is separated from the sarcolemma by an electronlucent zone about 40 nm in width (the lamina lucida). The cell membrane is involved in the formation of cell-to-cell junctions as described below.

The plasma membrane of each smooth muscle cell possesses inumerable small flask-shaped infoldings called caveolae (Fig. 8-2). These tend to be fairly uniform in size, measuring about 70 nm across and about 120 nm in length, the long axis being orthogonal to the cell surface. The basal lamina does not penetrate into the caveolae but extends as a continuous layer across their necks or stomata. The latter are about 35 nm at their narrowest part. The caveolae are not randomly distributed over the cell surface but tend to form rows parallel to the long axis of each cell. They are frequently observed in close association with elongated sacs of smooth endoplasmic reticulum (sarcoplasmic reticulum). Rows of caveolae are separated from each other by subsarcolelemmal accumulations of electron-dense material.

Each smooth muscle cell possesses a single centrally placed ovoid nucleus containing a peripheral zone of darkly staining chromatin beneath a double porous nuclear membrane.

Small oval mitochondria are scattered throughout the sacroplasm with a tendency to occur preferentially in regions immediately beneath the cell membrane. Other mitochondria occur in the conical-shaped regions at either pole of the cell nucleus. In these latter regions, elongated cisternae of both smooth and rough endoplasmic reticulum frequently occur together with poorly developed Golgi membranes. Very rarely, irregularly shaped lipid droplets and small dense glycogen granules may also be present. Lysosomes, residual bodies, and multivesicular bodies are also occasionally observed.

The sarcoplasm of each smooth muscle cell is packed with myofilaments, most of which are orientated parallel to the cell's long axis (Fig. 8-2). Small elongated electron-dense bodies occur at random among the myofilaments. Three distinct types of myofilament are present in ureteric smooth muscle cells, namely thick, thin, and intermediate. Thick (15 nm) and thin (5–7 nm) filaments are similar to the well-characterized filaments of striated muscles and are believed to consist of myosin and actin, respectively. Both the actin and myosin filaments are directly involved in the contraction process of the smooth muscle cells, possiblly by a mechanism that involves the sliding of one filament over the other in a manner similar to that which occurs in skeletal muscles. The thin filaments appear to be attached to the electron-dense bodies throughout the sarcoplasm and also to the cell membrane at the subsarcolemmal dense patches. The intermediate (10 nm) filaments possibly form an intracellular framework or cytoskeleton and are often found in close association with the electron-dense bodies, although it is not clear whether they are actually attached to them (5). The dense bodies and subsarcolemmal dense bands probably correspond to the Z-lines of striated muscle fibers.

In addition to myofilaments, longitudinally orientated cytoplasmic microtubules with diameters of 20–25 nm also occur in ureteric smooth muscle cells.

2.2. Cell-to-cell junctions

For the most part, each ureteric smooth muscle cell is separated from its neighbors by a gap of 100 nm or more that contains collagen fibrils, elastic fibers, and other extracellular material. However, in some areas adjacent cells form a more intimate relationship, giving rise to so-called cell-to-cell junctions. In the ureter, four different types of intercellular junctions have been described, namely *regions of close appro-*

←

Figure 8-1. Part of a muscle bundle from the human ureter, consisting of closely packed smooth muscle cells separated from one another by narrow connective tissue spaces. X 9600.

Figure 8-2. Ureteric smooth muscle cells in longitudinal section showing rows of flask-shaped caveolae and associated sacs of sarcoplasmic reticulum. Thick and thin myofilaments are visible in the sarcoplasm, while the outer aspect of each cell is covered by an amorphous basal lamina. X 56,000.

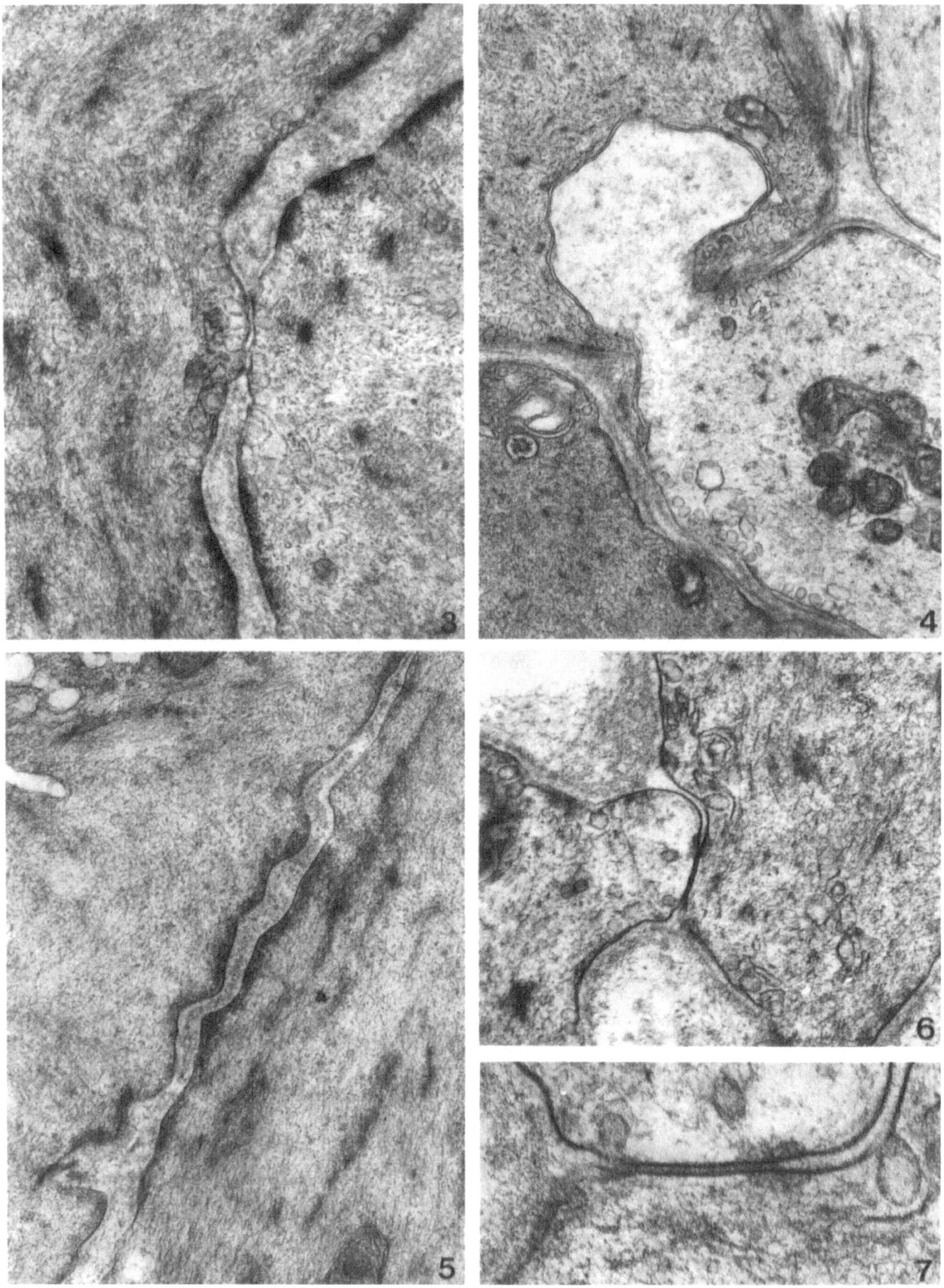
3
4
5
6
7

ach, *peg-and-socket* junctions, *intermediate* junctions, and *gap* junctions or nexuses (3).

2.2.1. Regions of close approach. At a region of close approach, the plasma membranes of neighboring smooth muscle cells converge to within 10–20 nm of each other (Fig. 8-3). Basal lamina material does not extend into the narrow intercellular cleft. Instead, the basal lamina of one cell is reflected back to become continuous with that of the adjacent cell. The apposing membranes of this type of junction may possess caveolae and/or electron-dense material on the cytoplasmic aspect. This is by far the commonest type of cell-to-cell junction observed between the smooth muscle cells of the human ureter (6), and as such it seems reasonable to postulate that this type of intercellular junction is responsible for the electrotonic propagation of peristaltic contraction waves from one cell to the next within a ureteric muscle bundle.

2.2.2. Peg-and-socket junctions. This type of junction consists of an elongated or bulbous projection from one cell that fits snugly into a depression in an adjacent cell (Fig. 8-4). At the interdigitation, basal lamina material is absent from the 10–20 nm gap separating the membranes of the two adjacent muscle cells. Occasionally the opposing cell membranes are more closely related in the narrowed stalk of the projection, the intercellular space measuring around 5 nm. Myofilaments are generally absent from the sarcoplasmic projection, giving it an electron-lucent appearance (Fig. 8-4). It has been suggested that this type of interdigitation provides a mechanical linkage between neighboring cells or may be an artifact due to adverse handling of the tissue prior to fixation (7). Alternatively, it may represent a special type of close approach and permit myogenic conduction (8).

2.2.3. Intermediate junctions. This type of junction consists of regions where the apposing plasma membranes lie approximately parallel to one another for distances up to 2.5 μm, separated by a gap of about 50 nm that contains a single basal lamina (Fig. 8-5). In addition, the sarcoplasm underlying the apposing membranes has an increased electron density identical to the plaque-like condensations that occur at other regions of the muscle cell membrane. It is not known whether the intermediate junctions have any functional significance or whether they simply represent regions where the subsarcolemmal electron-dense plaques of adjacent cells are by chance in register. Nevertheless, in these regions the close proximity of adjacent cells narrows the extracellular space such that the basal laminae become confluent. Intermediate junctions are commonly observed in ureteric smooth muscle.

2.2.4. Gap junctions. A gap junction is characterized by the extremely close apposition of the membranes of adjacent cells (Fig. 8-6). The ultrastructural appearance of gap junctions varies with the type of fixation employed during processing for electron microscopsy. Using glutaraldehyde fixation and block staining with aqueous uranyl acetate, a narrow gap of 2–3 nm in width is seen separating the apposing membranes, and the junction has therefore a seven-layered appearance (Fig. 8-7). With less adequate methods of fixation (as used in early fine-structural studies), this type of junction may appear as a five-layered structure, i.e., the outer leaflets of the two apposing membranes appear to be fused without an intervening gap. The gap junction is generally a

←

Figure 8-3. A region of close approach between two adjacent ureteric smooth muscle cells. A gap of about 20 nm separates the apposing membranes, while the basal lamina of one cell is reflected back to become continuous with that of its neighbor. X 35,200.
Figure 8-4. A peg-and-socket junction between smooth muscle cells of the human ureter. X 20,000.
Figure 8-5. An intermediate junction from the human ureter. The apposing membranes are separated by a minimum gap of 50 nm containing a single basal lamina. X 28,800.
Figure 8-6. A gap junction between neighboring ureteric smooth muscle cells. This type of cell-to-cell junction is extremely rare in ureteric muscle. X 35,200.
Figure 8-7. At high magnification, a gap of 2–3 nm is evident separating apposing membranes of the gap junction shown in Figure 8-6. X 390,000.

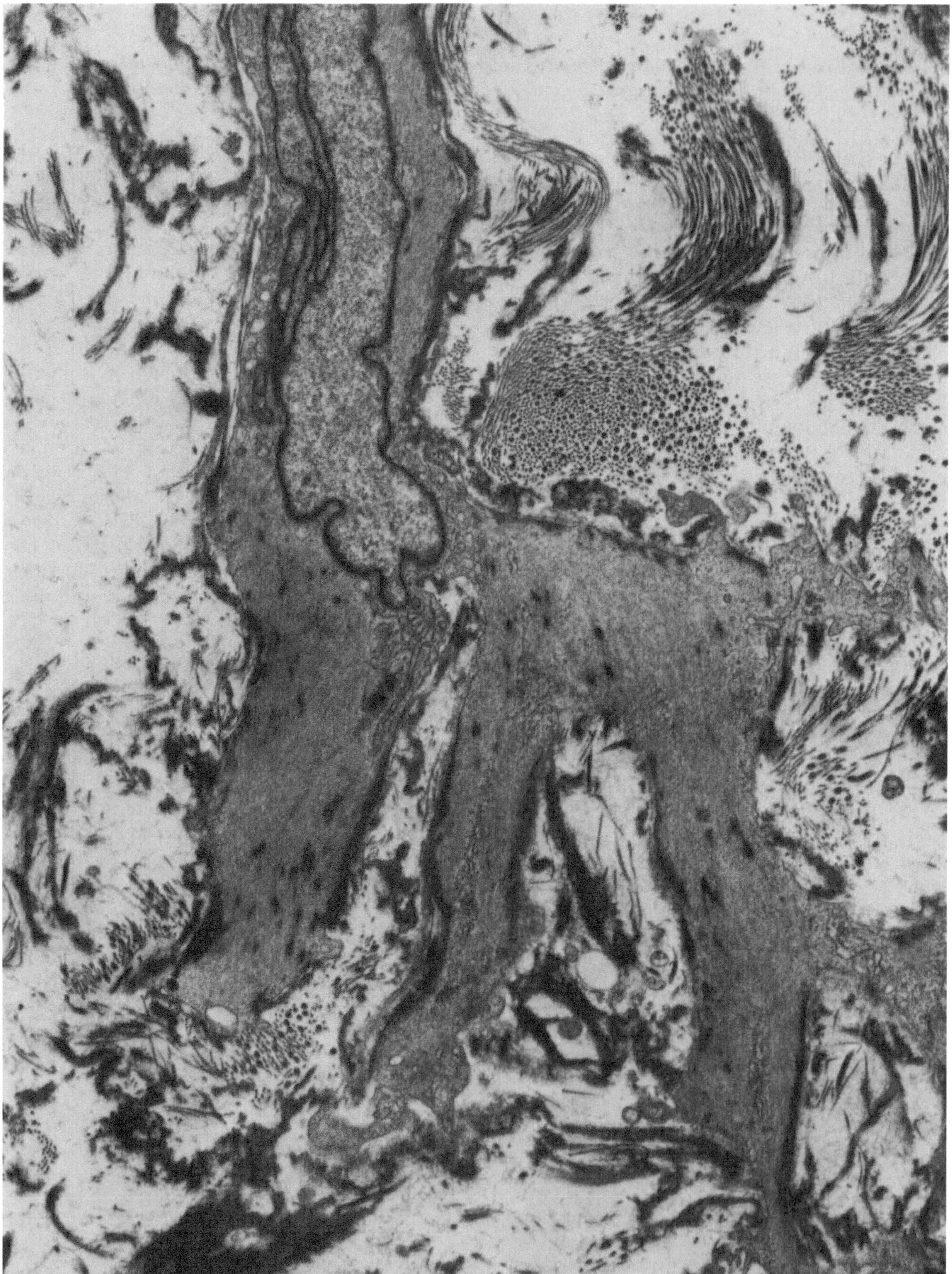

circular zone of cell-to-cell apposition at the periphery of which the basal lamina of one cell becomes continuous with that of the neighboring cell and does not extend into the gap. Junctions of this type are extremely rare in ureteric smooth muscle but are quite numerous in some other smooth muscles. By the use of tracers in such tissues, it has been shown that the minute gap between the membranes is accessible to extracellular substances and furthermore that the intercellular gap is occupied by regularly spaced discrete bridges between the apposing membranes. A narrow channel occurs within each of these bridges, allowing ions and small molecules to pass from one cell to the next. However, electronic spread of excitation from cell to cell does not appear to be dependent on the presence of large numbers of gap junctions (5) as exemplified by ureteric muscle.

3. The renal calices and pelvis

In various mammals including the human, the muscle coat of the renal calices and pelvis is composed of two morphological and histochemically distinct types of smooth muscle cell (9–12). One type is identical to that described for the ureter, while the other possesses a number of unusual features and is referred to as *atypical* smooth muscle.

3.1. Distribution of atypical smooth muscle cells in the renal calices and pelvis

In man, atypical smooth muscle cells occur in the region of attachment of each minor calyx to the renal parenchyma. These morphological distinctive cells are not arranged into compact bundles, but form a thin sheet of muscle that covers each minor caliceal fornix. These cells also extend across the renal parenchyma, which lies between the renal attachments of the minor calices. Thus, each minor calix is in effect connected to its neighbors by a thin layer of atypical smooth muscle. In the wall of each minor calyx, atypical smooth muscle cells are arranged longitudinally and form a discrete layer confined to the inner aspect of the muscle coat. This inner layer is closely applied to and interconnects with bundles of typical smooth muscle (see below). This arrangement continues throughout the walls of the major calices and renal pelvis. However, in the pelviureteric region this configuration ceases, and so the proximal ureter is devoid of a morphologically distinct inner layer of smooth muscle. Individually, atypical cells are separated from one another for much of their length by quantities of connective tissue. In addition, histochemical studies have shown that these cells differ from typical upper urinary tract smooth muscle in that they are devoid of non-specific cholinesterase (12). Although the physiological significance of this intracellular enzyme is not known at present, it is a useful means by which to distinguish the two types of smooth muscle cell in the light microscope.

3.2. Distribution of typical smooth muscle cells in the renal calices and pelvis

Typical spindle-shaped smooth muscle cells are grouped together into compact bundles that are first in evidence in the distal part of each minor calix. These bundles lie external to the atypical muscle cell layer and extend throughout the major calices and renal pelvis. In the pelvi-ureteric region these bundles are directly continuous with those that form the muscle coat of the ureter. In the major calices and renal pelvis, these muscle bundles are closely related on their inner aspects to the layer of atypical smooth muscle. Individual bundles lie in various directions, although the majority tend to be circularly disposed. These compact bundles of smooth muscle frequently branch and connect with adjacent muscle fascicles, thus forming a plexiform arrangement of intercommunicating muscle bundles. In the pelvi-ureteric region there is no localized thickening of muscle, and therefore a pelvi-ureteric sphincter does not exist anatomically (6). Typical smooth muscle cells forming the outer layer of the muscle

←

Figure 8-8. A branching atypical smooth muscle cell from the human renal calix. Bundles of collagen fibrils and densely stained elastic fibers surround the cell X 11,200.

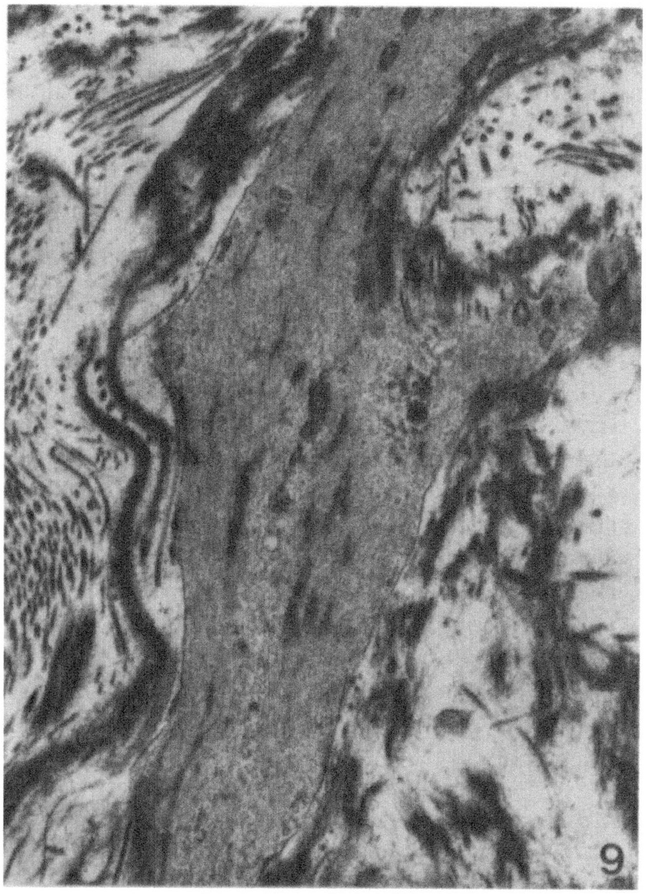
9

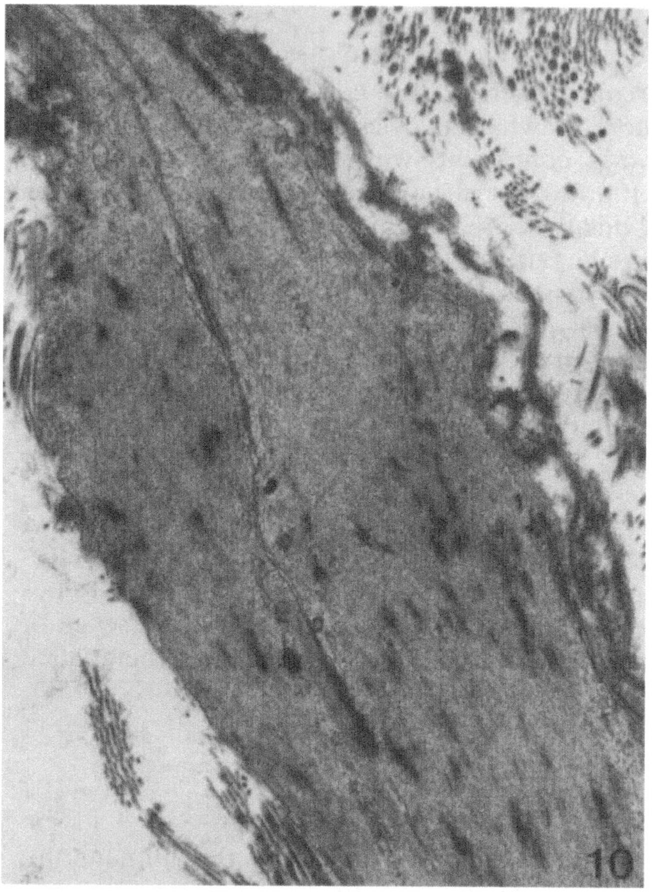
10

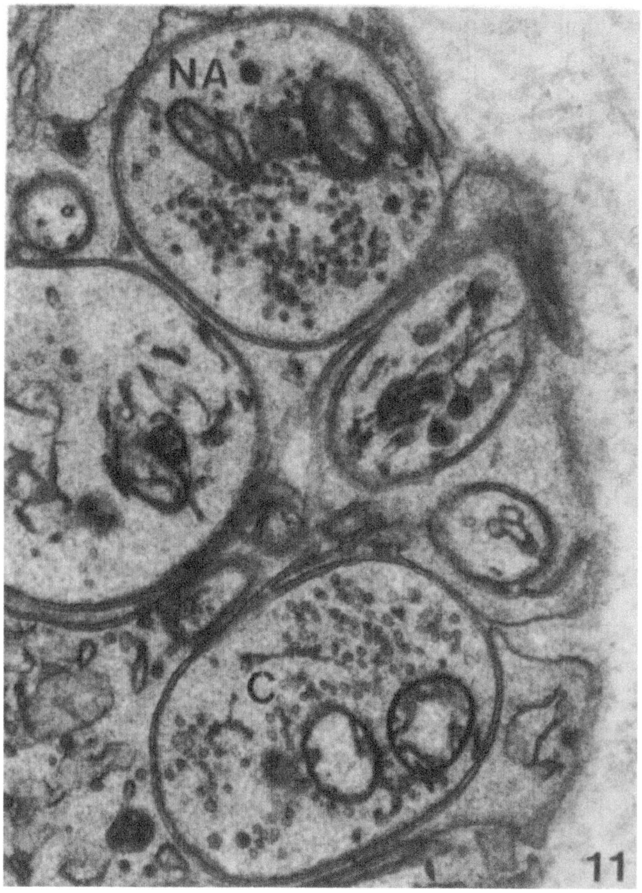
NA
C
11

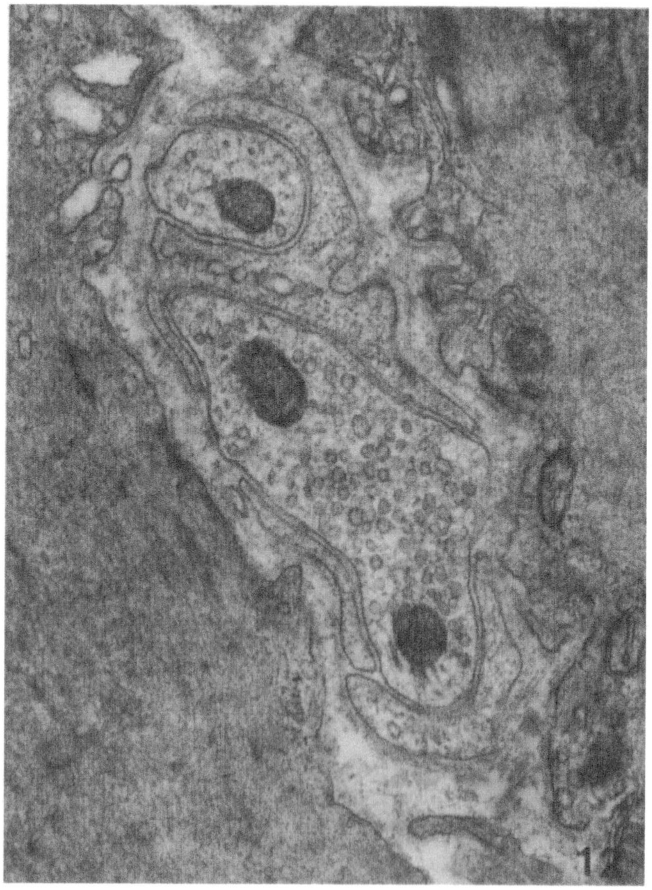
12

coat of the renal pelvis and major calices are rich in nonspecific cholinesterase and are thus easily distinguished from the atypical cell layer (12).

3.3. Fine structure of atypical smooth muscle cells

In the electron microscope, the atypical smooth muscle cells are readily identified because of their wide separation from one another by collagen and elastic fibers. Individual cells are extremely elongated and irregular in outline and often possess lateral protrusions or branches (Fig. 8-8). In addition, many cells possess rounded or angular projections of sarcoplasm that enhance their irregular appearance. Flask-shaped caveolae do not occur in such projections, but are present at other regions of the cells' surfaces. Each cell is surrounded by a basal lamina, which is often discontinuous over large areas of the sarcolemma (Fig. 8-9). The myofilaments of such cells are identical in type to those found in other upper urinary tract smooth muscle. However, within each cell the myofilaments are frequently arranged in elongated bundles separated by areas containing granular reticulum and small mitochondria. This arrangement contrasts with that of typical smooth muscle cells, in which the myofilaments generally occupy the major part of the sarcoplasm. Many of the atypical cells possess areas within their sarcoplasm that contain clusters of electron-dense glycogen granules.

Frequently an elongated sarcoplasmic projection from one cell extends out to form an intercellular junction with a similar protuberance from an adjacent cell. At the junctional region, the opposing cells membranes are separated by a gap of not more than 20 nm without any intervening basal lamina. Junctions of this type are similar to the regions of close approach that occur between ureteric smooth muscle cells. In addition, side-to-side apposition of adjacent cells form junctions of similar fine structure that can be traced for several microns in the plane of section (Fig. 8-10).

4. Innervation of the upper urinary tract

Autonomic nerve fibers occur in the muscle coat of the caliceal wall, the renal pelvis, and the ureter (3, 13). However, the majority of such nerves accompany small blood vessels that run through the muscle layer to supply a rich capillary plexus in the lamina propria. In addition to these perivascular nerves, a few autonomic fibers run independently among the smooth muscle bundles. The density of innervation gradually increases in a proximodistal direction so that the juxtavesical segment of each ureter is relatively richly innervated. Ganglion cells do not occur in the wall of the upper urinary tract except around the ureterovesical junctions.

Intramuscular nerves consist of bundles of axons supported by Schwann cells. The larger bundles contain up to 50 or more axons and mainly occur between the muscle bundles. Smaller nerve fibers containing around 5 to 10 axons occur within the muscle bundles of the ureter and renal pelvis. Many such axons possess swellings or varicosities along their length in which axonal vesicles and mitochondria accumulate (Fig. 8-11). These so-called axon terminals are often only partially ensheathed by neurilemmal (Schwann) cell cytoplasm and alternate with intervaricose regions that have a much narrower diameter.

Many workers now consider it possible to classify autonomic nerve fibers depending on the type of axonal vesicle they contain (14). Nerve terminals containing a large majority of small (45–60 nm diameter) agranular or electron-lucent vesicles together with a few large (70–100 nm diameter) granulated vesicles are considered to

←

Figure 8-9. Part of an atypical cell from the human renal pelvic wall. Large areas of the cell's surface are devoid of a basal lamina, while caveolae are relatively sparse. X 14,400.

Figure 8-10. Extensive regions of close approach are frequently seen between adjacent processes of atypical cells in the human renal calix. X 12,800.

Figure 8-11. A nerve bundle from the human ureter containing both cholinergic (C) and noradrenergic (NA) axons, distinguishable by their characteristic axonal vesicles. $KMnO_4$ fixation. X 28,400.

Figure 8-12. A neuromuscular synapse from the human ureter. The vesicle-packed axonal varicosities are only partially enclosed by neurolemmal cell cytoplasm X 32,000.

be cholinergic in type, while those containing mainly small (30–60 nm diameter) granulated or dense-cored vesicles are believed to be adrenergic in type (14). Adrenergic endings also contain a few large granular vesicles ranging in size from 60 nm to 120 nm (this range overlaps with that of the small vesicles). Both cholinergic and adrenergic nerve terminals (Fig. 8-11) have been observed in the muscle coat of the human ureter by electron microscopy (13, 15), thus confirming the results of earlier light microscopic studies that used histochemical techniques for the demonstration of acetylcholinesterase and noradrenaline (16). However, it must be emphasized that ureteric neuromuscular synapses (Fig. 8-12) are exceedingly sparse in comparison with many other autonomically innervated smooth muscles such as those of the urinary bladder or ductus deferens. In these organs, it has been estimated that almost every smooth muscle cell is directly innervated. In contrast, it seems likely that only a small proportion of ureteric smooth muscle cells are directly influenced by autonomic nerves.

Autonomic nerves in the wall of the upper urinary tract presumably have a modulatory function on the contractile activity of the muscle coat. However, it is generally believed that they are not directly responsible for the propagation of contraction waves. Indeed, there is considerable experimental evidence to support this view. Firstly, the electrical activity measured in the ureteric wall during the peristalsis, together with the rate of propagation of contraction waves, is characteristic of smooth muscle and not nervous activity. Secondly, the ratio of axon terminals to smooth muscle cells is extremely low. Thirdly, it has been shown that ureteric peristalsis continues in vivo in the presence of nerve-blocking agents such as tetrodotoxin and in vitro in denervated ureteric segments.

5. Ureteric peristalsis

It is well known that under normal conditions contraction waves originate in the proximal part of the upper urinary tract and propagate in an anterograde direction towards the bladder. However, the mechanism involved in the initiation of these contractile events has been the subject of much controversy in the past. On theory proposes that smooth muscle contraction is initiated by the stretching forces exerted by the luminal contents on the muscle coat contained within the walls of the renal calices and pelvis. However, there is now a considerable body of experimental evidence that demonstrates that the urinary tract possesses spontaneously active regions consisting of pacemaker muscle cells that initiate and exert a controlling influence on the peristaltic activity of the ureter (17, 18). From a morphological viewpoint, it seems likely that the atypical smooth muscle cells that occur at the attachment of each minor calix in the human and that are structurally distinct from those elsewhere may act as pacemaker sites. Similar atypical cells have been described in the upper urinary tracts of unicaliceal systems (9) and also in the multicalical system of the pig (11), where a similar pacemaking function has been proposed. In man, since each minor calix possesses such cells (and is linked across the renal parenchyma to other calices by similar cells), the number of pacemaker sites within a given system is related to the number of minor calices. It seems probable that the normal sequence of events begins with the initiation of a contraction wave at one of the several minor caliceal pacemaker sites. Once initiated, the contraction is propagated through the wall of the adjacent major calix and activates the smooth muscle of the renal pelvis. To what extent the inner layer of atypical cells acts as pacemaker (or as a preferential conduction pathway) remains to be determined. The proximal pacemaker site for successive contractions usually changes between the minor calices, although sometimes the same minor calix will initiate consecutive contractions before the site changes. Functionally, the proximal location of these pacemaker sites ensures that, once initiated, contraction waves are propagated away from the kidney, thereby avoiding undesirable pressure rises directed against the renal parenchyma. In addition, since several potential pacemaker sites exist, the initiation of contraction waves is unimpaired by partial nephrectomy because the minor calices spared by the resection remain in situ and continue their pacemaking function.

Each contraction wave extends across the renal

pelvis as far as the pelvi-ureteric junction, and it seems likely that the onward transmission into the ureter is dependent upon the volume of fluid contained within the renal pelvis. At high urine flow rates, every contraction wave reaching the pelvi-ureteric region is propagated as a ureteric contraction wave. At low flow rates, not all renal pelvic contractions are transmitted to the ureter. Only when a sufficient quantity of urine has accumulated in the renal pelvis does a pelvic contraction wave propagate distally beyond the pelviureteric region. Thus, the pelvi-ureteric region acts as a gate, allowing ureteric peristalsis to occur only when the volume of each bolus of urine propelled from the renal pelvis is above a critical amount.

In summary, ureteric peristalsis is apparently dependent upon two mechanisms within the proximal part of the urinary tract. Firstly, contraction waves in the renal pelvis are initiated by spontaneously active pacemaker sites located with the wall of each minor calix. Secondly, a regulating mechanism at the pelvi-ureteric region determines whether each contraction of the renal pelvis is propagated into the ureter. The latter event is related to urine flow and probably depends upon the stretching forces or tension generated in the wall of the pelvi-ureteric region. It is not yet known whether a malfunction of one or both of these mechanisms is involved in the etiology of functional obstruction of the upper urinary tract.

Contraction waves are thought to be propagated across the renal pelvis and along the ureter by means of myogenic conduction, resulting from electronic coupling of one muscle cell to its immediate neighbors.

In several other organs in which myogenic conduction is known to occur, adjacent smooth muscle cells are normally linked by means of the nexus, or gap junction. This specialized region is thought to provide a low resistance pathway, allowing electronic spread of excitation from one cell to another. It is surprising, therefore, that upper urinary tract smooth muscle is typified by a relative paucity of this type of cell-to-cell contact. However, regions of close approach (with a cell–cell gap of 10–20 nm) are extremely numerous between ureteric smooth muscle cells. Thus it seems probable that intercellular junctions of this type (rather than gap junctions) are responsible for the conduction of contraction waves from one ureteric smooth muscle cell to the next.

The direction of propagation is normally from the renal pelvis towards the bladder, as dictated by the pacemaker mechanism in the minor calices. Since muscle cells may conduct from one cell to the next in either direction, the direction of propagation may sometimes be reversed, resulting in retrograde contraction waves.

6. The urinary bladder

The muscle coat of the urinary bladder is formed of smooth muscle cells that make up the detrusor muscle. This muscle is often described as consisting of three layers; the muscle bundles of the outer and inner layers tend to be orientated longitudinally, while those of the middle layer are circularly disposed. However, the constituent muscle bundles frequently branch and reunite with one another to form an interlacing meshwork so that discrete layers are not readily discernible. Thus, from a functional viewpoint, the detrusor muscle comprises an integrated unit of interconnected muscle bundles which, on contraction, will cause a reduction in all dimensions of the bladder lumen (3, 19).

6.1. Fine structure of detrusor smooth muscle cells

Under the electron microscope, smooth muscle cells of the human urinary bladder are similar in appearance to those of the ureter. The cells are spindle-shaped, varying in length from 150 μm to 400 μm and from 6 μm to 8 μm in diameter (Fig. 8-13). An elongated nucleus occupies the widest part of each cell. The sarcoplasm is packed with myofilaments among which numerous electron-dense bodies are scattered. Organelles such as mitrochondria, Golgi membranes, and granular cisternae are relatively sparse and tend to cluster around either end of the elongated cell nucleus. The sarcolemma is characterized by rows of flask-shaped caveolae interspersed with subsarcolemmal electron-dense material. An electron-dense basal lamina surrounds each smooth muscle cell except at certain junctional regions.

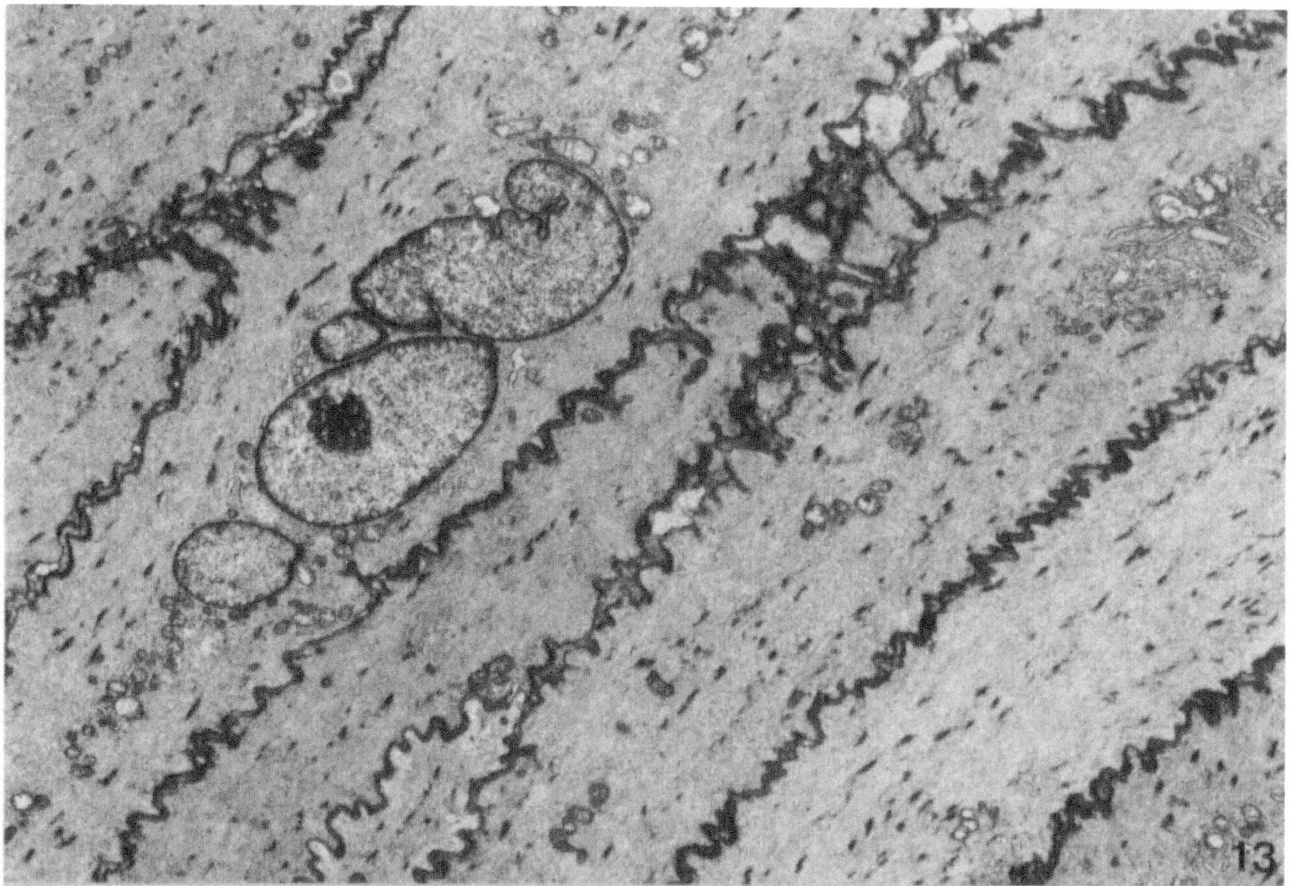
13

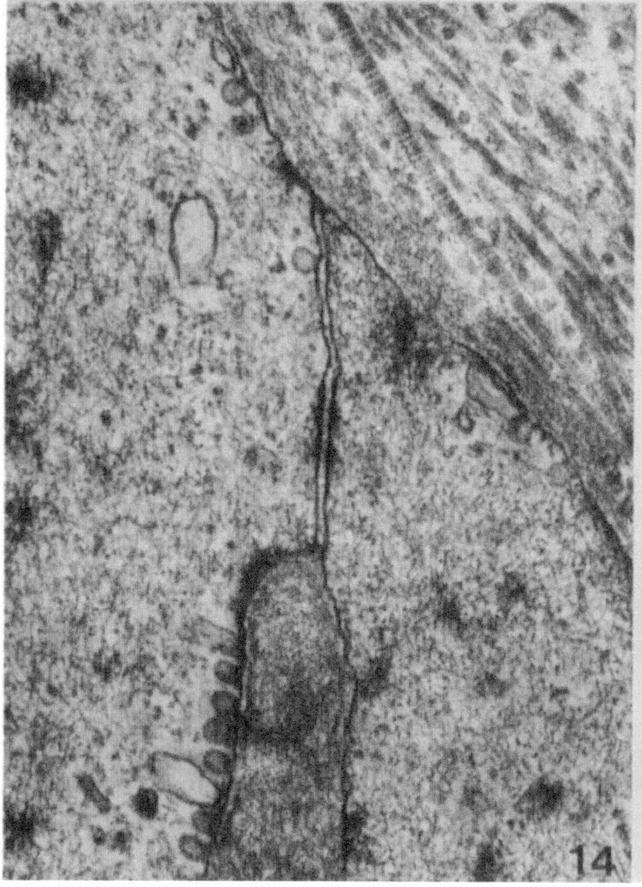
14

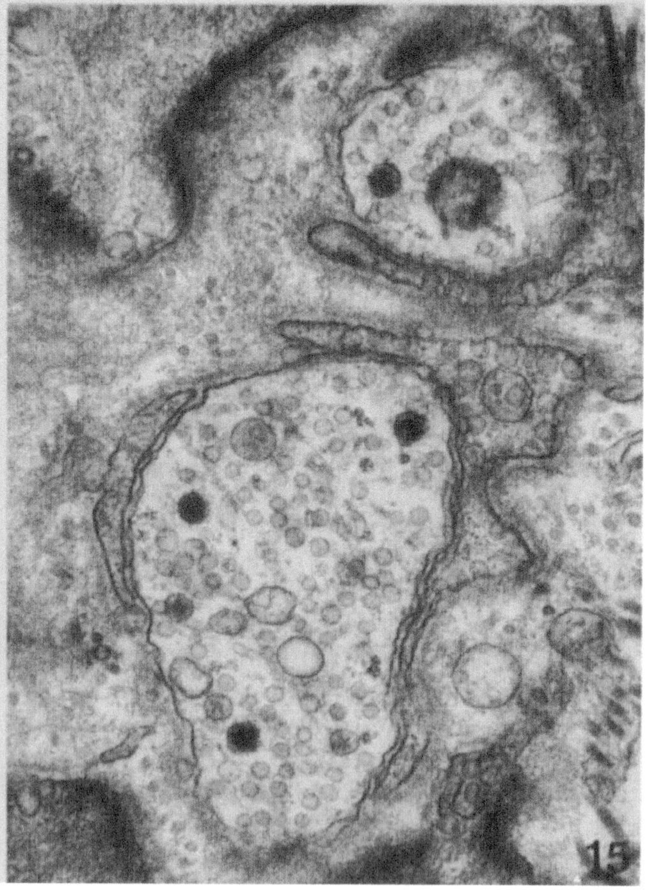
15

The most frequently observed type of junction between detrusor smooth muscle cells is the region of close approach (Fig. 8-14) at which an intercellular separation of 10–20 nm occurs over distances sometimes in excess of 1 μm . Junctions of the peg-and-socket and intermediate types are also present, although they are far less numerous than regions of close approach. True gap junctions (nexuses) are apparently absent from the detrusor muscle of humans and many other species that have been examined.

Since electrotonic spread of excitation occurs in the smooth muscle of the bladder wall, the regions of close approach may represent the morphological feature that enables this physiological event to take place in a similar manner to that in the ureter. Within each muscle bundle, the individual cells are closely packed together such that the basal lamina of one cell very often becomes confluent with that of its neighbors.

6.2. Innervation of the urinary bladder

The urinary bladder is profusely supplied with autonomic nerve fibers that form a dense plexus among the detrusor smooth muscle cells. The majority of these nerves contain acetylcholinesterase (20–22), and while they occur in profusion throughout the muscle coat of the bladder, some muscle bundles appear to be more richly innervated than others. In the electron microscope, the ratio of nerve axons to detrusor smooth muscle cells has been shown to be at least 1:1 (23). Most axonal varicosities lying adjacent to detrusor smooth muscle cells possess features characteristic of cholinergic nerve terminals (Fig. 8-15), i.e., they contain clusters of small (45–60 nm diameter) agranular vesicles together with occasional large (80–160 nm diameter) granulated vesicles and small mitochondria. Such terminal regions approach to within 20 nm of the muscle cells' surface and are either partially surrounded by or more often totally denuded of neurilemmal cell cytoplasm. Thus, the majority of the autonomic nerves innervating the detrusor muscle is considered to be excitatory cholinergic in type.

Unlike that of several other species (notably the cat), the human detrusor possesses an exceedingly sparse supply of sympathetic noradrenergic nerves (24). Although nerves of this type generally accompany the vascular supply to the bladder, they rarely extend among the smooth muscle cells of the detrusor.

In addition, it has been proposed that a third component occurs in the autonomic innervation of the urinary bladder (25). This nonadrenergic noncholinergic (NANC) nerve-mediated effect has been linked to several active substances, including vasoactive intestinal polypeptide, prostaglandins, and adenosine triphosphate, and it has been claimed that this NANC component represents a third type of effector nerve that provides a separate innervation to the bladder. Alternatively, it may be that other neurotransmitters are released by the cholinergic nerves that innervate the detrusor muscle. Under the electron microscope, axons containing a predominance of large granulated vesicles (80–160 nm diameter) together with occasional small agranular vesicles have been observed, although very infrequently, lying adjacent to detrusor smooth muscle cells. Whether such axons actually represent the proposed *peptidergic* type of autonomic effector nerve (the proportions of the two types of vesicle are reversed in a typical cholinergic nerve terminal) or whether they are merely chance sections through cholinergic axons has yet to be determined.

In addition, profiles containing a predominance of small mitochondria may occasionally be found among the smooth muscle cells of the bladder wall. It has been suggested that similar mitochondria-filled profiles in other tissues represent sensory nerve terminals (26). However, such profiles are relatively rare in the detrusor muscle of the bladder and may simply be sections

←

Figure 8-13. Closely packed detrusor smooth muscle cells from the human bladder wall. The cells have been fixed in the contracted state and consequently have extremely crenellated surfaces that interdigitate with one another. X 6400.

Figure 8-14. A region of close approach between adjacent detrusor smooth muscle cells. At such regions, the apposing membranes may possess subsarcolemmal accumulations of electron-dense material and/or caveolae. X 44,800.

Figure 8-15. A presumptive cholinergic axon terminal from human detrusor muscle. Numerous small agranular and occasional large granulated vesicles are characteristic of this type of axon. X 32,000.

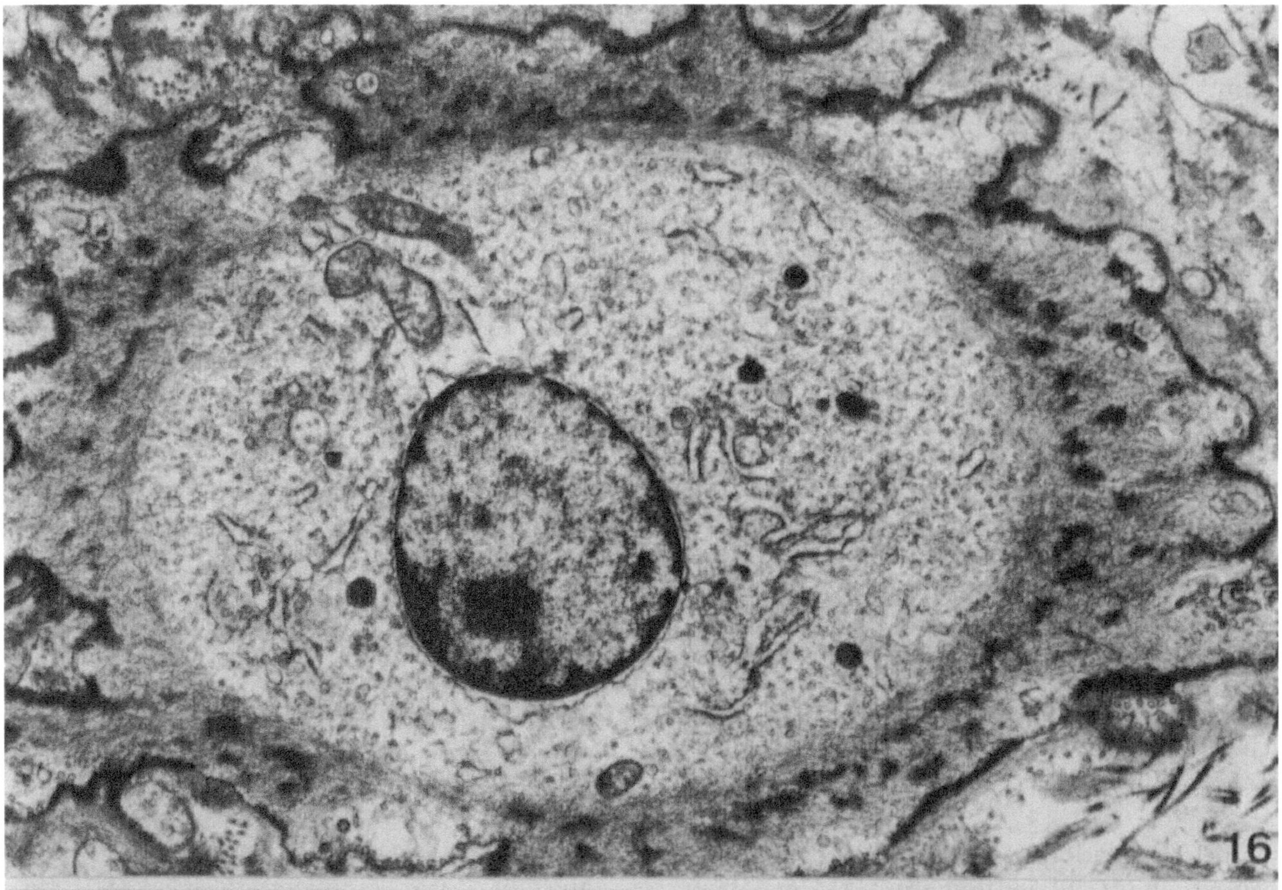
16

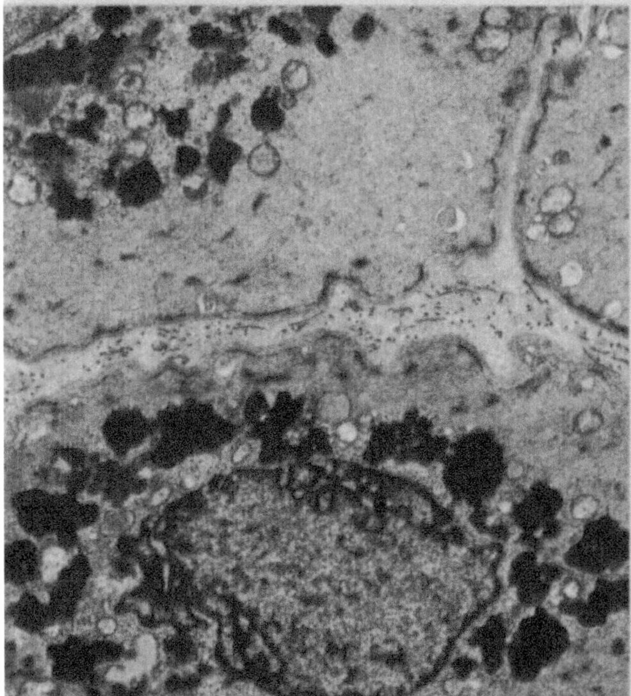
17

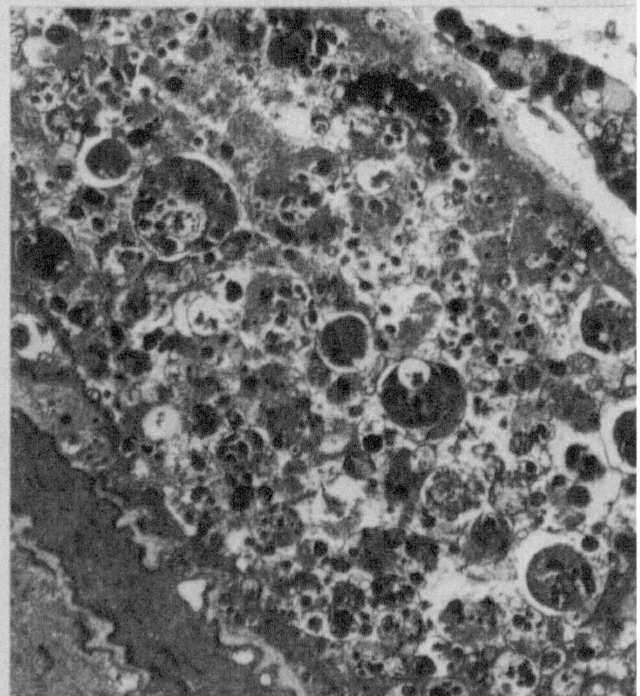
18

through mitochondria-rich areas of smooth muscle cells.

6.3. Intramural ganglia

Small clusters of autonomic ganglion cells occur throughout all regions of the human bladder wall, being especially numerous in the adventitia. These intramural ganglia contain from one to 20 or more acetylcholinesterase-positive, presumptive cholinergic neurons, similar to those occurring in the vesical plexus (27). Such neurons receive a preganglionic input from both cholinergic (excitatory) and noradrenergic (possibly inhibitory) nerve terminals (28).

The presence of two types of axosomatic terminals at the surface of the intramural ganglion cells has been confirmed by electron microscopy (29). Typical cholinergic preganglionic terminals contain numerous small agranular vesicles, while preganglionic noradrenergic terminals are distinguished by the presence of small, dense-cored vesicles.

Inhibition of detrusor muscle contraction may occur by inhibition of transmission to excitatory nerves within the intramural bladder ganglia, e.g., by the action of noradrenaline or adrenergic receptors on the cholinergic intramural neurons (30). In cats, it is known that sympathetic activity depresses bladder contractions both by an action on muscle (involving adrenoceptors) and an action to inhibit transmission in parasympathetic ganglia (also involving adrenoceptors) (31). However, in humans there is little direct sympathetic innervation of detrusor muscle, and therefore inhibition of ganglionic transmission appears to be the major mechanism of inhibition of detrusor smooth muscle in this species (23).

The ultrastructural features of the intramural ganglion cells are similar to those of other parasympathetic neurons that occur elsewhere. However, a number of unusual features have been described for the intramural neurons of the human bladder wall (32). First, the investing layer of satellite-cell cytoplasm is often incomplete, leaving large areas of the nerve-cell plasmalemma in direct contact with connective tissue. Second, groups of three or four nerve cells have been observed in close proximity to one another without an intervening layer of satellite cell cytoplasm. Nerve cells in this configuration thus form ephaptic connections with their neighbors over quite extensive areas of their surface. However, the functional significance of this arrangement is not clear. Third, many of the blood capillaries that course through the intramural ganglia have been shown to be fenestrated, and so adjacent nerve cells may be directly influenced by circulating hormones such as noradrenaline.

Electron microscopy has confirmed the presence of occasional small intensely fluorescent (SIF) cells in the intramural bladder ganglia. Cells of this type may be distinguished from ordinary ganglion cells by their content of numerous, large membrane-limited granules that are believed to represent amine storage sites.

6.4. Changes in the fine structure of urinary tract smooth muscle

It is well known that the intercellular connective tissue of the urinary tract may increase in amount in certain pathological conditions. This phenomenon is particularly marked in the bladders of patients with outflow obstruction (often due to prostatic hypertrophy). In such cases the detrusor muscle cells frequently become hypertrophied, and after longer times of obstruction many of the smooth muscle cells display an altered fine structure, the perinuclear region becoming filled with granular reticulum, mitochondria, and Golgi membranes (Fig. 8-16). Myofilaments and electron-dense bodies in these cells are confined to the cell periphery. In some instances, this apparent loss of myofilaments can be quite severe, and the cells begin to resemble fibroblasts except

←

Figure 8-16. A detrusor smooth muscle cell displaying an altered fine structure from a patient with bladder neck obstruction. The perinuclear region is filled with granular reticulum, while the myofilaments are confined to the cell's periphery. X 14,400.
Figure 8-17. An example of a detrusor myopathy. The sarcoplasm is packed with dense glycogen granules and numbers of large dense lysosomes. X 8200.
Figure 8-18. A smooth muscle cell from human detrusor muscle that is apparently undergoing spontaneous degeneration. The surrounding cells have a normal fine structure. X 6400.

that they still retain their covering of basal lamina. A similar alteration in fine structure has been described in the smooth muscle of the renal pelvic wall in cases of idiopathic hydronephrosis (33), where increased amounts of intercellular connective tissue also occur. Thus it appears that smooth muscle in both the upper and lower urinary tracts may react to obstruction by synthesizing connective tissue macromolecules and perhaps becoming less contractile in function.

In addition, urinary tract smooth muscle may display dramatic alterations in the fine structure due to unknown causes. Recently a case of detrusor muscle myopathy was reported (34) in which the smooth muscle cells of the bladder wall were packed with electron-dense glycogen granules and considerable numbers of lysosomes (Fig. 8-17). Finally, degeneration of individual smooth muscle cells in otherwise healthy detrusor muscle has also been observed in the electron microscope (Fig. 8-18).

References

1. Velardo JT: Histology of the ureter. In: The Ureter. H Bergman (ed), New York: Springer-Verlag, p 13–54, 1981.
2. Hanna MK, Jeffs RD, Sturgess JM, Barkin M: Ureteral structure and ultrastructure. I. The normal ureter. *J Urol* 116: 718–724, 1976.
3. Gosling JA, Dixon JS, Humpherson JR: Functional Anatomy of the Urinary Tract: An Integrated Text and Colour Altas. Edinburgh: Churchill Livingstone, 1983.
4. Notley RG: Electron microscopy of the lower ureter in man. *Br J Urol* 42: 439–445, 1970.
5. Gabella G: Structure of smooth muscles. In: Smooth Muscle: An Assessment of Current Knowledge. E Bulbring, AF Brading, AW Jones, T Tomita (eds), London: E Arnold, p 1–46, 1981.
6. Notley RG: Electron microscopy of the upper ureter and the pelvi-ureteric junction. *Br J Urol* 40: 37–51, 1968.
7. Merillees NCR: The nervous environment of individual smooth muscle cells of the guinea pig vas deferens, *J Cell Biol* 37: 794–817, 1968.
8. Henderson RM: Cell-to-cell contacts. In: Methods in Pharmacology, Vol 3, Smooth Muscle. EE Daniel DM Paton (eds), New York: Plenum Press, p 47–77, 1975.
9. Gosling JA, Dixon JS: Species variation in the location of upper urinary tract pacemaker cells. *Invest Urol* 11: 418–423, 1974.
10. Rizzo M, Pellegrini MSF, Riccardi RA, Penchietti R: Ultrastructure of the urinary tract muscle coat in man. *Eur Urol* 524: 171–177, 1981.
11. Dixon JS, Gosling JA: The fine structure of pacemaker cells in the pig renal calices. *Anat Rec* 175: 139–154, 1973.
12. Dixon JS, Gosling JA: The musculature of the human renal calices, pelvis and upper ureter. *J Anat* 135: 129–138, 1982.
13. Schulman, CC: Electron microscopy of the human ureteric innervation. *Br J Urol* 46: 609–623, 1974.
14. Burnstock G: Structure of smooth muscle and its innervation. In: Smooth Muscle. E Bulbring, AF Brading, AW Jones, T Tomita (eds), London: Edward Arnold, p 1–70, 1970.
15. Davis JE, Hagedorn JP, Bergmann LL: Anatomy and ultrastructure of the ureter. In: The Ureter. H Bergman (ed), New York: Springer-Verlag, p 55–70, 1981.
16. Duarte-Escalante O, Labay P, Boyarsky S: The neurohistochemistry of mammalian ureter: a new combination of histochemical procedures to demonstrate adrenergic, cholinergic and chromaffin structures in ureter, *J Urol* 101: 803–811, 1969.
17. Constantinou CE: Renal pelvic pacemaker control of ureteral peristaltic rate. *Am J Physiol* 226: 1413–1416, 1974.
18. Constantinou CE, Djurhuus JC: Urodynamics of the multicalceal upper urinary tract. In: Idiopathic Hydronephrosis. PH O'Reilly, JA Gosling (eds), London: Springer-Verlag, p 16–43, 1981.
19. Gosling JA: The structure of the bladder and urethra in relation to function. *Urol Clin North* Am 6: 31–38, 1979.
20. Mobley TL, Elbadawi A, McDonald DF, Schenk EA: Innervation of the human urinary bladder. *Surg Forum* 27: 505–506, 1966.
21. Elbadawi A: Neuromorphologic basis of vesicourethral function: 1. Histochemistry, ultrastructure and function of intrinsic nerves of the bladder and urethra. *Neurourol Urodynam* 1: 3–50, 1982.
22. McConnell J, Benson GS, Wood JG: Autonomic innervation of the urogenital system. Adrenergic and cholinergic elements. *Brain Res Bull* 9: 679–694, 1982.
23. Daniel FE, Cowan W, Daniel VP: Structural bases for neural and myogenic control of human detrusor muscle. *Can J Physiol Pharm* 61: 1247–1273, 1983.
24. Sundin T, Dahlstrom A, Norlen L, Svedmyr N: The sympathetic innervation and adrenoceptor function of the human lower urinary tract in the normal state and after parasympathetic denervation. *Invest Urol* 14: 322–328, 1977.
25. Ambache N, Zar MA: Non-cholinergic transmission by post-ganglionic motor neurons in the mammalian bladder. *J Physiol* 210: 761–783, 1970.
26. Iwayama T, Furness JB, Burnstock G: Dual adrenergic and cholinergic innervation of the cerebral arteries of the rat. *Circ Res* 26: 635–646, 1970.
27. Dixon JS, Gilpin SA, Gilpin CJ, Gosling JA: Intramural ganglia of the human urinary bladder. *Br J Urol* 55: 195–198, 1983.
28. de Groat WC, Booth AM: Inhibition and facilitation in parasympathetic ganglia of the urinary bladder. *Fed Proc* 39: 2990–2996, 1980.
29. Gilpin CJ: Fine structure of the intrinsic autonomic innervation of the human urinary bladder. M.Sc. thesis, Manchester University.

30. Fletcher TF, Bradley WF: Neuroanatomy of the bladder–urethra. *J Urol* 119: 153–160, 1978.
31. de Groat WC, Theobald RJ: Sympathetic inhibitor reflexes to the urinary bladder and ganglia evoked by electrical stimulation of vesical afferents. *J Physiol (Lond)* 259: 223–237, 1976.
32. Gilpin CJ, Dixon JS, Gilpin SA, Gosling JA: The fine structure of autonomic neurons in the wall of the human urinary bladder. *J Anat (Lond)* 137: 705–713, 1983.
33. Gosling JA, Dixon JS: The structure of the normal and hydronephrotic upper urinary tract. In: Idiopathic Hydronephrosis. PH O'Reilly, JA Gosling (eds), London: Springer-Verlag p 1–15, 1981.
34. Barnard RJ, Dixon JS, Gosling JA: Myopathy of detrusor smooth muscle. *Br J Urol* 59: 595–596, 1987.

Author's address:
Dr. John S. Dixon
Department of Cell & Structural Biology
University of Manchester
Stopford Building
Oxford Road
Manchester M13 9PT
England

CHAPTER 9

Smooth muscle in the male genital tract

GERHARD AUMÜLLER

1. Introduction

The male genital system is a ductal structure of considerable length consisting of different portions of highly specialized (secretory, absorptive, or motile) epithelial surfaces that interact with the intraluminal spermatozoa. During their transit through the ductal system, spermatozoa acquire their final step of maturation (1). While the functions of the epithelia in the male genital system are comparably well understood (2), the knowledge of the functional significance of the underlying motor elements is rather limited. It is generally presumed that the structure and function of myofibroblasts and smooth muscle cells surrounding the genital duct system are constructed in a way that is required for optimal function of the respective epithelium, i.e., intraluminal pressure, velocity in the passage of the intraluminal contents, retention or preservation of the geometrical configuration of the duct, speed of contraction, etc. Previous morphological studies have focused on the geometrical arrangement of muscle cells in the duct walls (3, 4, 5) and functional deductions have been made from the innervation patterns and densities of the smooth muscle cells. Also, the different histogenetic origin (Wolffian or Müllerian duct, urogenital sinus) has been taken into account (6). This was particularly important with respect to the pathogenetic mechanisms of certain pathological alterations such as benign prostatic hyperplasia. In the last few years, this pathological entity, previously known as prostatic adenoma, has been recognized to be primarily dependent upon a reactivation of the stroma. Considerable efforts have been focused on the question of the mechanism of induction of growth, proliferation, differentiation, and eventually hyperplasia of the epithelium as a consequence of stromal reactivation.

No definite interpretation of this and other questions in the cell biology of smooth muscle cells of the male genital system has been achieved as yet in spite of an enormous increase in knowledge on specific properties of smooth muscle cells, their subcellular elements, and their molecular components.

Recent observations on the distribution of smooth muscle cell-specific actins (7, 8), intermediate filaments (9, 10), and actin-binding proteins (11, 12), or the expression of growth factors (13, 14), have mostly been made in vascular or gastrointestinal smooth muscle. Only few studies regarding these recent topics in cell biology have been extended systematically to the different muscular components of smooth muscle in the male genital system (15, 16).

The present chapter therefore will present an overview of the regional morphology of contractile cellular components in the male genital system, starting in the testis and ending in penile urethra. The developmental changes in postnatal development, pubertal maturation, and senescent involution will be interpreted with regard to the general hormonal and metabolic situation. Finally, functional aspects, particularly with regard to pathological deviations, will be demonstrated focusing on the clinically most relevant example, that is, prostatic smooth muscle cells, the morphological substrate of benign prostatic hyperplasia.

2. Regional fine structure

2.1. Testis

The presence and distribution of contractile elements in the walls of the seminiferous tubules and along the ductus epididymidis is essential to an understanding of the intratubular hydrostatic pressure and of the transport of spermatozoa and fluid dynamics in the testis and epididymis. Johnson and Howards (17) have measured intratubular hydrostatic pressure in hamster seminiferous tubules and epididymal ducts. They found that although the pressure in the caput epididymidis was significantly higher than the pressure in the caudal tubules, the pressure in the seminiferous tubules was significantly lower than that in the caput. Therefore, the transport of sperm and fluid from the testis to the epididymis is most likely effected by intermittent elevations of intraseminiferous tubular pressure secondary to tubular and capsular contractions.

2.1.1. Capsule. Spontaneous contractions have been observed in the testicular capsule (18) as well as in seminiferous tubules (19). The occurrence of smooth muscle cells in testicular capsules has been described in various mammals (20). In cat and dog testis they are most numerous, and less prominent in rat and human. In the anterior part of the capsule, the number of cells is few; they may even be lacking. Posteriorly, as the capsule approaches and becomes continuous with the mediastinum, cells accumulate, particularly near the rete testis. Here they are packed quite closely, commonly in a parallel fashion, with occasional cell contacts in the form of close opposition of small cytoplasmic processes. The cells are generally flat, sometimes with branching processes. Their nuclei are elongated, often with irregular outlines. Most of the cytoplasm is occupied by tightly packed myofilaments and interlocking dense bodies (Fig. 9-2). Organelles are located mainly at the poles of the nuclei, including mitochondria, rough endoplasmic reticulum, free ribosomes, and a Golgi apparatus. Caveolae close to the surface are often continuous with the plasmalemma. A basal lamina is associated with the cell surface. Often it appears incomplete, with a close association of both collagen and elastic material.

The majority of capsular cells obviously responsible for testicular capsular contractions in vitro (21) are myofibroblasts (22). These cells show ovoid nuclei and marginally condensed chromatin. Indentations of the nuclear surface are rarely observed (Fig. 9-1). Cell organelles accumulate at the nuclear poles. Abundant cisternae of endoplasmic reticulum are seen, often distended and replete with a fine granular content. Free ribosomes, polyribosomes, a few multivesicular bodies, lysosomes, and mitochondria are found close to the prominent Golgi apparatus. The majority of vesicles is attached to the cell surface in a manner similar to the caveolae in smooth muscle.

A considerable portion of the cells contain bundles of 6–8 nm thin filaments. These are usually situated near the plasma membrane and are most prominent in cytoplasmic processes. Condensed areas resembling the dense bodies of smooth muscle cells are interspersed in the filament bundles. Filaments insert in plaques of electron-dense material that are attached to the inner zone of the plasma membrane. The cells lack a continuous basal lamina, but basal-lamina-like material can be found close to their surface in circumscribed areas.

The myofibroblasts of the testicular capsule develop elongated ramified processes containing only few organelles but prominent bundles of filaments. The processes of neighboring cells reach each other. Specialized contacts seem to be absent. Often, the plasma membranes of two cells run parallel at a distance of 8–12 nm, but no marked structural differentiation is seen in the intercellular space. Extracellular connective tissue consists predominantly of collagen and microfibrils and occasionally of some elastic material. The mode of mechanical linkage of myofibroblasts with fibrillar material of the extracellular material is uncertain. Microfibrils, frequently arranged to bundles, approach the cells at the dense plaques. Perhaps these have a structure similar to the fibronexus observed at other locations (23).

2.1.2. Seminiferous tubule. Clermont (24) described contractions of rat seminiferous tubules in vitro as traveling over short distances and moving in the direction of the rete testis. The cellular substrate of these contractions has been identified in the peritubular myofibroblasts. These are present in the lamina propria of the seminiferous tubules of man (25–29), mouse (30, 31), monkey (28), rat (32, 33), dog (34), swine (35, 36), sheep (37), snake (38), and several other vertebrates, where they are arranged in a species-specific manner (28, 39). The boundary tissue of the seminiferous tubule of the rat consists of four different layers: 1) an inner noncellular layer comprising various amounts of collagen sandwiched between two basement membranes; 2) the inner cellular layer of contractile cells, i.e., myofibroblasts; 3) the outer noncellular layer containing scattered collagen fibrills; and 4) the outer layer of very flat cells without fine filaments, probably fibroblasts and referred to as the endothelium of peritubular lymphatic vessels by some authors.

While in ultrathin sections the appearance of the peritubular myofibroblasts has been described as stellate (26, 28), in the scanning electron microscope, after disclosing their surface by collagenase treatment (33), peritubular myofibroblasts are identified as a layer of flat squamous (down to 1 μm thick) cells (Fig. 9-3). They are thin, attenuated (with the exception of the nucleus bulging slightly at the central portion) cells of various shape, ranging from rectangular to hexagonal or polygonal and arranged close to each other, as seen in freeze-fracture replicas (Fig. 9-4).

In the human testis, the outer aspect of the tubular basal lamina faces a number of layers (usually not more than six) of myofibroblasts and intercellular spaces, mostly occupied by collagen fibers. The existence of elastic fibers has been denied by Bustos-Obregon and Holstein (26), but confirmed by Hermo et al. (28). In human peritubular myofibroblasts, a discontinuous basement-membrane-like structure is seen, while in the hamster it is continuous, 40–80 nm thick, and particularly rich in alkaline phosphatase (40, 41). Cross-sectioned myofibroblasts are thin, elongated cells replete with bundles of filaments measuring 8 nm, which are particularly abundant in the peripheral zone of the cytoplasm and anchored to dense plaques at the plasma membrane (Figs. 9-5–9-7). Here, numerous caveolae or vesicles are found. Neighboring cells are in close contact (intermediate junction type, intercellular space of about 15 Å). Mitochondria and glycogen granules are found intermingled with short profiles of rough endoplasmic reticulum in the cytoplasm. Also, smooth membranous inclusions are seen. Whether or not these are related to phagosomes, observed in testicular smooth muscle cells in urodela (42), is not clear. The nucleus is elongated, rich in peripherally condensed chromatin and sometimes of irregular outline. The Golgi zone is polarized towards on extremity of the cytoplasm facing the nucleus, sometimes containing some electron-dense material. The size of the Golgi apparatus seems to be hormone-dependent. In the blinded hamster, the Golgi apparatus of peritubular myofibroblasts becomes much more prominent (40) than in normal cells. Arrays of vesicles extend from the poles of the Golgi stacks up to the plasmalemma and fuse with it, whereas the alkaline phosphatase-containing vesicles are believed to be involved in the formation of the alkaline phosphatase-rich basal laminae of the peritubular tissue. Using heavy meromyosine (HMM) decoration of partly extracted porcine or human peritubular cells, Toyama (36) was able to demonstrate the presence of actin in these cells (Fig. 9-8). The periodicity of bound HMM complexes was 35 nm. Individual filaments showed arrowheads that pointed in the same direction, but opposing polarity of the HMM-decorated filaments was also observed. Thicker filaments (10 nm) observed by Toyama (36) have been identified as myosin through the use of immunohistochemical methods (29, 43). Immunohistochemistry has likewise revealed the presence of both vimentin and desmin (15, 44) in human and rat peritubular cells. In addition to these two intermediate filament proteins, the peritubular cells express a nonerythroid α-spectrin immunoanalogue (15). This characteristic feature distinguishes rat peritubular myofibroblasts from most other smooth muscle cells that lack nonerythroid α-spectrin immunoreactivity (45).

Recent studies on peritubular cells cultured in vitro (44) have shown that these cells secrete proteins that are characteristic for this cell type.

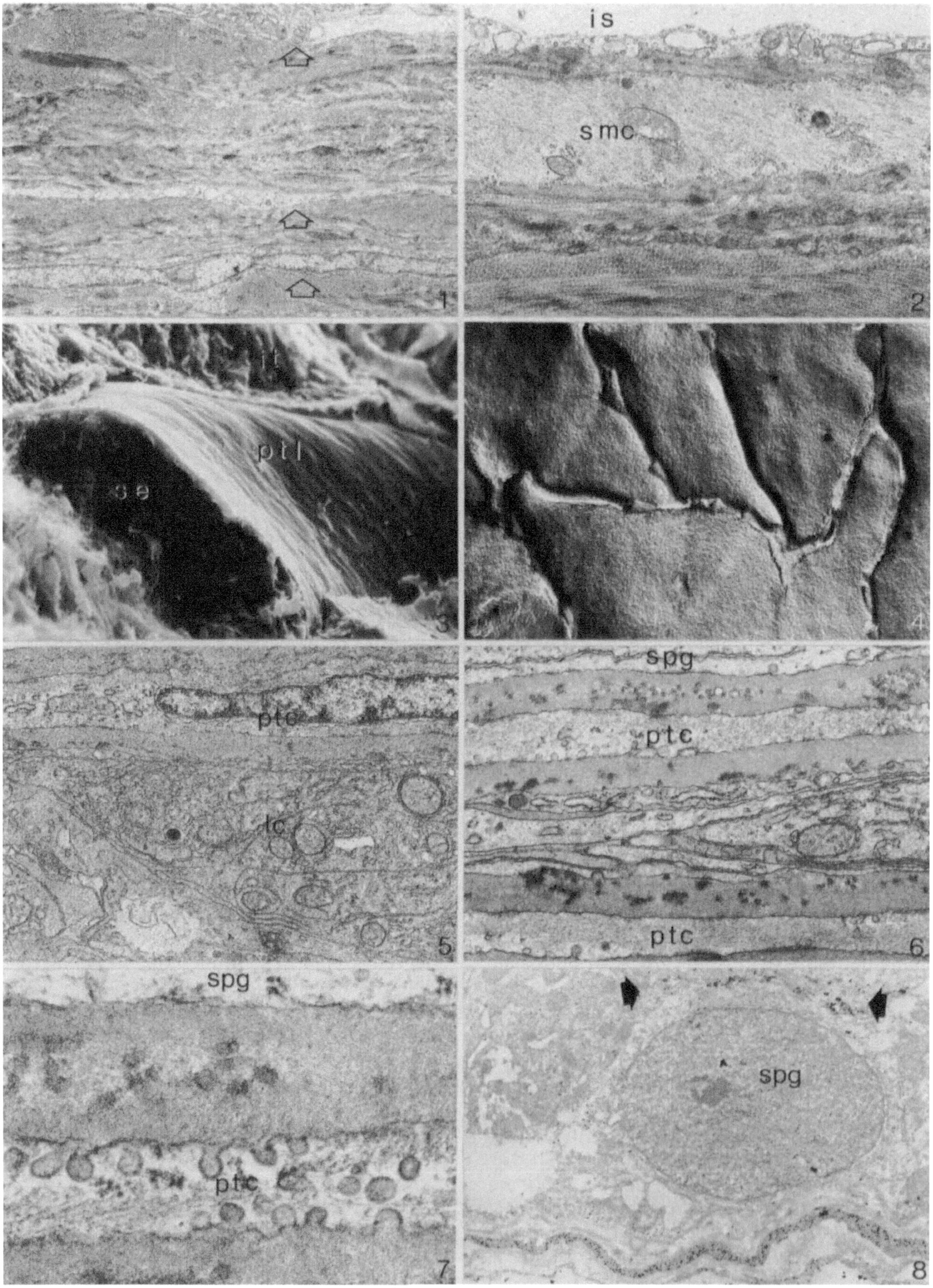
1
is
smc
2
ptl
se
3
4
ptc
lc
5
spg
ptc
ptc
6
spg
ptc
7
spg
8

The predominant secreted protein was designated P 40 (M_r 40000); it was found also in incubation media of cultured seminiferous tubular cells, but was absent in incubation medium of cultured Sertoli cells or in the incubation medium of seminiferous tubular segments after enzymatic removal of their peritubular cell wall. Among additional proteins produced by peritubular cells in vitro, fibronectin could be of particular interest (46), since it could reflect the adaptation of cultured cells to an inert substrate upon which they are plated.

2.2. *Epididymis*

During passage through the epididymis, sperm achieve functional maturity, developing both the capacity for forward motility and for effecting fertilization of the ovum (47). The passage through the epididymis allows the interaction of the epididymal epithelium with the sperm surface, resulting in the remodeling of the shape of the acrosome, increased disulfide bonding of certain sperm structures, and other changes in the structural and biochemical properties of the plasma membrane (2).

Sperm passage through the epididymal duct is effected by active contractions of the duct wall regulating the duration of contact between intratubular spermatozoa and the surrounding epididymal epithelium (48).

Peristaltic movements characterize the contractions of the epididymal tubules in vivo (49), while the distal cauda and vas deferens show brief, forceful nerve-mediated reflex contractions during ejaculation. These differences in contractility are correlated with changes in the complex architecture of the tubular wall in the various epididymal segments (50).

In the human epididymis (51), there is a continuous increase in the amount of tubular contractile cells starting with circularly arranged smooth muscle cells in the ductuli efferentes and ductus epididymidis at the proximal caput. Scanty strands of longitudinally and obliquely oriented smooth muscle bundles form an additional incomplete outer muscle layer around the ductus epididymidis of the corpus. Myofibroblasts are predominantly found around the excretory ducts from the ductuli efferentes to the midcauda (52, 53).

At the transition of the corpus and cauda epididymidis, ordinary large smooth muscle cells are interspersed between the myofibroblasts, forming a composite thick subepithelial muscle coat. More distally, the two-layered muscle coat of the deferential portion of the ductus epididymidis acquires a third longitudinally oriented layer, a pattern of construction that is retained in the vas deferens.

Based on previous findings of Holstein (50), Baumgarten et al. (51) distinguish three types of contractile cells in the human epididymis: 1) contractile cells of medium electron density containing exclusively thin filaments (6 nm), 2) dark contractile cells containing bundles of thin and single thick filaments (14 nm), and 3) light contractile cells with loosely dispersed, interweaving thin and thick filaments (Figs. 9-9–9-13). In addition, ordinary smooth muscle cells occur in the wall of the cauda epididymidis and throughout the vas deferens. These contain an abundance of thin filaments of uniform size (Figs. 9-14, 9-15). Frequent interweaving occurs between small bundles of myofilaments, causing a more or less regular distribution pattern of dispersed dense bodies. A similar regular pattern of dense patches is observed at the inner aspect of the plasma membrane, which alternates with areas where caveolae are numerous. Cell organelles accu-

←

Figures 9-1–9-8. Myofibroblasts and smooth muscle cells in the rat testis. (1) In the capsule only very few, thin myofibroblasts (arrows) are present (X 3000). (2) Smooth muscle cell (smc) in the testicular capsule of the rat close to its inner aspect (is) (X 10,000). (3) Survey scanning electron micrograph of a seminiferous tubule of the rat testis exposing the peritubular layer (ptl), the inerstitial tissue (it) and the seminiferous epithelium (se) (X 300). (4) Freeze-etch replica of peritubular cells apposed in flat interlocking extensions (X 21,000). (5) A peritubular cell (ptc) of the rat testis neighboring a Leydig cell (lc) (X 10,800). (6) Alternating distribution of peritubular cells (ptc) and acellular connective tissue underneath a spermatogonium (spg) (X 17,100). (7) At high magnification, the peritubular cell (ptc) facing a spermatogonium (spg) shows numerous clear vesicles (X 45,000). (8) Immunohistochemical demonstration of actin in a peritubular cell using the immunogold technique. Immunoreactive actin is also visible at the Sertoli cell junction (arrows) above a spermatogonium (spg) (X 5000).

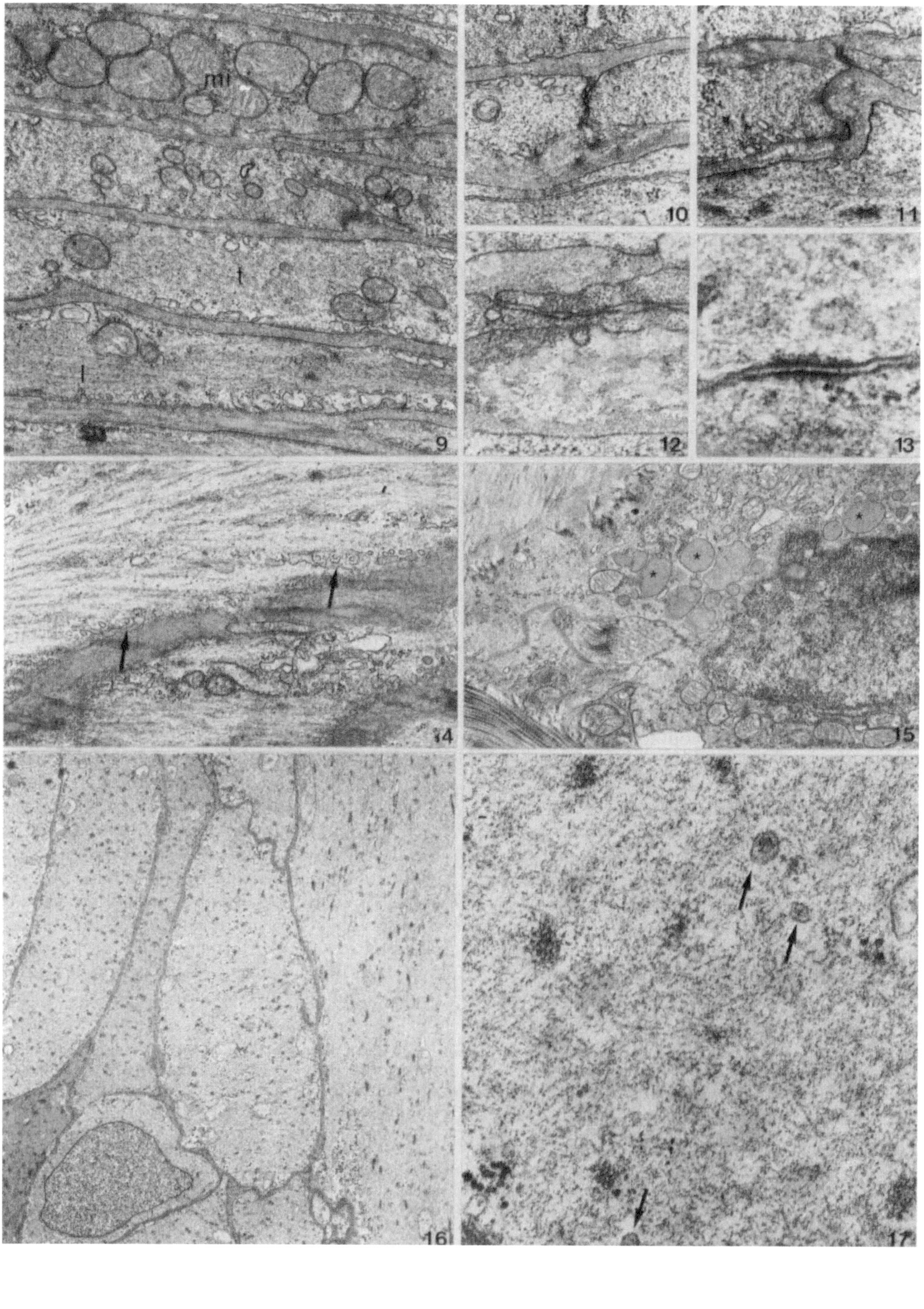
mi
9
10
11
12
13
14
15
16
17

mulate in the proximity of the nucleus, but are also irregularly distributed all over the cell. Fingerlike processes protrude from the cells, sometimes forming contacts of an intermediate type with neighboring cells. Infrequently, bulbous protrusions of one muscle cell are seen enclosed by crescentlike portions of an adjacent cell.

A generally similar distribution of contractile cells was described in the rat epididymis by Francavilla et al. (54). Here, flat cells with light cytoplasm are disposed in two to three over-lapping layers around the epithelium. These cells contain exclusively thin filaments (5–6 nm in diameter) that are concentrated at the periphery of the cell. In the distal caput and corpus, these cells are surrounded by two to three layers of electron-dense (dark) cells, which are replaced by smooth muscle cells along the cauda. The electron density of these cells seem to depend on the dense arrangement of microfilament bundles containing mostly thin filaments intermingled in a lattice like fashion with thick ones (11–12 nm in diameter). In the human epididymis, increased density of dark myofibroblasts was thought to result from accumulated membranes of the endoplasmic reticulum (51). These membranes are often found in concentric arrays around individual mitochondria or clusters of ribosomes. They are arranged in longitudinally oriented lamellar complexes filling large areas of the cytoplasm. At the very ends of these complexes, small vesicles are found intermingled with glycogen.

Another type of filamentous structure is scattered in the cytoplasm of these dark cells, appearing as a tubule of 14–15 nm in diameter surrounded by a halo (51, 55). In human epididymis, a third type of contractile cell is found with particularly electron-translucent cytoplasm and only loosely arranged strands of microfilaments. These are often running obliquely, interweaving with longitudinally oriented filaments. A certain number of these filaments measure about 14 nm in diameter. At places, individual myofilaments seem to change their diameter along their length from 14 nm to 6 nm and the reverse. Sometimes changes occur at regular intervals, producing the impression of textural periodicity.

An electron-dense basement membrane regularly surrounds both the dark cells and the large smooth muscle cells, but is discontinuous around the light cells. The thickness of the basement membrane increases after castration (56).

Large areas of apposition are visible between neighboring cells, but no junctional specializations of the plasma membrane have been observed by these authors. The intercellular space contains collagen and elastic fibers. The number of the latter increases towards the outer cell layers, being particularly high in the cauda between the smooth muscle cells. Immunohistochemically, Francavilla et al. (54) have found fibronectin scattered around the contractile cells mainly in the cauda, where elastic fibers are particularly numerous. This supports the contention that fibronectin may allow contractile cells to transfer their mechanical activity to elastic fibers and collagen (which lack an active contractile function), thus facilitating a homogeneous and rapid transmission of the contraction to the entire tubular wall.

2.3. Vas deferens

The human vas deferens consists of two portions, the vasal segment and the ampulla. The former is cylindrical in shape, measuring about 40 cm in length with an external diameter of 2–4 mm; its structure resembles that of the cauda epididymidis (57). The latter, only 5 cm in length, is

←

Figures 9-9–9-15. Myofibroblasts and smooth muscle cells in the rat epididymis. (9) Different forms of myofibroblasts in the caput epididymidis. One cell contains numerous large mitochondria (mi). Note the transverse (t) or longitudinal (l) orientation of the microfilaments (X 17,000). (10–13) Different forms of intermediate type junctions observed between epididymal myofibroblasts (10: X 28,000, 11: X 25,000, 12: X 60,000, 13: X 80,000). (14) Smooth muscle cell from the distal portion of the rat epididymis with a peculiar type of surface vesicles (arrows; X 20,000); (15) Granule (asterisk) containing smooth muscle cell from the cauda epididymidis (X 12,000).

Figures 9-16 and 9-17. Smooth muscle cells from the vas deferens of the rat. (16) Survey electron micrograph showing the high density in the arrangement of smooth muscle cells (X 4000). (17) Surface vesicles containing dense-core material (arrows) in smooth muscle cells of the vas deferens (X 60,000).

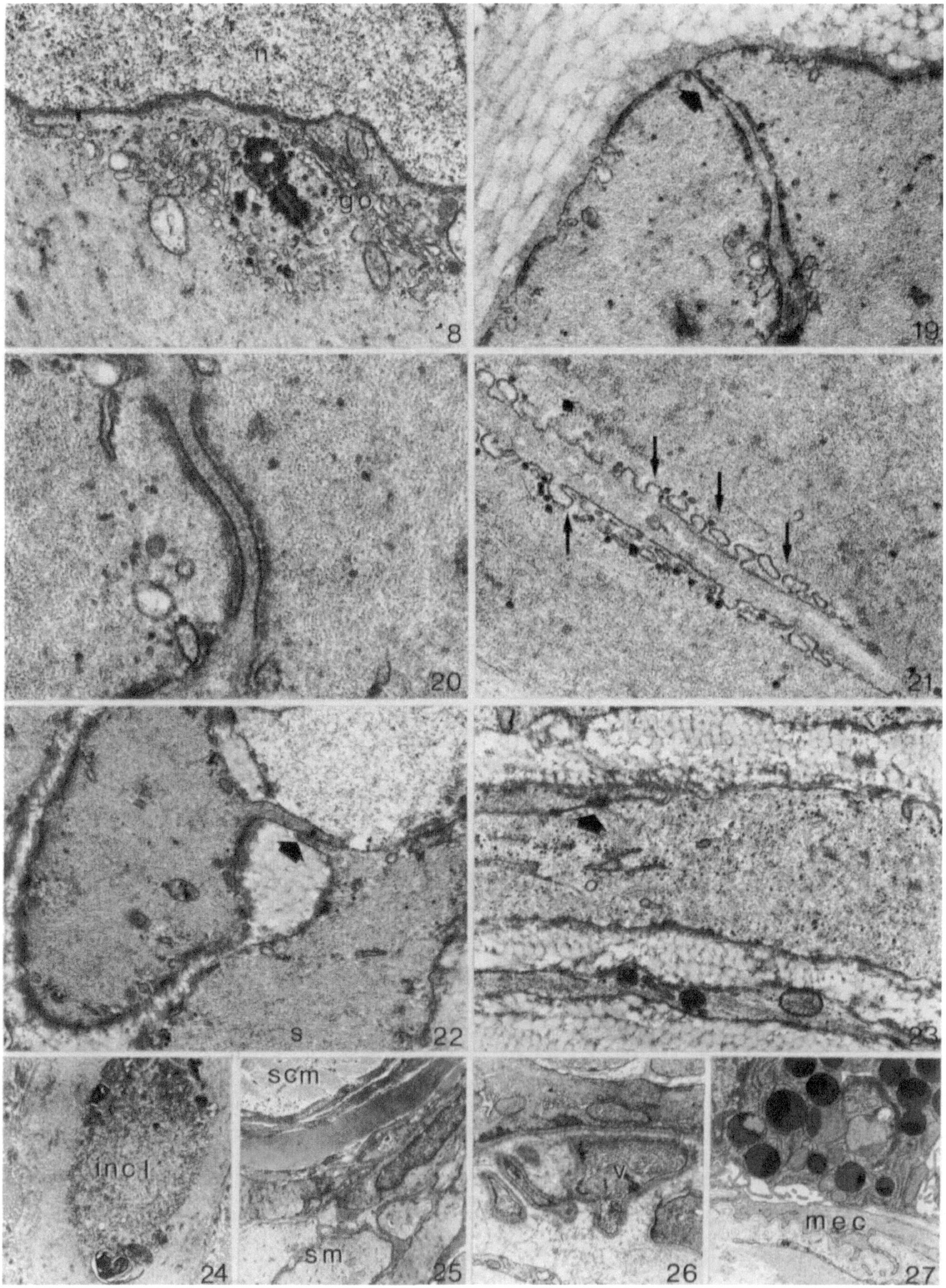

n
go
18
19
20
21
s
22
23
incl
24
scm
sm
25
v
26
mec
27

dilated and fusiform, and its structure resembles that of the seminal vesicles (58). Smooth muscle makes up about 92%–99% of the vas deferens cross-sectional area (59). The outer longitudinal muscle layer composes 32% to 60% of the total vas deferens cross-sectional area, whereas the inner longitudinal plus and circular muscle layers make up 39% to 59% of the total vas deferens cross-sectional area (59).

Although there are several studies on the ultrastructure of the vas deferens in the rat (60, 61, 62), mouse (63), guinea pig (64, 65, 66), rabbit (67), and human (51, 57, 68, 69), the fine structure of the smooth muscle in the deferential wall has not been intensively studied. More detailed observations have been recently made in smooth muscle cells of the rat vas deferens (70) (Figs. 9-16, 9-17). In addition to the ultrastructural features already described in the epididymis section, vesicular and tubular membranous structures containing an electron-opaque material were found in the smooth muscle cells. Similar structures were also found in a subfraction of microsomes of vas deferens smooth muscle, which was shown to be rich both in plasma membrane and in putative endoplasmic reticulum markers. Treatment of the tissues with calcium-free Krebs solution containing EGTA prior to fixation eliminated almost completely the presence of these dense-cored membranous structures (DMSs). Tracer studies using horseradish peroxidase suggested that some of the DMS may be continuous to the extracellular space and may originate from infolding of the plasma membrane. The authors suggest that these structures may be involved in the regulation of intracellular calcium. In the canine vas deferens, differences in cell shape and cell contacts occur between proximal and distal portions of the vas deferens (Figs. 9-18–9-23).

2.4. Seminal vesicles

The secretions of the seminal vesicles are added to the ejaculate subsequent to the contractions of the prostate and the vas deferens (71), effecting a coagulation of the seminal fluid that is moderate in humans and strong in rodents (*copulatory plug*) (72).

Similar to the vas deferens, smooth muscle cells of the human seminal vesicles form different layers, the exact arrangement of which is controversial (73). Previous studies of Gall (4) and Düllmann (74) in monkey seminal vesicle walls, indicating three layers, have been challenged. Instead, the different layers (ranging between two and ten) should be regarded as flat, interlacing ribbons of different length and thickness, arranged in a curved or spiral or helical course. Secondary and tertiary ramifications originate from these flat interlacing ribbons, particularly in the subepithelial layer, forming basketlike aggregations of smooth muscle cells around individual glandular structures.

The ultrastructure of smooth muscle cells in human seminal vesicles is largely similar to that of the distal cauda portion of the epididymis or the vas deferens. A particular feature, also observed in prostatic smooth muscle, is presence of knoblike protrusions from the cells that are in close contact with neighboring cells, bulging into cuplike depressions of the adjacent cell. At these locations, the intercellular space is narrowed to ≈20 nm. Several surface vesicles, often in a trifoillike arrangement, are found underneath the plasma membranes of either cell.

In human seminal vesicle smooth muscle cells, signs of degeneration are often encountered. An early event is the appearance of glycogen particles scattered throughout the cytoplasm and accumu-

←

Figures 9-18–9-23. Smooth muscle cells in the canine vas deferens (18–20: distal portion; 21–23: ampullary portion). (18) Golgi area (go) with a pair of centrioles close to the nucleus (n) (X 21,000). (19) Gap junction (arrow) between smooth muscle cells (X 40,000). (20) Symmetric arrangement of dense patches at the plasma membranes of adjacent smooth muscle cells (X 81,000). (21) Peculiar type of surface vesicles (arrows) in ampullary smooth muscle cells (X 60,000). (22) Thin, overlapping extensions of neighboring smooth muscle cells (s) forming a focal contact (arrow) (X 32,000). (23) Thin layer of myofibroblasts in between the layers of smooth muscle and of epithelium: some cells are connected by intermediate junctions (arrow) (X 25,000).

Figures 9-24–9-27. Smooth muscle cells in the seminal vesicle and the penile urethra. (24) In aged humans, some smooth muscle cells contain amorphous inclusions (incl) derived from deteriorated cytoplasmic organelles (X 6000). (25) Interlacing bundles of striated (scm) and smooth (sm) muscle cells in the rat urethra (X 1200). (26) Smooth muscle cells containing numerous vesicles (v) in a urethral artery (X 5000). (27) Myoepithelial cell (mec) from the bulbocavernous gland of the rat. (X 3500).

lating on the poles of the elongated nucleus.

The increase in glycogen is accompanied by an increase in number of surface vesicles of the cells. In more advanced stages, their cytoplasm is characterized by a very prominent accumulation of glycogen, the cisternae of rough endoplasmic retriculum become dilated, and desquamation of ribosomes from the membranes is seen. This leads to a continuous reduction of cytoplasmic organelles and a replacement by amorphous material (Fig. 9-24).

2.5. *Prostate gland*

The secretions of the prostate are among the first portions of the ejaculate to be expelled from the posterior urethra (71). Because (at least in the rat), the prostate's contents have components that delay semen coagulation, these secretions are hypothesized to be essential in preventing premature semen coagulation, which soon would obliterate the urethra. Because of its strategic situation at the juncture of the urinary and seminal pathways and its particular propensity to develop benign hyperplasia or even malignant transformation, the prostate gland has attained considerable interest of morphologists and endocrinologists. Nonetheless, the fibromuscular stroma of the adult prostate has received little attention, although several ultrastructural studies on the human (73, 75–79) canine (80, 81) and rodent prostate (82–86) exist.

In the human prostate, more or less thick bundles of smooth muscle cells extend radially from the composite musculature of the urethra and merge peripherally into the prostatic capsule, which is made up of an outer vascular, intermediate fibrous, and inner muscular layer. Secondary bundles form a sometimes circular and sometimes oblique or tangential interlobular or periductal layer, which is continuous with thin tertiary bundles that are arranged in a basketlike manner around the acini (5). The ultrastructure of prostatic smooth muscle cells is rather identical in various species and locations within the gland. The cytoplasm of these cells is occupied chiefly by fine filaments (6 nm in diameter) that are mainly oriented parallel to the long axis of the cell. Spindle-shaped dense bodies are scattered through the course of the filaments. The latter extend into dense plaques subjacent to the plasma membrane. The arrangement and distribution of cell organelles, is nearly identical with that in smooth muscle of the seminal vesicles. Surface vesicles (caveolae) have been found arranged in clusters separated from each other by a smooth cell surface on freeze-etch replicas. Each cell is surrounded by a basal lamina about 50 nm in thickness. At some locations on the surface of a cell, a projection of one smooth muscle cell protrudes into a cup-depression in an adjacent cell. At these locations, the external laminae surrounding the cells are absent and extracellular space between the two apposed plasma membranes is narrowed to 15–20 nm, forming intermediate-type junctions. These are more frequent in rat prostate as compared to the human prostate. Intermediate junctions are particularly frequent between smooth muscle cells close to or within the muscle layer of the prostatic urethra. Here, they are often intermingled with a dense network of elastic fibers.

In the rat, bundles of unmyelinated nerve processes are numerous in prostatic stroma, and the distance to accompanying muscle cells ranges from 50–500 nm. At certain points, axon varicosities that contain aggregations of numerous small clear vesicles 30–60 nm in diameter, some dense-core vesicles 15–20 nm in diameter, and rare large vesicle 100 nm in diameter make closer contact with smooth muscle cells. In some instances, the axons lie on the unindented surface of the muscle cell and sometimes in a shallow groove in its surface. In other cases, deep indentations are found in smooth muscle cells surrounding an axon. The plasma membrane of the axon is separated from that of the muscle cell by a space 15–20 nm wide. No membrane specialization at these points of contact have been observed, although myofilaments usually are absent from the underlying cytoplasm (83).

Experimental studies in the rat and the dog have demonstrated that the ultrastructure of prostatic smooth muscle cells is strongly hormone-dependent which is important with respect to the pathogenesis of benign prostatic hyperplasia (87).

2.6. *Urethra and external genitalia*

2.6.1. Urethra. The male urethral sphincter is a striated muscle in contact with the urethra from the base of the bladder to the perineal membrane.

The individual muscle fibers, 25% to 30% smaller than the fibers of associated muscles (88), are of both the fast- and slow-twitch muscle fiber type (89). During accelerated growth of the prostate during puberty, the sphincter is displaced, with atrophy of the overlaying muscle by increased infiltration of prostatic stroma and vasculature. In this area dense network of both smooth and striated muscle can be seen (73) (Fig. 9-25). Smooth muscle cells in this area make several points of contact and are innervated by peptidergic nerves, the essential transmitter being vasoactive intestinal polypeptide (90).

2.6.2. Penis. Erection is a process under parasympathetic control, although the failure of atropin to block erection is difficult to understand. The discovery of vasoactive intestinal polypeptide (VIP) in the corpora cavernosa of men (90) led to the suggestion that this was the active neurotransmitter substance. VIP is a potent arterial vasodilator, and the intracavernous injection of papaverine or α-adrenoceptor-blocking agents induces vasodilation and erection.

A still controversial question is whether or not the so-called polster arteries or their corporal smooth muscle activity is necessary for erectile function.

Myoendothelial cells, clusters of smooth muscle cells within the intima of large penile arteries, forming primarily longitudinally oriented ridges, were believed to increase and decrease in size, thus controlling the blood flow through the corporal vessels. According to McConnel et al. (91), these intimal pads are located mostly at branching points of the vessels, which are never innervated but instead are arteriosclerotic lesions at various stages of development. The authors therefore refute the polster theory of erection.

At the ultrastructural level, Fujimoto and Takeshige (92) have studied in the rabbit the so-called helicine arteries, branches of the deep penile artery, which redivide into clusters of 3–5 spiral arteries.

These lack the internal elastic lamina and have a relatively thick muscular coat arranged in concentric layers. After redivision, the media cells appear as so-called epithelioid cells. These contain filaments (6–9 nm in diameter), limited in number and oriented irregularly throughout the cytoplasm. Dense bodies are rare or even absent. The plasma membrane is studded with numerous caveolae. The extracellular basal lamina is of varying thickness; often it is lacking, and apposing cell membranes are connected by desmosome-like attachments. Cytoplasmic organelles such as endoplasmic reticulum, ribosomes, and mitochondria never accumulate in the nuclear region, but are dispersed throughout the cytoplasm (Figs. 9-26, 9-27).

Unlike those of the penile arteries, the walls of the cavernous veins are composed preferentially of a collagenous stroma interspersed throughout with small isolated groups of smooth muscle cells (93). These display a moderately scalloped outline. Glycogen granules are present throughout the cytoplasm. Occasional caveolae are observed at the cell membrane. The basal lamina appears as a narrow band along the cell membrane. Changes in penile blood flow, effecting either stasis or high-flow priaprism, result in considerable changes in the ultrastructure of trabecular smooth muscle cells. The ratio of trabeculae to smooth muscle, which indicates the amount of contractile tissue in the trabeculae normally ranges between 0.45 and 0.70 but drops to between 0.22 and 0.55 in patients with priaprism (94). In stasis priaprism lasting more than 12 hours, the trabecular smooth muscle cells focally display degenerative alterations. The perinuclear portion of cytoplasm, normally a small area containing mitochondria, profiles of rough endoplasmic reticulum, ribosomes, and the Golgi apparatus, is considerably increased in size, displacing the reduced mass of contractile filaments to the periphery. In more progressive stages, most trabecular smooth muscle cells undergo necrosis or are at least in various stages of transformation into fibroblast-like cells, but are still surrounded by a basement membrane. The alterations are similar to those observed in the media wall of blood vessels under pathological conditions, such as reduced O_2-tension and altered wall pressure.

2.6.3. Scrotum. The tunica dartos of the scrotum was recognized early on as particularly important for thermoregulation in the human testis, and its influence on spermatogenesis is well documented (95, 96). There is one study that has demonstrated an intricate arrangement of smooth muscle cells, myofibroblasts, and connective tissue within scrotal corium and subcutis (95). In the corium, myofibroblasts occur, displaying an ovoid, somewhat compressed nucleus surrounded by a rich multitude of cytoplasmic constituents and relatively few microfilaments inserting in attachment plaques on the plasma membrane. At these points a basement membrane is seen close to the plasma membrane. A thin layer of microfilaments interweaves with neighboring collagen bundles.

The bundles of musculature in the corium and subcutis, consisting of varying number of smooth muscle cells of typical ultrastructure, are closely aggregated, sometimes in a contracted state. The cells are surrounded by a basement membrane, bundles of filaments sometimes gluded together with elastin and more distant from the tapering ends of the smooth muscle cells ramifying within a network of collagen fibrils. Only the ordinary smooth muscle cells of the tunica dartos receive an adrenergic innervation. Myofibroblasts are obviously not influenced by the sympathetic nervous system.

The myomotor innervation of the tunica dartos constitutes the final efferent link in thermoregulatory reflex pathways, the initial afferent link being the sensory axons from the skin. These nerve fibers, when passing the different layers of the scrotum, may associate with the afferent adrenergic axon. This at least would explain the presence of myelinated axons in almost all nerve bundles in the tunica dartos.

3. Developmental changes

3.1. Pubertal maturation

The peritubular myofibroblasts will be discussed here in detail, since several articles exist considering comparative aspects, histochemical data, and experimental alterations of this particular cell type. These articles render a multitude of details on the developmental plasticity of these cells observed under pathological conditions (97).

Comparing tubular contractility, histochemical differentiation of phosphatases, ultrastructure of the tubular wall, and maturation of the germinal epithelium in rats during postnatal development, Kormano and Hovatta (98) observed histochemically demonstrable alkaline phosphatase and 5′-nucleotidase activities appearing from the 10th day onwards. The tubules began to contract by day 15, when myofilaments first were observed in the peritubular cells. Contractions of the tubules reached adult values at 40 days, preceding completion of spermatogenesis by about 10 days.

The transformation of human peritubular fibroblasts into myofibroblasts during puberty follows the same structural pattern as observed in the rat (99). During the first year, the tubules are surrounded by a basement membrane, a collagenous layer and a third zone, consisting of one to two layers of fibroblasts. The more peripherally located fibroblasts seem to advance in cellular differentiation. These types of cells persist up to about the 13th year. During onset of puberty, the fibroblasts start to divide, forming a three- to six-layered zone. The more peripherally located cells still display the features of undifferentiated fibroblasts, while the cells facing the basal lamina of the tubule develop the characteristics of myofibroblasts; i.e., microfilaments appear as well as dense bodies, dense plaques, and surface vesicles. This differentiation is accompanied by characteristic changes of the connective tissue. The development of the epididymal myofibroblasts generally seems to follow the same developmental pattern as described for seminiferous peritubular cells.

There are quite a number of studies on postnatal development of the epididymis (e.g., 100, 101, 102), but the maturation of the tubule wall has only been given specific attention in a recent article by Francavilla et al. (55). Maturation of the genital ducts starts in their distal portion (vas deferens and cauda epididymidis) one week after birth and an additional week later in the more cranial portions. Peritubular contractile cells (and epithelium) are structurally mature 35 days after birth. The cytodifferentiation of the peritubular contractile cells is accompanied by a progressive increase in immunoreactivity against smooth muscle actin and is spatially and temporally related to the appearance of contractile filaments. These appear first in the cells just beneath the epithelium, and progressively spread throughout distant cells. An immunoreaction for myosin, on the other hand, is already present in the peritubular contractile cells of one-day-old rats, and it does not change thereafter.

The differentiation of the peritubular cells is associated with changes of the peritubular matrix in that fibronectin immunoreactivity, present in punctate aggregates surrounding the peritubular cells in newborn animals, is gradually removed during postnatal development. This could be related to the anatomical shaping of the tubule wall, where the architecture of the wall may be predetermined by a transitory scaffold of a fibronectin-rich exoskeleton that ensures the correct organization and alignment of peritubular cells. During differentiation of the peritubular cells, the irregular masses of surrounding matrix are replaced by a continuous basement membrane, which apparently interacts with cell surface components that in turn modulate the arrangement of the cytoskeleton (55).

3.2. Senescent involution

With advancing age, testicular involution takes place, which morphologically encompasses a variable degree of hypospermatogenesis with fibrosis of the peritubular and interstitial tissue (103). Using a stereological evaluation of electron micrographs of testes from 28 men aged 20 to 48 years and 28 men aged 50 to 90 years, Johnson et al. (104) found significant age-related reductions in total volume of seminiferous tubules and of seminiferous epithelium and in length of tubules. The volume density and thickness of boundary tissue increased with age. The volume of boundary tissue per man and the volume density of myofibroblasts in the boundary tissue did not vary with age. The number of myofibroblasts per cross section of seminiferous tubule increased in older men. This thickening was not due to an increase in boundary tissue, but resulted from a reduction in the length of the seminiferous tubule.

Involution of the seminiferous tubules may lead to 1) light or marked hypospermatogenesis, 2) maturation arrest at spermatocyte level, 3) arrested maturation at spermatogonium levels, and eventually 4) the formation at sclerosed tubules. It has been assumed that the increase in thickness of the tunica propria impedes metabolic exchange with the tubular lumen, effecting the degeneration of intratubular cells (105). Alternatively, it has been suggested that tubular hyalinization is secondary to the destruction of germ cells and that the fibroblasts of the tubular wall synthesize collagen fibers, allowing a replating of the tubules (106). The exact role and alteration of peritubular myofibroblasts in this process remains undetermined. Vascular alterations seem to be the major cause for tubular degenerative changes (107, 108).

There are a number of experimental studies that have considered the role of myofibroblasts during testicular damage. Haider et al. (97) in a case of varicocele found deep invaginations of the lamina propria, sometimes containing a myofibroblast reaching into the wall of the seminiferous tubules. The myofibroblasts lacked Ca^{++}-ATP'ase activity. They therefore suggested impaired transport processes and contractility in the tubular wall.

Cryptorchidism is another pathological condition affecting the structure of the peritubular cells (109). As early as seven days after cryptorchidism, the tunica propria is widened due to an increase in the width of the extracellular space. There are increased quantities of collagen and ground substance within the basement membrane surrounding the tubules as well as lining the surface of myofibroblasts. With increased duration of the cryptorchid state, remarkable convolutions of the myofibroblasts and their basement-membrane-type lining is observed. These layers of ground substance become less closely apposed to the surface of the myofibroblasts, and collagen accumulates within the widened extracellular spaces.

Another mechanism influencing the functioning and morphology of the peritubular cells is the local hormonal situation. Hovatta and Koskimies (110) have observed that the contractility of rat seminiferous tubules is not affected by cyproterone acetate or progesterone, since their levels, although systematically administered, were obviously too low to replace testosterone within testicular cells. Low doses of testosterone, on the other hand, and estradiol, drastically diminishing gonadotrophin secretion, totally abolished the contractility of the seminiferous tubules. While testosterone did not significantly alter the ultrastructure of peritubular cells, after estradiol treatment the basement-membrane-type layer of the tubules was wrinkled and folded. The nuclei of the myoid cells protruded into the seminiferous epithelium. The rough endoplasmic reticulum was sparse, and the few mitochondria seen were small. Occasionally small electron-dense granules were found in the cytoplasm of the myofibroblasts, but microfilaments had disappeared.

The few examples presented indicate that the causes of involution of the seminiferous tubules and the concomitant alterations of the peritubular tissue, including the myofibroblasts, are certainly multiple. They are generally related to the aging of somatic tissue, and are specifically dependent upon testicular temperature, hormonal situation, vascular perfusion, and metabolic state.

4. Functional Aspects

4.1. Innervation

Generally speaking, the semen-transporting duct system consists of differently constructed subdivisions that are characterized by an opposite motility behavior under resting conditions (51). The proximal portion, starting with the seminiferous tubules, exhibits spontaneous local, slow, rhythmic, migrating contractions not unlike peristaltic movements. Spontaneous contractility depends on the inherent properties of the contractile cells and on the pattern of innervation (high sensitivity to low amounts of endogenous catecholamines) (51). The intermediate portion, i.e., the distal cauda of the epididymis, the vas deferens, and the accessory sex glands, remains quiescent unless involved in nerve-mediated, brief, forceful contractions. The complete quiescence of densely innervated smooth muscle, e.g., in the vas deferens, has been suggested to depend on genuine properties of smooth muscle cells themselves (distribution of α- and β-adrenoceptors) rather than on complete inhibition of nervous activity and transmitter release. A still more complex situation exists in the distal portion of the seminal transport system, where the prostatic and spongy urethral smooth muscle is surrounded by skeletal muscle that develops clonic contractions during semen emission, governed by parasympathetic neurons.

The male genital tract receives a dual autonomic innervation: sympathetic from the least thoracic and lumbar roots via the hypogastric nerves, and parasympathetic via the pelvic nerves from the sacral roots (for review, see 111). While the testis is sparsely innervated, the density of both adrenergic and cholinergic innervation increases towards the proximal end of the genital tract, being highest in the vas deferens where the smooth muscle is extremely densely innervated.

The exceptionally rich adrenergic innervation of the vas deferens originates from short adrenergic neurons (112). In castrated animals, abundant small noradrenergic vesicles can be isolated from the vas deferens. The biochemical studies of Fried et al. (113) suggest that noradrenaline is synthesized in large dense-cored vesicles, and readily released, while the noradrenaline subsequently taken up enters the small dense-core vesicles. Basbaum and Heuser (114) on the other hand, have shown that noradrenaline is released from small dense-core vesicles by exocytosis in the mouse vas deferens. The membrane of these vesicles is recycled by the varicosities to form new vesicles within a short period of time; these then become loaded with transmitter.

Noradrenaline has long been regarded as the sole motor neurotransmitter in the vas deferens, though it seems to be only partly responsible for the smooth muscle contraction induced by electrical stimulation (115). Other neurotransmitters could also be involved in the neurogenic response, e.g., purines (116) and neuropeptides such as NPY, recently co-localized in dopamine-β-hydroxylase-containing neurons of guinea pig vas deferens and seminal vesicles (117, 118). Stjernquist et al. (118) suggest that NPY does not act as a neurotransmitter, but has an inhibitory effect on neurally induced contractions. It could perhaps act before the site of the neuromuscular junction by modulating the release of noradrenaline or another hitherto unknown transmitter effecting motoric activity of the vas deferens.

The picture becomes still more complicated by the presence of other neuropeptides (substance P, vasointestinal polypeptide, gastrin-releasing peptide, and enkephalin) in the vas deferens, the seminal vesicles, and/or the prostate in a species- and tissue-specific manner (see 118). It is believed that the neuropeptides in the nerves of the vas deferens and the seminal vesicles participate in a complex way for the intrinsic neural regulation of sperm transport in this portion of the male internal reproductive system. This may be effected either through direct smooth muscle action or by modulating the action of classical transmitters.

4.1.1. Prostate. In most species studied, a more or less dense network consisting of both adrenergic and cholinergic nerves (119, 120) seems to innervate the smooth muscle coats and septa as well as blood vessels in the prostate. The human prostate obviously receives a considerably less intense adrenergic innervation than most laboratory animals (120), e.g., the rat (121). There, adrenergic nerves are often seen in close contact with the smooth muscle cells surrounding the prostatic alveoli and secretory ducts. The adrenergic innervation is about proportional to the thickness of the muscular layer. This neuromuscular organization is thought to be of importance in the emptying mechanism of the prostate. Nerve fibers containing vasointestinal polypeptide (VIP) and met- or leu-enkephalin are also described in the human prostate (122). VIP-containing nerves were detected mainly in association with the epithelium, while nerves containing enkephalins seem to be related to smooth muscle. Alm et al. (123) suggested that VIP-containing nerves could be characteristic of sphincters, since they were numerous surrounding the ducts of the prostate at their openings to the urethra. Certainly in this region the innervation pattern is particularly complicated, because it represents the center, where muscular activities governing voiding, ejaculation, and erection are coordinated.

4.2. *Contractility*

According to Ohkawa (124) the nature of the neuromuscular transmission in the smooth muscle cell of the prostate gland seems to be similar to that the vas deferens and the seminal vesicle (of the guinea pig) (125, 126). In all three organs, excitatory junction potentials occur spontaneously (in the circular layer) and can be evoked by stimulation of the hypogastric nerve or by field stimulation. Their mean amplitude and frequency is 2.6 mV and 26.6 per minute, respectively (126). Pharmacological studies indicate that these excitatory junction potentials are induced by the action of neurotransmitters released from the nerve endings in the tissue and that the synapse is α-excitatory adrenergic.

The exclusive role of noradrenaline as a motor neurotransmitter in the vas deferens is doubtful (118). Also, there are differences between the seminal vesicles and the vas deferens. Studying the effects of norepinephrine (NE) and NPY on the smooth muscle of these organs in vitro (in guinea pig), Stjernquist et al. (118) found that NE inhibited the response to electrical nerve stimulation increased the basic tension in the vas deferens, and contracted the smooth muscle of the seminal vesicle, but had no effect on the contractile response to transneural stimulation in the latter organ. NPY had similar effects on the vas deferens and the seminal vesicle in that it inhibited the electrically induced contractions and had no effect on the basic tension. An experimental confirmation was achieved by analyzing the supersensitivity of the deferens after castration to in vitro electrical stimulation (127, 128). After castration, the vas deferens had increased spontaneous activity, i.e., spontaneous depolarization activity and a decreased resting membrane potential.

Also, the relationship between phasic and tonic components of contractile activity had changed. The maximum contractile response to electrical stimulation, norepinephrine, ATP, acetylcholine, and histamine increased. In the hamster vas deferens, these changes developed slowly after castration, reaching a maximum at eight weeks. Supersensitivity was apparently not due to increased postsynaptic adrenergic sensitivity, decreased neuronal uptake of catecholamine, decreased presynaptic feedback by prostaglandin or adrenergic agonist, or alteration in transmitter release. In contrast, the adrenergic component (tonic component) of the contractile response to field stimulation was lost after castration, while the nonadrenergic phasic component remained intact. According to Belis and Longhurst (128), the neurogenic response after castration may have a greater dependence on a purinergic component. An additional, perhaps decisive, component in the nonspecificity and slow development of supersensitivity may be the effect of castration upon smooth muscle cell membrane. Sexual development and increasing testosterone levels during maturation alter calcium distribution or binding within vas deferens smooth muscle. Perhaps postcastration changes of smooth muscle, such as reductions in cell volume (129), sarcoplasmic reticulum, and contractile filaments, increase in rough endoplasmic reticulum and surface vesicles, and changes in the extracellular matrix may alter the intermediately exchangeable calcium of the smooth muscle cells, the most important being the sarcoplasmic reticulum (66).

4.3. Hormone dependence of smooth muscle differentiation

Cellular differentiation of smooth muscle cells due to hormonal challenge is a well-known phenomenon, e.g., in uterine muscle (130, 131). Burghardt et al. (132) have shown certain structure–activity relationships and a dose dependence in the ability of a number of steroidal and nonsteroidal estrogen-receptor-binding ligands to affect the formation and internalization of gap junctions in hypophysectomized rat myometrial cells. Cellular differentiation of male genital smooth muscle cells is likewise dependent on the presence of an effector hormone, which in this case is testosterone.

Rohr and Bartsch (87, 133, 134) have shown in a series of studies using stereological methods that estrogens, in the absence of androgens, are able to transform prostatic and seminal vesicle (129) smooth muscle cells into *activated* cells. The concept of activated smooth muscle developed from the earlier observations of Chamley-Campbell et al. (135) on vascular smooth muscle cells, where at least two different phenotypic states of smooth muscle, dependent on age, were observed. In the developing organism, smooth muscle cells have a fibroblastlike appearance, divide, and secrete extracellular matrix components; at this stage they are referred to as being in *synthetic* phenotype. In the adult, the smooth muscle cells become highly differentiated and specialized, and contract in response to chemical and mechanical stimuli; at this stage they are referred to as being in a *contractile* state. However, the differentiation of the cells under certain pathological conditions, such as arteriosclerosis, is reversible and results in the appearance of a modified, fibroblastlike cell type. The transforming process includes a reorganization of the cytoskeleton (136) and changes in the expression of contractile proteins (137, 138) and intermediate filament proteins (8). Concomitantly, rough endoplasmic reticulum and Golgi apparatus proliferate at the expense of myofilaments (139). As a result, the cells loose their ability to contract, start to secrete extracellular matrix components, and divide (140). Similar observations have been made in prostatic smooth muscle cells under estrogenic challenge (87).

Biochemical studies on separated stromal and epithelial components of the prostate (141, 142) found a much higher content of estrogen receptor in the stroma relative to the epithelium, and also — particularly under conditions of benign prostatic hyperplasia — increased activity of 5α-reductase, the enzyme responsible for reducing the relatively inactive androgen testosterone to the highly active dihydrotestosterone (DHT). The advent of immunocytochemical demonstration of the estrogen receptor (143) made it possible to directly visualize the estrogen receptor in the canine prostate (144). The estrogen receptor was detected in nuclei of the mucosal epithelium and submucosal cells of the prostatic urethra, where the intensity was highest in the region of the verumontanum. Specific estrogen receptor immunoreactivity was also present in prostatic stroma, perhaps in smooth muscle cells, with a higher staining intensity in the peri-urethral region of the prostate than in the periphery.

Indirect evidence for a hormonal response of prostatic smooth muscle cells (in a pattern strictly dependent upon its location within the prostate, either close to the urethra, or intermediate or subjacent the capsule) has been found in different endocrine studies (145–148).

An ultrastructural study devoted to phenotypic alterations of canine prostatic smooth muscle after a six-month long-term-treatment with androgens and estrogens (and/or anti-androgens and/or anti-estrogens) has been performed by Aumüller et al. (149) is castrated dogs (Figs. 9-28–9-33). Compared to normal conditions, in the castrated canine prostate the size of the individual smooth muscle cell is clearly reduced, along with a decrease in microfilaments and dense bodies. The arrangement of the cells is condensed; they form thick bands situated between broad strands of connective tissue. Androgen substitution (in this case 3α-androstenediol), even in the presence of estrogen and anti-estrogen, is capable of reversing the atrophic changes.

In the case of diminished androgen levels and increased estrogen levels, signs of metabolic and structural alteration develop, initially in form of clusters of glycogen surrounding the perinuclear zone. In castrated animals treated simultaneously with androstenediol, cyproterone acetate (an anti-androgen), and estradiol, an enormous accumulation of lipid occurred in the perinuclear zone of the smooth muscle cells, replacing a great proportion of cytoplasmic organelles and myofilaments. Similar alterations occurred in the adjacent fibroblasts. Estrogen was identified as the compound inducing structural and functional dedifferentiation of prostatic smooth muscle cells in castrated animals treated exclusively with estradiol. Most cells showed fatty degeneration and only few cells in the contractile state remained. Estrogen-mediated dedifferentiation of prostatic smooth muscle cells was also observed in castrated dogs treated with an androgen that it partly metabolized to estrogen by the enzyme aromatase (150). This was dose-dependent. In initial stages of the treatment, alterations in smooth muscle cells were observed, resembling those of the synthetic state of vascular smooth muscle. It is tempting to speculate that a changed endocrine situation in the aged human leads to an increased number of activated or synthetic smooth muscle cells, effecting certain epithelial–stromal interactions usually operating during the formation of the gland and resulting in benign prostatic hyperplasia (151, 152, 153).

4.4. Epithelial–stromal interactions

Embryonic development, morphogenesis, and expression of functional activity of the male genital system is governed by androgens produced in the fetal testis. In a pioneering series of thorough and elegant studies, Cunha (153) used a heterotypic (or homotypic) recombination system of embryonic epithelia and mesenchyme to explore the possible role of mesenchyme in transmitting morphogenetic signals aroused by androgens to the epithelium. Prostatic organogenesis only occurred in response to androgens, when epithelium of the urogenital sinus was combined with homotypic or heterotypic mesenchyme of urogenital origin (152). Epithelium of the embryonic seminal vesicles only expressed androgen-induced morphogenesis when combined with mesenchyme of either the urogenital sinus or the seminal vesicle and not with nontarget integumental mesenchyme. Obviously, the morphogenetic effects of androgen upon urogenital epithelium are mediated through unique properties of the urogenital mesenchyme that are not present in mesenchyme from other organ systems (153). The mechanisms of these tissue interactions are still unknown; they might operate through cell-to-cell contract, cell–extracellular matrix interactions, spatial distribution of glycosaminoglycans in the basal lamina, or remodeling patterns of the extracellular matrix. The possible significance and molecular action of fibroblasts and particularly of smooth muscle cells of urogenital origin in altering, conditioning, or contributing to the extracellular matrix still await experimental analysis (153).

Recent studies of Cunha's group on the inductive potency of the urogenital mesenchyme have shown that mesenchyme of the cranial portion of the urogenital sinus is the actual glandular inductor, while mesenchyme of the caudal portion acts primarily as an inductor of the prostatic urethra (154). Within the prostatic complex proper of the mouse, considerable differences exist, in that distal ducts are definitely more androgen-dependent and androgen-sensitive than those of the proximal regions (155–157). This may be explained as a result of corresponding regional differences in the inductive activities within the developing prostate.

Whether these observations in the mouse can also be applied to the developing human prostate (158) and to pubertal growth of the human prostate (159) remains to be established. Concerning the expression of abnormal epithelial features within the urogenital tract, such as benign prostatic hyperplasia, these may also be linked to altered stromal characteristics (151). The recent findings of an interdependence between synthesis of platelet-derived growth factor, heparinlike glycosaminoglycans, and vascular smooth muscle growth (13, 14) should encourage upcoming

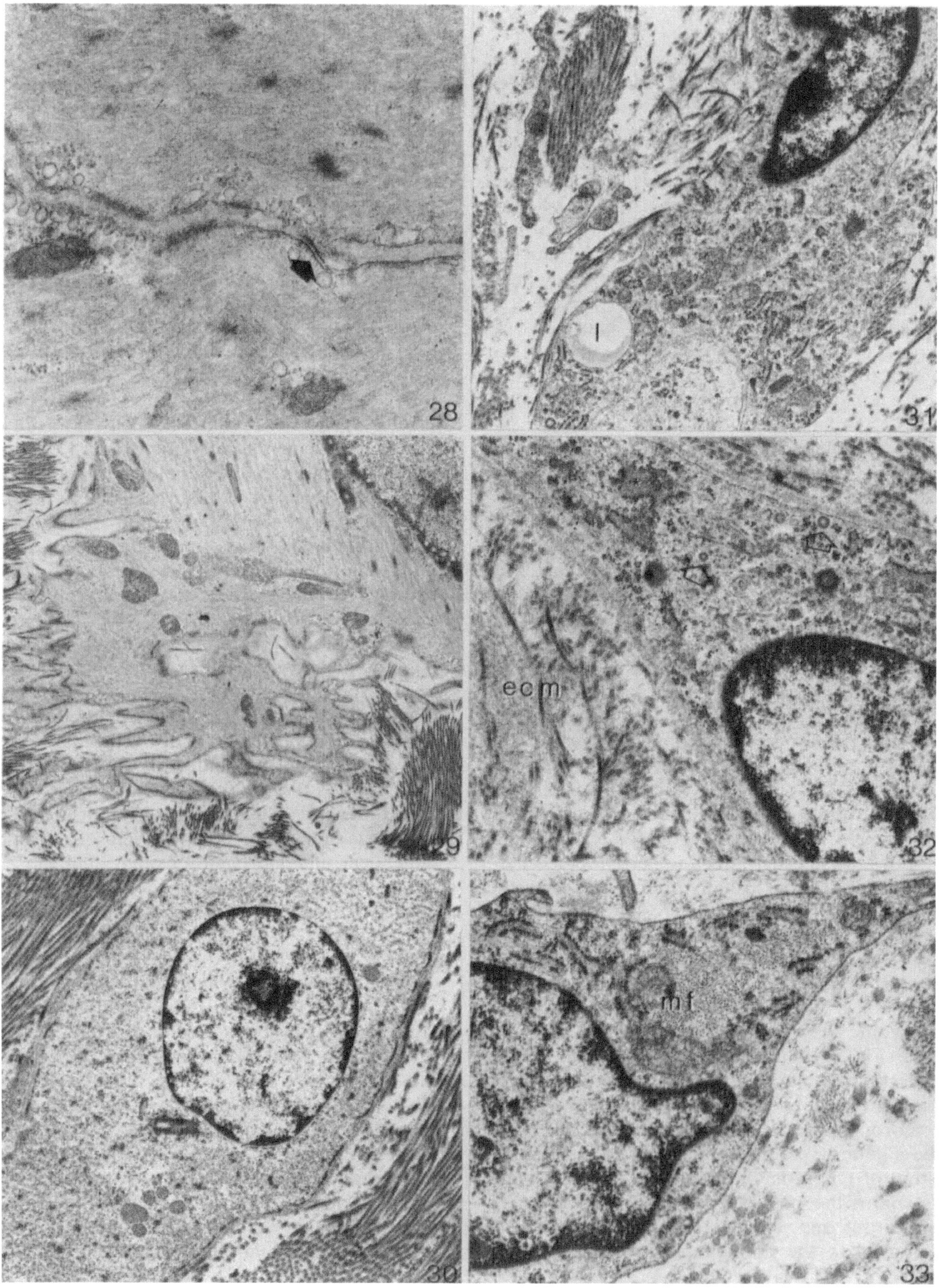
28
31
l
29
ecm
32
30
mf
33

scientific efforts to find experimental support for a hypothesis about the role of epithelial–stromal interactions in the control of gene expression in the prostate, recently advanced by Tenniswood (160). This hypothesis proposes the existence of three factors — two growth factors, namely a stromally derived growth factor (SDGF) and an epithelially derived growth factor (EDGF), and one inhibiting factor, namely epithelially derived inhibiting factor (EDIF) — that together modulate gene expression in the prostate during development. The hypothesis also attempts to explain the etiology of certain prostatic decreases: if, for example, the production of SDGF and EDGF is not regulated in a coordinated manner, the overproduction of one or the other would be expected to lead to hyperplastic structures that are either predominantly epithelial (if SDGD is in excess) or stromal (if EDGF is in excess). In the normal adult gland, the constitutive expression of EDIF by the epithelial cells would repress SDGF gene expression in the stromal cells. This would prevent replication in both cell types, enabling them to express continually the genes for steroid metabolism and secretion. In this hypothesis, stromal cells, especially smooth muscle cells, have been taken into account as a morphologically and functionally stable and differentiated cellular population. As has been shown above, this is not the case (as likewise it is not the case for the epithelium). Instead, there are considerable phenotypic alterations of the smooth muscle cells, depending on the hormonal situation, reflecting altered functional activities of the cells. It seems tempting to speculate that an estrogen-induced shift of smooth muscle cells from a contractile to a synthetic state would initiate the production of a stromally derived growth factor or another imbalance in the system, effecting partially uncontrolled growth (as observed) either of smooth muscle cells or glandular structures during development of BPH-formation.

4.5. Significance of smooth muscle cells of the male genital tract in reproductive biology and medicine

Transport of spermatozoa from their production site within the seminiferous tubules through the rete testis and the efferent ductules into the epididymal duct is one of the major functions of peritubular myofibroblasts that is effected without detailed control of the nervous system. Changes in the reactivity and functioning of the peritubular cells will result in altered thickness and metabolic activity of the peritubular tissue, which in turn will affect the intratubular cells. Furthermore, the transport process will be impaired, resulting in changes of sperm number and maturation.

The smooth muscle cells of the intermediate and distal portions of the seminal transporting system are the substrates of erection and ejaculation. These functions require a spatially and temporally highly differentiated and regulated innervation and contraction pattern that is under the strict control of the autonomous nervous system.

Hence, it is conceivable that vascular, metabolic, and endocrine disorders may disturb this highly regulated system, resulting in reduced or damaged sperm production and/or disturbances of erection and ejaculation. The recent advances in plastic surgery of the male genital ducts have been prompted, inter alia, by certain patients who had undergone vasectomy and wanted to become refertilized. In addition to the changes observed within the epithelium of vas deferens and

←

Figures 9-28–9-33. Phenotypic modulation of rat and canine prostatic smooth muscle cells after androgen deprivation or estrogen challenge. (28) Smooth muscle cells from the lateral prostate of an intact rat. Arrow points to a gap junction (X 35,000). (29) Fourteen days after castration, the cells are shrunken and have acquired a highly irregular outline (X 7100). (30) Prostatic smooth muscle cell from a castrated dog, long-term treated with an androgen/anti-androgen plus estrogen/ anti-estrogen regimen. The cell shows some fixation artifacts. As a sign of slight activation, the amount of surrounding connective tissue is increased (X 8000). (31) Activated prostatic smooth muscle cell from a castrated and estrogen-treated dog. Note the proliferated endoplasmic reticulum and a lipid droplet (1) (X 9000). (32) Activated prostatic smooth muscle cell from a castrated and estrogen-treated dog. The amount of extracellular matrix (ecm) and connective tissue is increased. The cells contain several coated vesicles (arrows) and profiles of endoplasmic reticulum with electron-dense contents (asterisk) (X 18,000). (33) Activated prostatic smooth muscle cell from a castrated and estrogen-treated dog. Some residual microfilaments (mf) are seen (X 30,000).

epididymis (161), degenerative effects and found in the distal portions of the vas deferens, preferentially with respect to the autonomic innervation (162). It is possible that the consequences of partial denervation may play a crucial role in those patients in whom infertility persists despite evidence of satisfactory mechanical continuity achieved by vasovasostomy. This may also apply for more elaborate plastic surgical interventions such as vasoepididymostomoses (163).

Another clinically important aspect of male genital smooth muscle is the development of benign prostatic hyperplasia, which is observed more frequently the older patients are. As has been described in the preceding section, at present only hypotheses are available to explain the pathogenesis of this disease (164); therefore in most cases it can be cured only by surgical intervention.

5. Conclusions

Three portions of the male genital duct system can be distinguished with respect to the contractile elements surrounding its wall. The first portion includes the seminiferous tubules and procedes to the rete testis, the efferent ductules, and the proximal portion of the epididymal duct. It is motile elements are myofibroblasts, spontaneously contractile flat cells wrapped around the tubules, that allow a slow and continuous transport of spermatozoa at low intraluminal pressure and extensive contact with the epithelial investments. The second portion originates in the distal cauda, includes the ductus deferens, its ampulla, and the seminal vesicles, and terminates in the prostatic portion of the urethra. In its most distal portion it still contains a thin layer of myofibroblasts that are gradually replaced by definite fibroblasts. These are surrounded by an enormous concentration of regularly arranged and densely innervated smooth muscle cells that are responsible for a rapid and forceful transportation of semen and seminal fluids into the posterior urethra. Here the third, terminal portion of the duct system starts. It is characterized by an intimate combination of smooth muscle cells, cavernous veins, and arteries with modified muscle cells in the media. In addition, skeletal muscle fibers are arranged around the proximal segment of this portion, allowing the jetlike ejection of semen in spite of the high pressure elicited by the adjacent rigid corpora cavernosa. In addition to fine structural differences concerning the contractile apparatus, the intermediate filaments, and the contact with the extracellular matrix, myofibroblasts and contractile smooth muscle as the two basic motor cell types of the male genital system differ with respect to innervation, contraction physiology, surface receptors, and plasticity to hormonal stimuli. There is increasing evidence of species differences and tissue specificity of smooth muscle cells. The most meticulously studied cell type is the smooth muscle cell of the vas deferens. It contains the α-adrenoceptor, but the exact mechanism of stimulation–contraction coupling, and its modification by peptidergic, cholinergic, and/or purinergic mechanisms remain to be elucidated. Hormonal alterations such as testosterone deprivation or estrogen stimulation result in characteristic morphological transformations of the cells that are responsible for altered electrophysiological properties.

The recent observation of growth factors (such as platelet-derived growth factor (PDGF) in vascular smooth muscle) has prompted the design of hypotheses on prostatic growth, where the participation of stromal components, such as smooth muscle cells, plays a significant role.

References

1. Bedford JM: Significance of the need for sperm capacitation before fertilization in eutherian mammals. *Biol Reprod* 28: 108–120, 1983.
2. Olson GE: Changes in the sperm surface during maturation in the epididymis. In: Ultrastructure of Reproduction. Gametogenesis, Fertilization and Embryogenesis. van Blerkom J, Motta PM (eds), Boston: Martinus Nijhoff, p 97–109, 1984.
3. Goerttler K: Die Konstruktion der Wand des menschlichen Samenleiters und ihre funktionelle Bedeutung (als Beispiel eines eigenartigen, unbekannten Förderungsmechanismus des Inhalts in einem glattmuskeligen Rohr). *Morph Jahrb* 74: 550–580, 1934.
4. Gall F: Die Muskulatur der glandula vesiculosa. *Z Mikr Anat Forsch* 57: 590–612, 1951.
5. Aumüller G: Zur Gefäß- und Muskelarchitektur der menschlichen Prostata. *Z Anat Entw Gesch* 135: 88–100, 1971.

6. Suzuki Y, Lamb JC, McLachlan JA: Age-dependent morphological changes in the seminal colliculus in male mice. *Anat Embryol* 158: 1–12, 1979.
7. Gown AM, Vogel AM, Gordon D, Lu PHL: A smooth muscle-specific monoclonal antibody recognizes smooth muscle actin isozymes. *J Cell Biol* 100: 807–813, 1985.
8. Skalli O, Ropraz P, Trzeciak A, Benzonana G, Gillessen D, Gabbiani G: A monoclonal anitbody against α-smooth muscle actin: a new probe for smooth muscle differentiation. *J Cell Biol* 103: 2787–2796, 1986.
9. Kjörell H, Thornell LE, Lehto VP, Virtanen I, Whalen RG: A comparative analysis of intermediate filament proteins in bovine heart purkinje fibres and gastric smooth muscle. *Eur J Cell Biol* 44: 68–78, 1987.
10. Barsky SH, Green WR, Grotendorst GR, Liotta LA: Desmoplastic breast carcinoma as a source of human myofibroblasts. *Am J Pathol* 115: 329–333, 1984.
11. Wilkins JA, Risinger MA, Lin SH: Studies on proteins that co-purify with smooth muscle vinculin: identification of immunologically related species in focal adhesions of nonmuscle and Z-lines of muscle cells. *J Cell Biol* 103: 1438–1494, 1986.
12. Siliciano D'Angelo J, Craig SW: Properties of smooth muscle meta-vinculin. *J Cell Biol* 104: 473–482, 1987.
13. Majack RA, Coates Cook S, Bornstein P: Platelet-derived growth factor and heparin-like glycosaminoglycans regulate thrombospondin synthesis and deposition in the matrix by smooth muscle cells. *J Cell Biol* 101: 1059–1070, 1985.
14. Sjölund M, Hedin N, Sejersen TH, Heldin CH, Thyberg J: Arterial smooth muscle cells express platelet-derived growth factor (PDGF) A chain mRNA, secrete of PDGF-like mitogen, and bind exogenous PDGF in a phenotype and growth state-dependent manner. *J Cell Biol* 106: 403–413, 1988.
15. Virtanen J, Kallajoki M, Närvänen O, Paranko J, Thornell LE, Mietinen M, Lehto V-P: Peritubular myoid cells of human and rat testis are smooth muscle cells that contain desmin-type intermediate filaments. *Anat Rec* 215: 10–20, 1986.
16. Aumüller G, Habenicht UF, El Etreby MP: Pharmacologically induced ultrastructural and immunohistochemical changes in the prostate of castrated dogs. *Prostate* 11: 211–218, 1987.
17. Johnson AL, Howards SS: Intratubular hydrostatic pressure in testis and epididymis before and after vasectomy. *Am J Physiol* 228: 556–564, 1975.
18. Holstein AF, Weiss C: Über die Wirkung der glatten Muskulatur in der Tunica albuginea im Hoden des Kaninchens; Messungen des interstitiellen Druckes. *Z Ges Exp Med* 142: 334–337, 1967.
19. Roosen-Runge EC: Motions of the seminiferous tubules of rat and dog. *Anat Rec* 109: 413 (abstr), 1951.
20. Leeson TS, Cookson FB: The mammalian testicular capsule and its muscle elements. *J Morph* 144: 237–254, 1974.
21. Bell C, McLean JR: The autonomic innervation of the rat testicular capsule. *J Reprod Fertil* 32: 253–258, 1973.
22. Gorgas K, Böck P: Myofibroblasts in the rat testicular capsule. *Cell Tissue Res* 154: 533–541, 1974.
23. Singer JJ, Kazazis DM, Kawka DW: Localization of the fibronexus at the surface of granulation tissue myofibroblasts using double-label immunogold electron microscopy on ultrathin frozen sections. *Eur J Cell Biol* 38: 94–101, 1985.
24. Clermont Y: Contractile elements in the limiting membrane of the seminiferous tubules of the rat. *Exp Cell Res* 15: 438–440, 1958.
25. Böck P, Breitenecker G, Lunglmayr G: Kontraktile Fibroblasten (Myofibroblasten) in der Lamina propria der Hodenkanälchen vom Menschen. *Z Zellforsch* 133: 519–527, 1972.
26. Bustos-Obregón E, Holstein AF: On structural patterns of the lamina propria of human seminiferous tubules. *Z Zellforsch* 141: 413–425, 1973.
27. De Kretser DM, Kerr JB, Paulsen CA: The peritubular tissue in the normal and pathological human testis. An ultrastructural study. *Biol Reprod* 12: 317–324, 1975.
28. Hermo L, Lalli M, Clermont Y: Arrangement of connective tissue components in the walls of seminiferous tubules of man and monkey. *Am J Anat* 148: 433–446, 1977.
29. Cavallotti C, Carpino F, Familiar G, Re M, Vicari A: Myosinlike microfilaments in the human normal and pathological testis. *Acta Anat* 99: 220–227, 1977.
30. Gardner PJ, Holyoke EA: Fine structure of the seminiferous tubule of the swiss mouse. 1. The limiting membrane, Sertoli cell, spermatogonia and spermatocytes. *Anat Rec* 150: 391–404, 1964.
31. Bressler RG, Ross MH: Differentiation of peritubular myoid cells of the testis: effects of intratesticular implantation of newborn mouse testes into normal and hypophysectomized adults. *Biol Reprod* 6: 148–159, 1972.
32. Dym M, Fawcett DW: The blood-testis barrier in the rat and the physiological compartmentation of the seminiferous epithelium. *Biol Reprod* 3: 308–326, 1970.
33. Murakami M, Hamasaki M, Okita S, Abe J: SEM surface morphology of the contractile cells in the rat seminiferous tubules. *Experientia* 35: 1099–1101, 1979.
34. Connell CJ, Christensen AK: The ultrastucture of the canine testicular interstitial tissue. *Biol Reprod* 12: 368–382, 1985.
35. Dierichs R, Wrobel KH: Licht- und elektronenmikroskopische Untersuchungen an den peritubulären Zellen des Schweinehodens während der postnatalen Entwicklung. *Z Anat Entwickl Gesch* 143: 49–64, 1973.
36. Toyama Y: Actin-like filaments in the myoid cell of the testis. *Cell Tissue Res* 177: 221–226, 1977.
37. Bustos-Obregón E, Courot M: Ultrastructure of the lamina propria in the ovine seminiferous tubule. *Cell Tissue Res* 150: 481–492, 1974.
38. Unsicker K, Burnstock G: Myoid cells in the peritubular tissue (lamina propria) of the reptilian testis. *Cell Tissue Res* 163: 545–560, 1975.
39. Bustos-Obregón E: Ultrastructure and function of the lamina propria of mammalian seminiferous tubules. *Andrologia* 8: 179–185, 1976.
40. Gravis CJ: Testicular involution after optic enucleation: ultrastructure and alkaline phosphatase cytochemistry of

the peritubular tissue. *Am J Anat* 151: 213–226, 1978.
41. Chapin RE, Phelps JL, Miller BE, Gray TJB: Alkaline phosphatase histochemistry discriminates peritubular cells in primary rat testicular cell culture. *J Androl* 8: 155–161, 1987.
42. Bergmann M, Schindelmeiser J, Greven H: Indications for a phagocytic capacity of smooth muscle cells in the testicular wall of Salamandra salamandra (L) amphibia, urodela. *Acta Zool* 63: 81–83, 1982.
43. Gröschel-Stewart U, Unsicker K: Direct visualization of contractile proteins in peritubular cells of the guinea pig testis using antibodies against highly purified actin and myosin. *Histochemistry* 51: 315–319, 1977.
44. Kierszenbaum AL, Crowell JA, Shabanowitz RB, Dephilip RM, Tres LL: Protein secretory patterns of rat Sertoli and peritubular cells are influenced by culture conditions. *Biol Reprod* 35: 239–251, 1986.
45. Lehto V-P, Virtanen I: Immunolocalization of a novel cytoskeleton-associated polypeptide of Mr 230000 daltons (p 230). *J Cell Biol* 96: 703–716, 1983.
46. Tung PS, Skinner MK, Fritz JB: Fibronectin synthesis is a marker for peritubular cell contaminants in Sertoli cell-enriched cultures. *Biol Reprod* 30: 199–211, 1984.
47. Bedford JM, Calvin N, Cooper G: The maturation of spermatozoa in the human epididymidis. *J Reprod Fertil Suppl* 18: 199–213, 1973.
48. Hamilton DW: Structure and function of the epithelium lining the ductuli efferentes, ductus epididymidis and ductus deferens in the rat. In: Handbook of Physiology, Section 7, Vol 5, Male Reproduction System. Washington, DC: American Physiological Society, p 259–301, 1975.
49. Risley PL The contractile behavior in vivo of the ductus epididymidis and vasa efferentia in the rat. *Anat Res* 130: 471–478, 1958.
50. Holstein A-F: Morphologische Studien am Nebenhoden des Menschen (Zwangl. Abhandl. Geb. norm. pathol. Anat; W. Bargmann, W. Doerr, Hrsg., Heft 20), Stuttgart: Thieme, 1969.
51. Baumgarten HG, Holstein A-F, Rosengren E: Arrangement, ultrastructure and adrenergic innervation of smooth musculature of the ductuli efferentes, ductus epididymidis and ductus deferens of man. *Z Zellforsch* 120: 37–79, 1971.
52. Ramos AS, Dym M: Ultrastructure of the ductuli efferentes in monkey. *Biol Reprod* 17: 339–349, 1977.
53. Hoffer AP, Greenberg J: The structure of the epididymis, efferent ductules and ductus deferens of the guinea pig: A light microscope study. *Anat Rec* 190: 659–677, 1978.
54. Francavilla S, De Martino C, Scorza Barcellona P, Natali PG: Ultrastructural and immunohistochemical studies of rat epididymis. *Cell Tissue Res* 233: 523–537, 1983.
55. Francavilla S, Moscardelli S, Properzi G, De Matteis MA, Scorza Barcellona P: Postnatal development of epididymis and ductus deferens in the rat. *Cell Tissue Res* 249: 257–265, 1987.
56. Delongeas J-L, Gelly J-L, Leheup B, Grignon G: Influence of testicular secretions on differentiation in the rat epididymis: ultrastructural studies after castration, efferent duct ligation and cryptorchidism. *Exp Cell Biol* 55: 74–82, 1987.
57. Vendrely E: Structure and histophysiology of the human vas deferens. *Prog Reprod Biol Med* 12: 8–17, 1985.
58. Riva A, Testa-Riva F, Usai E, Cossu M: The ampulla ductus deferentis in man, as viewed by SEM and TEM. *Arch Androl* 8: 157–164, 1982.
59. Cohen J, Forster E, Gillenwater JY: Quantitative age related histologic changes in the human vas deferens. *Invest Urol* 16: 305–306, 1979.
60. Friend DS, Farquhar MG: Functions of coated vesicles during protein absorption in the rat vas deferens. *J Cell Biol* 35: 357–376, 1976.
61. Hamilton DW, Cooper TG: Gross and histological variations along the length of the rat vas deferens. *Anat Rec* 190: 795–810, 1978.
62. Kennedy SW, Heidger PM Jr.: Fine structural studies of the rat vas deferens. *Anat Rec* 194: 159–180, 1979.
63. Yamauchi A, Burnstock G: Post-natal development of smooth muscle cells in the mouse vas deferens. A fine structural study. *J Anat (Lond)* 104: 1–15, 1969.
64. Merrilees NCR, Burnstock G, Holman ME: Correlation of fine structure and physiology of the innervation of smooth muscle in the guinea pig vas deferens. *J Cell Biol* 19: 529–550, 1963.
65. Furness JB, Iwayama T: The arrangement and identification of axons innervating the vas deferens of the guinea-pig. *J Anat* 113: 179–196, 1972.
66. McGuffee LJ, Little SA, Skipper BJ: Localization of calcium in vas deferens using Ca EM autoradiography: relationship to species and the effect of ^{45}Ca removal. *Anat Rec* 217: 321–327, 1987.
67. McGuffee LJ, Wheeler-Clark ES, Skipper BJ, Little SA: The cellular distribution of calcium in freeze-dried rabbit vas deferens using EM autoradiography. *Anat Rec* 211: 117–125, 1985.
68. Popovic NA, McLeod DG, Borski AA: Ultrastructure of the human vas deferens. *Invest Urol* 10: 266–277, 1973.
69. Hoffer AP: The ultrastructure of the ductus deferens in man. *Biol Reprod* 14: 425–443, 1976.
70. Robert MK, Lee W, Kwan CY, Daniel EE: Dense-cored membranous structures in smooth muscle cells of the vas deferens of the rat. *Cell Tissue Res* 235: 43–49, 1984.
71. Tauber PF, Zaneveld LJD, Propping D, Schumacher GFB: Components of human split ejaculates. I. Spermatozoa, fructose, immunoglobulines, albumin, lactoferrin, transferrin and other plasma proteins. *J Reprod Fertil* 43: 249–267, 1975.
72. Williams-Ashman HG: Transglutaminases and the clotting of mammalian seminal fluids. *Mol Cell Biochem* 58: 51–61, 1984.
73. Aumüller G: Prostate gland and seminal vesicles. In: Handbuch der mikroskop. Anatomie des Menschen VII/6. (A Oksche Berlin-New York-Heidelberg: Springer, L Vollrath (eds), p 1–380, 1979.
74. Düllmann J: Konstruktionsanalytische Untersuchungen am Ureter und deri Glandula vesiculosa des Rhesusaffen. *Acta Anat* 68: 344–360, 1967.
75. Kirchheim D, Bacon RL: Elektronenmikroskopische

Untersuchungen der normalen Prostata, der Prostatahypertrophie und des Prostatacarcinoms. *Urologe* 5: 292–305, 1968.
76. Brandes D, Kirchheim D, Scott WW: Ultrastructure of the human prostate: normal and neoplastic. *Lab Invest* 13: 1541–1560, 1964.
77. Oberholzer M, Ochsenbein A, Rohr H, Bartsch G, Ehrsham R: Calculating mean volumes of the single smooth muscle cells in human prostate. *Mikroskopie (Wien)* 37: 279–281, 1980.
78. Robel P, Eychenne B, Blondeau JP, Picard-Groyer M-T, Baulieu E-E, Bruner-Lorand J, Hechter D: Characteristics of separated epithelial and stromal subtractions of prostate: II. Human prostate. *Prostate* 5: 255–268, 1984.
79. Aumüller G: Fine structure of monkey (Macaca mulatta) male accessory sex glands, juvenile and adult. *Z Mikrosk Anat Forsch* 90: 545–556, 1976.
80. Aumüller G, Stofft E, Tunn U: Fine structure of the canine prostatic complex. *Anat Embryol* 160: 327–340, 1980.
81. Timms BG, Chandler JA, Sinowatz F: The ultrastructure of basal cells of rat and dog prostate. *Cell Tissue Res* 173: 543–554, 1976.
82. Flickinger CJ: The fine structure and development of the seminal vesicles and prostate in the fetal rat. *Z Zellforsch* 109: 1–14, 1970.
83. Flickinger CJ: The fine structure of the interstitial tissue of the rat prostate. *Am J Anat* 134: 107–126, 1972.
84. Dahl E, Kjaerheim A, Tveter K: The ultrastructure of the accessory sex organs of the male rat. Effects of an antiandrogenic compound, SKF 22,340. *Lab Invest* 33: 62–71, 1975.
85. Ichihara I, Kallio M, Pelliniemi LJ: Light and electron microscopy and of the ducts and their subepithelial tissue in the rat ventral prostate. *Cell Tissue Res* 192: 381–390, 1978.
86. Toma JG, Buzzell GR: Fine structure of the ventral and dorsal lobes of the prostate in the young adult syrian hamster, Mesocricetus auratus. *Am J Anat* 181: 132–140, 1988.
87. Rohr HP, Krisl J, Holliger O, Oberholzer M, Bartsch G: Stereological analysis of the dog prostate (analytical model). *Urol Res* 9: 193–199, 1981.
88. Oelrich TM: The urethral sphincter muscle in the male. *Am J Anat* 158: 229–246, 1980.
89. Tokunaka S, Murakami N, Fujii H, Okamura K, Miyata M, Hashimoto H, Yachiku S: Coexistence of fast and slow myosin isozymes in human external urethral sphincter. A preliminary report. *J Urol* 138: 659–662, 1987.
90. Willis W, Ottesen B, Fahrenkrug J, Sundler F, Wagner G: Vasoactive intestinal polypeptide as a possible neurotransmitter in penile erection. *Acta Physiol Scand* 113: 545–549, 1981.
91. McConnell J, Benson GS, Schmidt WA: The vasculature of the human penis: a reexamination of the morphological basis for the polster theory of erection. *Anat Rec* 203: 475–484, 1982.
92. Fujimoto S, Takeshige Y: The wall structure of the arteries in the corpora cavernosa penis of rabbits; light and electron microscopy. *Anat Rec* 181: 641–658, 1975.
93. Melman A, Bressler RS, Henry DP, Macadoo VK: Ultrastructure of human penile erectile tissue in patients with abnormal norepinephrine content. *Invest Urol* 19: 46–48, 1981.
94. Spycher MA, Hauri D: The ultrastructure of the erectile tissue in priapism. *J Urol* 135: 142–147, 1986.
95. Holstein AF, Orlandini GE, Baumgarten HG: Morphological analysis of tissue components in the tunica dartos of man. *Cell Tissue Res* 154: 329–344, 1974.
96. Hodson N: The nerves of the testis, epididymis, and scrotum. In: The Testis. AD Johnson, WR Gomes, NL Vandemark (eds), New York-London: Academic Press, p 47–99, 1970.
97. Haider SG, Passia D, Servos G, Hettwer H: Electron microscopic evidence for deep invaginations of the lamina propria towards the seminiferous tubule lumen in a patient with varicocele. *Int J Androl* 9: 27–37, 1986.
98. Kormano M, Hovatta O: Contractility and histochemistry of the myoid cell layer of the rat seminiferous tubules during postnatal development. *Z Anat Entwickl Gesch* 137: 239–248, 1972.
99. Seguchi H, Hadziselimovic F: Morphologie der peritubulären Strukturen des Tubulus seminiferus bei Kindern. Eine elektronenmikroskopische Studie. *Z Mikrosk Anat Forsch* 88: 1149–1160, 1974.
100. Alexander NJ: Prenatal development of the ductus epididymidis in the rhesus monkey. The effects of fetal castration. *Am J Anat* 135: 119–134, 1972.
101. Sun EL, Flickinger CJ: Development of cell types and of regional differences in the postnatal rat epididymis. *Am J Anat* 154: 27–56, 1979.
102. Arya M, Vanha-Perttula T: Postnatal development of lectin-binding pattern in rat testis and epididymis. *Acta Anat* 127: 100–109, 1986.
103. Paniagua R, Nistal M, Amat P, Rodriguez MC, Martin A: Seminiferous tubule involution in elderly men. *Biol Reprod* 36: 939–947, 1987.
104. Johnson L, Petty CS, Neaves WB: Age-related variation in seminiferous tubules in men. A stereologic evaluation. *J Androl* 7: 316–322, 1986.
105. Hadziselimovic F: Cryptorchidism. Ultrastructure of normal and cryptorchid testis development. *Adv Anat Embryol Cell Biol* 53: 1–74, 1977.
106. Söderström KO: Tubular hyalinization in human testis. *Andrologia* 18: 97–103, 1986.
107. Hatakeyama S, Takizawa T, Kawahara Y: Focal atrophy of the seminiferous tubules in the human testis. *Acta Pathol Jpn* 29: 901–911, 1979.
108. Vrzgulova M: Changes in the lamina propria of the seminiferous tubules after ischaemia in the testis of rams. *Zool Jb Anat* 101: 407–424, 1979.
109. Kerr JB, Rich KA, de Kretser DM: Effects of experimental cryptorchidism on the ultrastructure and function of the Sertoli cell and peritubular tissue of the rat testis. *Biol Reprod* 21: 823–838, 1979.
110. Hovatta O, Koskimies AJ: Functional and structural aspects of the rat seminiferous tubules after treatment with exogenous cyproterone acetate, testosterone, progesterone and oestradiol. *Int J Androl* 1: 61–75, 1978.

111. Vaalasti A: Autonomic innervation of the prostate. *Acta Universitatis Tamperensis Ser A* 113: 1–30, 1980.
112. Sjöstrand NO: The andrenergic innervation of the vas deferens and the accessory male genital glands. An experimental and comparative study of its anatomical and functional organization in some mammals including the presence of adrenalin and chromaffin cells in these organs. *Acta Physiol Scand Suppl* 257: 1–82, 1965.
113. Fried G, Lagercrantz H, Hökfelt T: Improved isolation of small noradrenergic vesicles from rat seminal ducts following castration. A density gradient centrifugation and morphological study. *Neuroscience* 3: 1271–1291, 1978.
114. Basbaum CB, Heuser JE: Morphological studies of stimulated adrenergic axon varicosities in the mouse vas deferens. *J Cell Biol* 80: 310–325, 1979.
115. Ambache N, Zar MA: Evidence against adrenergic motor transmission in the guinea-pig vas deferens. *J Physiol* 216: 359–389, 1971.
116. Meldrum LA, Burnstock G: Evidence that ATP acts as a cotransmitter with noradrenaline in sympathetic nerves supplying the guinea pig vas deferens. *Eur J Pharmacol* 92: 161–163, 1983.
117. Stjernquist M, Håkanson R, Leander S, Owman Ch, Sundler F, Uddman R: Immunohistochemical localization of substance P vasoactive intestinal polypeptide and gastrin-releasing peptide in vas deferens and seminal vesicle, and the effect of these and eight other neuropeptides on resting tension and neurally evoked contractile activity. *Regul Pept* 7: 67–86, 1983.
118. Stjernquist M, Owman Ch, Sjöberg NO, Sundler F: Coexistence and cooperation between neuropeptide Y and norepinephrine in nerve fibers of guinea pig vas deferens and seminal vesicle. *Biol Reprod* 36: 149–155, 1987.
119. Owman C, Sjöstrand NO: Short adrenergic neurons and catecholamine-containing cells in vas deferens and accessory male genital glands of different mammals. *Z Zellforsch* 66: 300–320, 1965.
120. Baumgarten HG, Falck B, Holstein AF, Owman C, Owman T: Adrenergic innervation of the human testis, epididymis, ductus deferens and prostate: a fluorescence microscopic and fluorimetric study. *Z Zellforsch* 90: 81–95, 1968.
121. Vaalasti A, Hervonen A: Innervation of the ventral prostate of the rat. *Am J Anat* 154: 231–244, 1979.
122. Vaalasti A, Linnoila I, Hervonen A: Immunohistochemical demonstration of VIP (Met^5) – and (Leu^5) – enkephalin immunoreactive nerve fibres in the human prostate and seminal vesicles. *Histochemistry* 66: 89–98, 1980.
123. Alm P, Alumets J, Brodin E, Håkanson R, Nilsson G, Sjöberg NO, Sundler F: Peptidergic (substance P) nerves in the genitourinary tract. *Neuroscience* 3: 419–425, 1978.
124. Ohkawa H: Sympathetic neuromuscular transmission in the smooth muscle of guinea-pig prostate gland. *Int J Fertil* 28: 68–77, 1983.
125. Ohkawa H: Evidence for adrenergic transmission in the circular smooth muscle of the guinea pig seminal vesicle. *Tohoku J Exp Med* 134: 141–158, 1981.
126. Ohkawa H: Excitatory junction potential recorded from the circular smooth muscle of the guinea-pig seminal vesicle. *Tohoku J Exp Med* 136: 89–102, 1982.
127. Abreu LC, Picarelli ZP, Valle JR: Contractile capacity of seminal vesicles from rats in different hormonal conditions. *Res Commun Chem Pathol Pharmacol* 27: 57–71, 1980.
128. Belis JA, Longhurst PA: Hormonal influence on the neurogenic response of the hamster vas deferens. *J Urol* 133: 729–732, 1984.
129. Bruengger A, Mariotti A, Rohr HP, Bartsch G, Stahel W, Wiederkehr P, Carmichael SW, Mawhinney MG: Androgen and estrogen effect on guinea pig seminal vesicle muscle: A combined stereological and biochemical study. *Prostate* 9: 303–310, 1986.
130. Kelly RE, Verhage HG: Hormonal effects on the contractile apparatus of the myometrium. *Am J Anat* 161: 375–382, 1981.
131. Merk FB, Kwan PWL, Leav I: Gap junctions in the myometrium of hypophsectomized estrogen treated rats. *Cell Biol Int Rep* 4: 287–293, 1980.
132. Burghardt RC, Gaddy-Kurten D, Burghardt RL, Kurten RC, Mitchell PA: Gap junction modulation in rat uterus III. Structure-activity relationships of estrogen receptor-binding ligands on myometrial and serosal cells. *Biol Reprod* 36: 741–751, 1987.
133. Rohr HP, Oberholzer M, Bartsch G, Keller M: Morphometry in experimental pathology (methods, baseline data, and applications). *Int Rev Pathol* 54: 233–325, 1976.
134. Bartsch G: Stereology, a new quantitative morphological approach to study prostatic function and disease. *Eur Urol* 3: 85–91, 1977.
135. Chamley-Campbell J, Campbell GR, Ross R: The smooth muscle cell in culture. *Physiol Rev* 59: 1–61, 1979.
136. Palmberg L, Sjölund M, Thyberg J: Phenotype modulation in primary cultures of arterial smooth-muscle cells: reorganization of the cytoskeleton and activation of synthetic activities. *Differentiation* 29: 275–283, 1985.
137. Gabbiani G, Kocher O, Bloom WS, Vandekerckhove J, Weber K: Actin expression in smooth muscle cells of rat aortic intimal thickening, human atheromatous plaque, and cultured rat aortic media. *J Clin Invest* 73: 148–152, 1984.
138. Larson DM, Fujiwara K, Alexander RW, Gimbrone MA Jr: Myosin in cultured vascular smooth muscle cells: immunofluorescence and immunochemical studies of alteration in antigenic expression. *J Cell Biol* 99: 1582–1589, 1984.
139. Chamley JH, Campbell GR, McConnell JD, Gröschel-Stewart U: Comparison of vascular smooth muscle cells from adult human, monkey and rabbit in primary culture and in subculture. *Cell Tissue Res* 177: 503–522, 1977.
140. Thyberg J, Palmberg L, Nilsson J, Ksiazek J, Sjölund M: Phenotype modulation in primary cultures of arterial smooth muscle cells on the role of platelet-derived growth factor. *Differentiation* 25: 156–167, 1983.
141. Cowan RA, Cowan SK, Grant JK, Elder HY: Biochemi-

cal investigations of separated epithelium and stroma from benign hyperplastic prostatic tissue. *J Endocrinol* 74: 111–120, 1977.
142. Krieg M, Klötzl G, Kaufmann G, Voigt KD: Stroma of human benign prostatic hyperplasia: preferential tissue for androgen metabolism and oestrogen binding. *Acta Endocrinol* 96: 422–432, 1981.
143. Greene GL: Application of immunochemical techniques to the analysis of estrogen receptor structure and function. In: Biochemical Actions of Hormones. G Litwack (ed), New York: Academic Press, 207–239, 1984.
144. Schulze H, Barrack ER.: Immunocytochemical localization of estrogen receptors in spontaneous and experimentally induced canine benign prostatic hyperplasia. *Prostate* 11: 145–162, 1987.
145. Huttunen E, Romppanen T, Helminen HJ: Testosterone action on the ventral prostate lobe of the castrated rat as assessed with a stereologic morphometric method. *Am J Anat* 165: 199–209, 1982.
146. Leav J, Merk FB, Ofner P, Goodrich G, Kwan PWL, Stein BM, Sar M, Stumpf WE: Bipotentiality of response to sex hormones by the prostate of castrated, or hypophysectomized dogs. Direct effects of estrogen. *Am J Pathol* 93: 69–91, 1978.
147. Tunn UW, Schüring B, Senge T, Neumann F, Schweikert HU, Rohr HP: Morphometric analysis of prostates in castrated dogs after treatment with androstanediol, estradiol and cyproterone acetate. *Invest Urol* 18: 289–292, 1980.
148. Funke PJ, Tunn UW, Senge T, Neumann F: Effects of the antioestrogen tamoxifen on steroid induced morphological and biochemical changes in the castrated dog prostate. *Acta endocrinol* 100: 462–472, 1982.
149. Aumüller G, Funke PJ, Hahn A, Hoffbauer G, Tunn U, Neumann F: Phenotypic modulation of the canine prostate after long-term treatment with androgens and estrogens. *Prostate* 3: 361–373, 1982.
150. Aumüller G, Habenicht UF, El Etreby MF: Pharmacologically induced ultrastructural and immunohistochemical changes in the prostate of the castrated dog. *Prostate* 11: 211–218, 1987.
151. McNeal JE: Origin and evolution of benign prostatic enlargement. *Invest Urol* 15: 340–345, 1978.
152. Cunha GR: Tissue interactions between epithelium and mesenchym of urogenital and integumental origin. *Anat Rec* 172: 529–542, 1972.
153. Cunha GR, Chung LWK, Shannon JM, Reese BA: Stromal–epithelial interactions in sex differentiation. *Biol Reprod* 22: 19–42, 1980.
154. Sugimura Y, Norman JT, Cunha GR, Shamon JM: Regional differences in the inductive activity of the mesenchyme of the embryonic mouse urogenital sinus. *Prostate* 7: 253–260, 1985.
155. Sugimura Y, Cunha GR, Donjacour AA: Morphogenesis of ductal networks in the mouse prostate. *Biol Reprod* 34: 961–971, 1986.
156. Sugimura Y, Cunha GR, Donjacour AA: Morphological and histological study of castration-induced degeneration and androgen-induced regeneration in the mouse prostate. *Biol Reprod* 34: 973–983, 1986.
157. Sugimura Y, Cunha GR, Donjacour AA, Bigsby RM, Brody JR: Whole-mount autoradiography study of DNA synthetic activity during postnatal development and androgen-induced regeneration in the mouse prostate. *Biol Reprod* 34: 985–995, 1986.
158. Kellokumpu-Lethinen P, Santti R, Pelliniemi LJ: Correlation of early cytodifferentiation of the human fetal prostate and Leydig cells. *Anat Rec* 196: 263–273, 1980.
159. Aumüller G, Seitz J, Bischof W: Immunohistochemical study on the initiation of acid phosphatase secretion in the human prostate. *J Androl* 4: 183–191, 1983.
160. Tenniswood M: Role of epithelial–stromal interactions in the control of gene expression in the prostate: An hypothesis. *Prostate* 9: 375–385, 1986.
161. Flickinger CJ: Fine structure of the rabbit epididymis and vas deferens after vasectomy. *Biol Reprod* 13: 50–60, 1975.
162. Dixon JS, Gilpin CJ, Gilpin SA, Gosling JA, Grant JFB: The effects of vasectomy on the autonomic innervation of the human vas deferens. *J Urol* 137: 1014–1016, 1987.
163. Kelâmi A: Atlas of Operative Andrology. Berlin–New York: De Gruyter, 1980.
164. Aumüller G: Morphologic and endocrine aspects of prostatic function. *Prostate* 4: 195–214, 1983.

Author's address:
Prof. Gerhard Aumüller
Department of Anatomy and Cell Biology
Philipps-University
D-3550 Marburg
Federal Republic of Germany

CHAPTER 10

Ultrastructure of smooth muscle tissue in the female reproductive tract: uterus and oviduct

SHINGO FUJII, IKUO KONISHI,
HIDETAKA KATABUCHI & HITOSHI OKAMURA

1. Introduction

The uterus is a hollow organ consisting of an upper, primarily muscular part, the corpus uteri, and a lower part, predominantly connective tissue, the cervix. The oviducts open into the upper and lateral angles of the uterus, constituting a conduit between the endometrial and peritoneal cavities. The body of the uterus is composed of three layers of smooth muscle cells (myometrium): outer and inner longitudinal layers and a circular intermediate layer accompanied by a rich vasculature between the layers (1). The oviduct is also composed of three layers of smooth muscle cells (myosalpinx), as well as the myometrium, but on the whole, the muscle elements are thinner than those of the uterus.

The oviducts and uterus are specifically designed for reproductive functions. The oviducts constitute a conduit between the ovaries and uterus. They bring ova and spermatozoa into proximity, furnish the environment for fertilization and early cleavage, and deliver the preimplantation embryo into the uterine cavity (2). Among these tubal functions, the transportation of gametes and the embryo is mainly conducted by a contractility of the smooth muscle cells of the oviduct (2). In contrast, the uterus fulfills a much greater complexity of normal functions than perhaps any other organ in the human body. In pregnancy, the uterus must enable the fertilized ovum to be implanted in its wall to provide for the supply of vital nutrients to the growing fetus, and must develop enough activity to expel the viable fetus at the end of a fixed period of time and subsequently return to the prepregnant state (3). The successful performance of these functions requires a rapid and enormous increase in the size and weight of the organ and considerable differentiation of its tissue. This enormous increase occurs in the myometrium and is almost entirely caused by an increase in the dimensions of the smooth muscle cells (hypertrophy), although some cell division (hyperplasia) does occur in early pregnancy (3). After menopause, with the waning of ovarian hormonal support, not only the endometrium but also the myometrial smooth muscle cells show atrophy. Consequently, the cells of the myometrium, although similar in structure to smooth muscle cells of extrauterine origin, have the unique ability to respond to ovarian and placental hormonal stimuli (4).

In order to approach the unique smooth muscle of the female genital tract, we will first present the ultrastructural features of the development of smooth muscle in the human fetal uterus and oviduct, and then discuss the ultrastructural changes of the smooth muscle cells during the reproductive period and pregnancy, and after menopause.

2. Smooth muscle of the uterus (the myometrium)

2.1. Development of smooth muscle in the human fetal uterus

Late in the fifth to sixth week of embryonic life, the coelomic epithelium invaginates at several

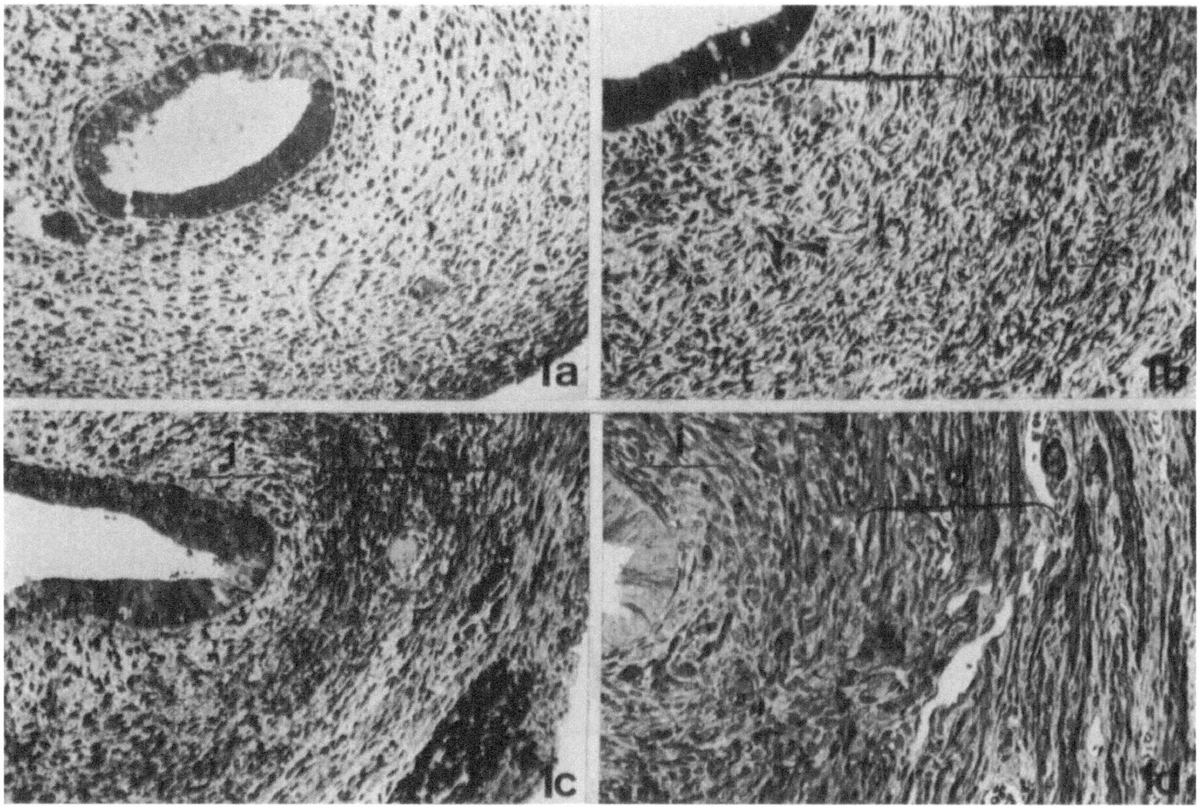

Figure 10-1. Transverse sections of the human uterine corpora at 12 weeks (a), 16 weeks (b), 20 weeks (c), and 31 weeks (d) of gestation. Mesenchymal cells arrange themselves into an outer (o) and inner (i) layer at 16 weeks. The outer layer, which increases in thickness with advancing age, develops into smooth muscle. S: serosa. X 100. (Reproduced by permission of Konishi et al.: *J Anat* 139: 239–252, 1984.)

points on the lateral surface of the urogenital ridge, and coalesces to form a tube termed the paramesonephric duct. The paired ducts extend caudally, and by the end of the seventh week of embryonic life, the ducts fuse to form a single structure. The fused paramesonephric ducts give rise to the body of the uterus, the cervix, and the upper vagina (5). Differentiation of the mesenchymal cells accompanied by the paramesonephric ducts results in the formation of the tubular muscular structure of the uterus and oviduct.

In light — microscopic studies, the smooth muscle is reported to appear in the wall of the genital canal between 18 and 20 weeks, and to be well developed by approximately 24 weeks (6–8). However, a study of the prenatal development of uterine smooth muscle by light and electron microscopy in specimens obtained from ten human fetuses between 12 and 40 weeks of gestation produced a slightly different point of view (9).

At 12 weeks of gestation (Fig. 10-1a) (9), the mesenchymal cells are round or stellate, about 10 μm in length, and contain large round nuclei with condensed nuclear chromatin near the nuclear membrane, which are distributed sparsely in the uterine mesenchyme (Fig. 10-2a). Mitochondria, rough-surfaced endoplasmic reticulum (rER), and free ribosomes are scarce in the cytoplasm, and intracytoplasmic filaments are not observed. Intercellular junctions between the cells are negligible. Collagen fibrils are sparse in the matrix. Ultrastructurally, the uterine mesenchymal cells remain undifferentiated at this stage.

By 16 weeks (9), two layers of mesenchymal cells are delineated: the cells near the serosa (the outer layer: myometrium) are most abundant and elongated, whereas the cells toward the lumen (the inner layer: endometrial stroma) are sparse and round in shape (Fig. 10-1b).

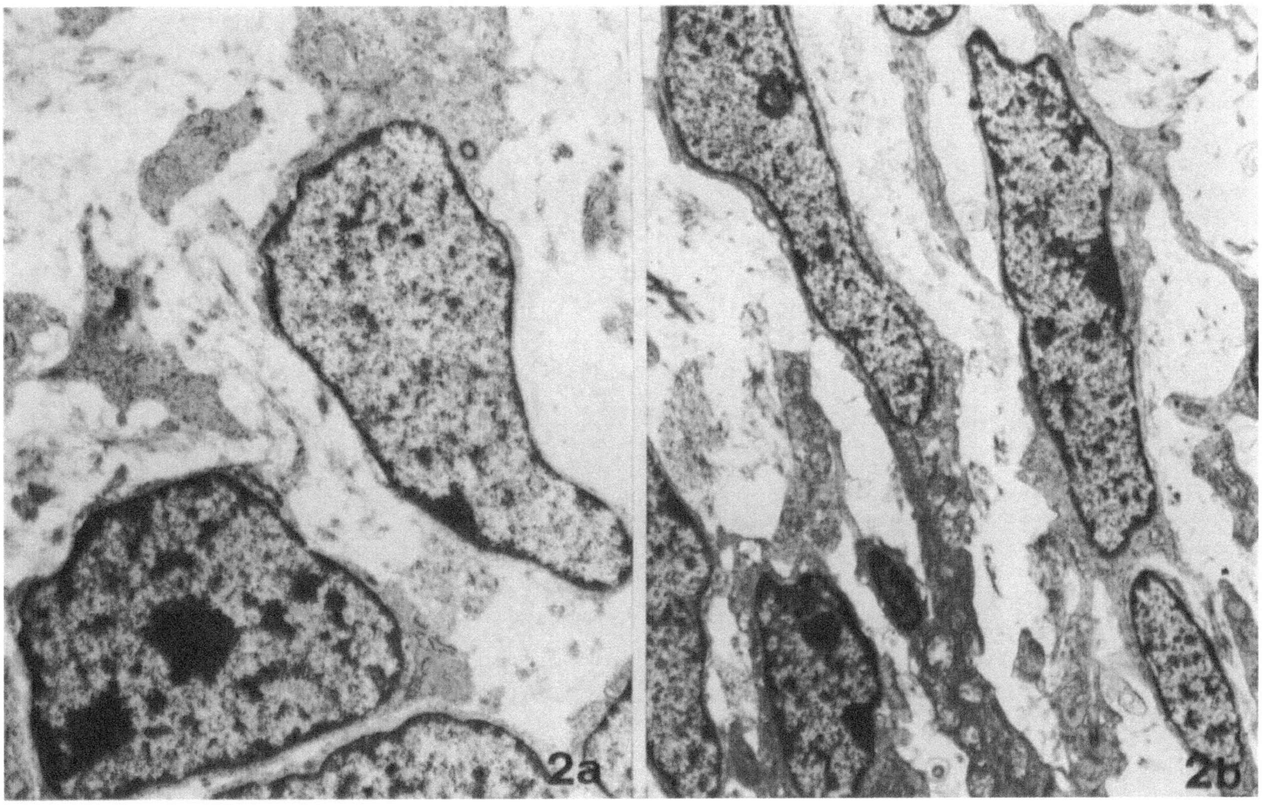

Figure 10-2. (a) Electron micrograph of the body of the fetal uterus at 12 weeks of gestation. Mesenchymal cells have large nuclei with marginally condensed chromatin and cytoplasm with poorly developed organelles. X 9000. (b) Outer layer of the body of the fetal uterus at 14 weeks of gestation. Mesenchymal cells are slightly elongated, but cytoplasmic filaments with dense bodies are not present. X 5000.

2.1.1. Development of the outer layer of the fetal uterine wall (the myometrium). From 14 to 16 weeks (Fig. 10-1b) (9), elongated cells, about 10–20 μm in length and having oval nuclei with condensed chromatin along their margin, are observed (Fig. 10-2b). Cytoplasmic organelles are not well developed; a few filaments but no dense bodies are present in some of these cells. Tiny vesicles exist along the cell membrane, but vesicles are smaller in number than the surface vesicles of typical smooth muscle cells. Single cilia occasionally protrude into the matrix of these cells. A few intercellular contacts exist, but desmosomelike junctions are rare.

From 18 to 20 weeks of gestation (Fig. 10-1c) (9), the cells are even more elongated than those at 14–16 weeks, measuring about 20–40 μm in length, and are greater in number. The nucleus is oval and the nuclear chromatin is dispersed within the nuclear matrix. The nucleocytoplasmic ratio is reduced. Intracytoplasmic organelles such as mitochondria, rER, and Golgi apparatus are well developed. Free ribosomes are especially numerous. Intracytoplasmic filaments with few dense bodies are observed in some portions of the cytoplasm. These filaments are about 6–8 nm in diameter (Figs. 10-3a, 10-3b). Surface vesicles along the cell membrane have increased in number by 20 weeks (Fig. 10-3b). However, no external lamina or dense plaques can be identified along the cell membrane. There are more intercellular contacts and a few desmosomelike junctions. These fine features are characteristic of immature smooth muscle cells, especially since a few myofilaments are present. These immature smooth muscle cells first appear at 18 weeks and increase by 20 weeks. At 20 weeks of gestation, filaments are more abundant in cells located near the subserosal vascular networks than in cells near the inner layer.

At 26 weeks of gestation (9), the number of

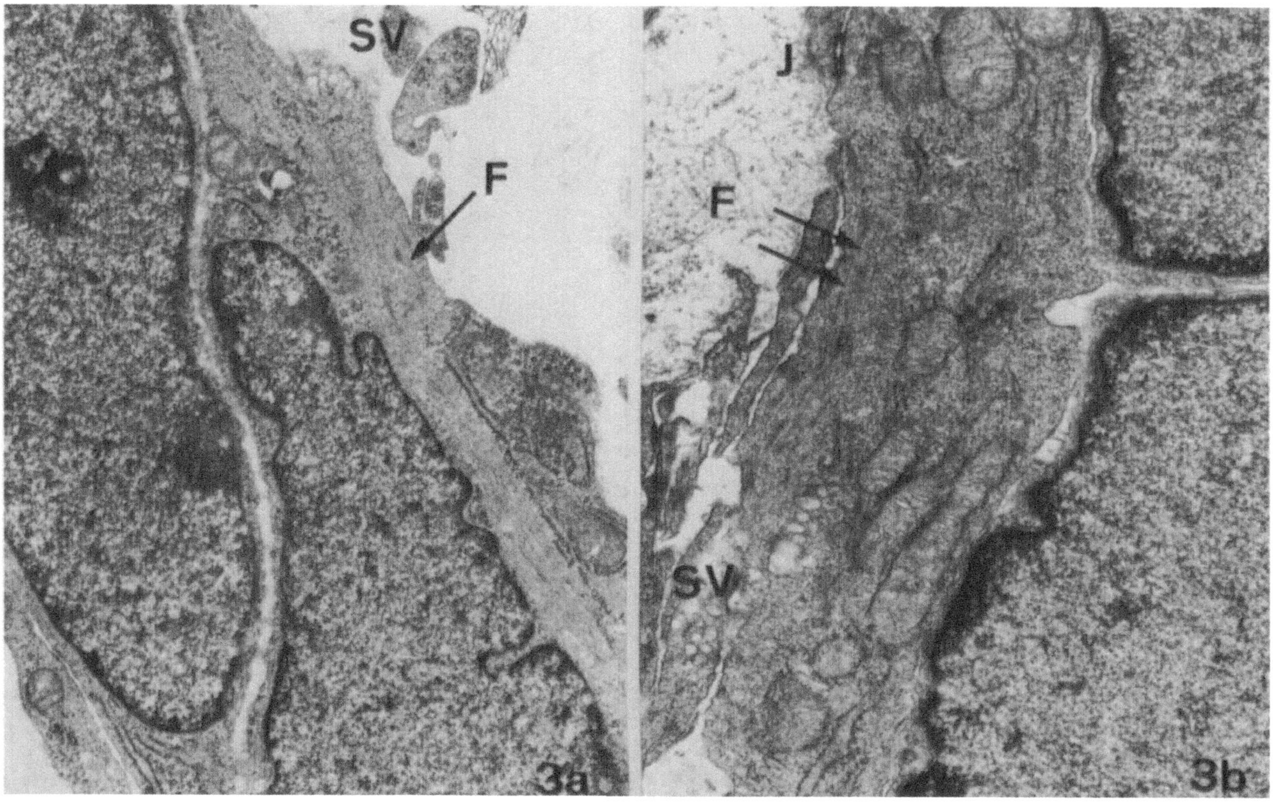

Figure 10-3. (a) Mesenchymal cells in the outer layer of the body of the fetal uterus at 18 weeks of gestation contain oval nuclei with dispersed chromatin and a few intracytoplasmic filaments (F). Several surface vesicles (SV) are present, but external lamina or dense plaques are not present along the cell membrane. X 14,000. (b) Mesenchymal cells in the outer layer of the fetal uterus at 20 weeks of gestation demonstrating well-developed cytoplasmic organelles, such as free ribosomes, rER, mitochondria, and Golgi apparatus. Note that there are a few filaments (F) with dense bodies and many surface vesicles (SV) of the cell membrane, and intercellular contacts with desmosomelike junctions (J). X 19,500.

elongated cells increases markedly. The cytoplasm of these cells is occupied mostly by filaments with dense bodies (Fig. 10-4). Cytoplasmic organelles are located mainly in the perinculear region. Surface vesicles are well developed, and there are some dense plaques along the cell membrane. Intercellular contacts with several desmosomelike junctions are prominent; however, development of the external lamina is incomplete. Nuclear indentations are not observed. Therefore, these cells exhibit the ultrastructural characteristics of smooth muscle cells apart from the appearance of the external lamina and nuclear indentation.

At 31 weeks (Fig. 10-1d) or 40 weeks (9), bundles of cells like smooth muscle cells are obvious. By 31 weeks of gestation, the cells are even more elongated, being 50 μm or more in length, and form bundles. These cells have all the ultrastructural characteristics of smooth muscle cells, including abundant filaments with dense bodies, dense plaques along the cell membrane, numerous surface vesicles, and an external lamina (Fig. 10-5). Intracytoplasmic organelles are limited to the perinuclear region. Intercellular contacts are not as prominent as at 26 weeks. However, the oval nuclei in these cells are not indented, and nuclear chromatin is evenly dispersed throughout the nuclear matrix.

2.1.2. Development of the inner layer of the fetal uterine wall (the endometrial stroma) (Fig. 10-1a-d). From 14 to 16 weeks (9), the cells are stellate or round in shape, and have features similar to cells in the 12-week fetus.

At 18–20 weeks (9), the cells are spindle-shaped, 10–20 μm in length, and resemble fibroblasts. Intracytoplasmic organelles are moderately developed and collagen fibrils are more obvious

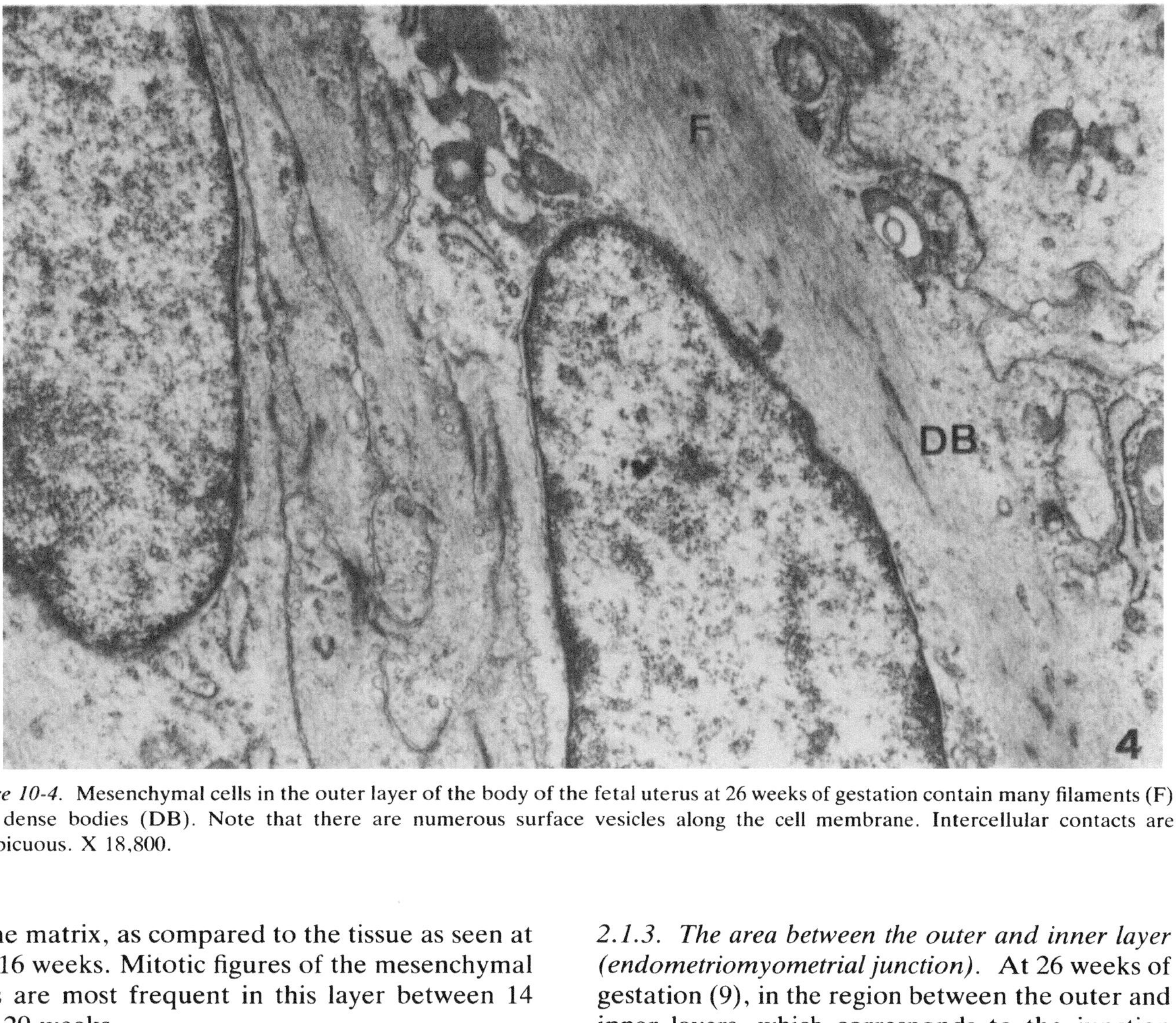

Figure 10-4. Mesenchymal cells in the outer layer of the body of the fetal uterus at 26 weeks of gestation contain many filaments (F) with dense bodies (DB). Note that there are numerous surface vesicles along the cell membrane. Intercellular contacts are conspicuous. X 18,800.

in the matrix, as compared to the tissue as seen at 14–16 weeks. Mitotic figures of the mesenchymal cells are most frequent in this layer between 14 and 20 weeks.

At 26 weeks of gestation (9), two morphologically distinct mesenchymal cells exist. One type is spindle-shaped, resembling the fibroblasts observed in this layer at 18–20 weeks. The other type is round, resembling predecidual cells, with abundant cytoplasm, and is observed in the vicinity of the blood vessels. It contains well-developed rER and Golgi apparatus in the cytoplasm, surface vesicles, and small cytoplasmic processes projecting toward the matrix. External laminalike materials partially envelop these cells.

At 31 or 40 weeks (9), in addition to fibroblast-like cells, cells with abundant cytoplasm and well-developed organelles resembling predecidual cells are usually located around blood vessels, as observed at 26 weeks.

2.1.3. The area between the outer and inner layer (endometriomyometrial junction). At 26 weeks of gestation (9), in the region between the outer and inner layers, which corresponds to the junction between the myometrium and endometrial stroma in the adult, there are a number of spindle-shaped cells that contain a few intracytoplasmic filaments and well-developed organelles. These cells are ultrastructurally similar to cells in the outer layer at 18–20 weeks; therefore, at this stage, immature smooth muscle cells exist in this region.

At 31 or 40 weeks of gestation (9), this area is several cells thick. These cells have a few filaments with dense bodies characteristic of immature smooth muscle cells.

Collectively, until 16 weeks of gestation, cytoplasmic filaments with dense bodies characteristic of smooth muscle cells are not identified in the mesenchymal cells of the uterus. Spindle-shaped cells, containing a few myofilaments scattered in

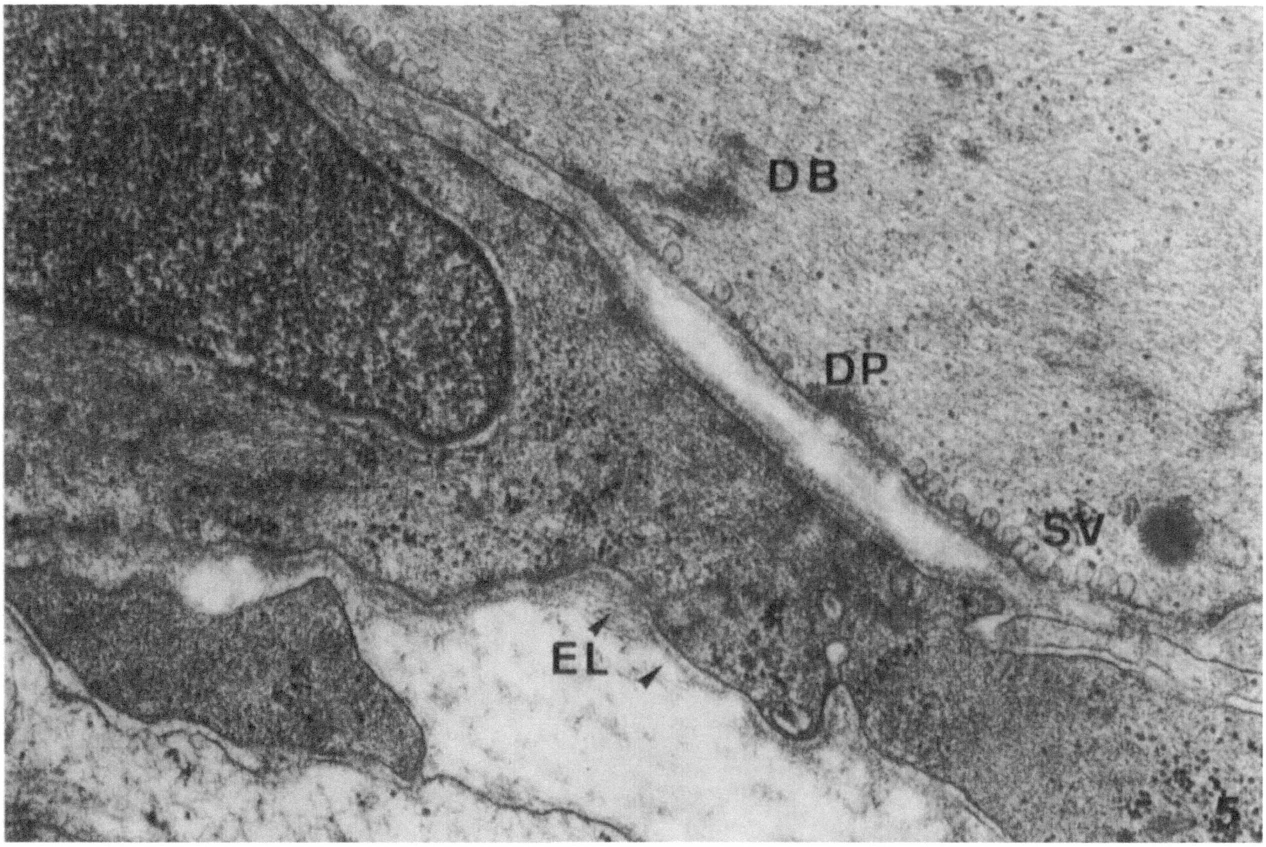

Figure 10-5. The cells in the outer layer of the body of the fetal uterus at 31 weeks of gestation have numerous filaments with dense bodies (DB). Dense plaques (DP), surface vesicles (SV), and an external lamina (EL) are well developed. X 32,500.

the cytoplasm and well-developed organelles such as mitochondria, free ribosomes, granular endoplasmic reticulum, and Golgi membranes, first appear in the outer layer of the uterus at 18 weeks, when the fetus has a crown–rump length of 145 mm. These cells are interpreted as immature smooth muscle cells, since they have a form intermediate between undifferentiated mesenchymal cells and mature smooth muscle cells. Similar features of developing smooth muscle cells have been reported in studies on the perinatal development of rabbit myometrium (10), rat ureter (11), and mouse ductus deferens (12). Other ultrastructural characteristics of smooth muscle cells develop later; surface vesicles of the cell membrane begin to increase at about 20 weeks, dense plaques along the cell membrane appear by 26 weeks, and an external lamina is almost complete by 31 weeks. Although nuclear indentation is not observed, the cells in the outer layer at 31 weeks exhibit all the other features of mature smooth muscle cells. Therefore, in the human fetal uterus, it is considered that smooth muscle differentiation begins at 18 weeks of gestation, and that by 31 weeks, the myometrium is formed in the outer layer of the wall of the uterus, and is clearly distinguishable from the inner layer corresponding to the endometrial stroma.

Uterine smooth muscle cells originate from undifferentiated mesenchymal cells, as observed at 12 weeks of gestation. The myometrial layer increases in thickness with advancing age; nevertheless, mitotic figures in mesenchymal cells are detected mainly in the inner layer from 14 weeks. Moreover, immature smooth muscle cells are identified in the region between the myometrial and endometrial stromal layers both at 26 and 31 weeks, when bundles of almost mature smooth muscle cells are already formed. These observations imply that undifferentiated mesenchymal cells that develop into smooth muscle cells may exist in the inner layer of the fetal uterus and that smooth muscle differentiation may occur in the junctional area between the myometrial and endometrial stromal layers. This view of the histogenesis of fetal uterine smooth muscle is consistent with the observation that uterine smooth muscle is newly produced by endometrial stroma at the endometriomyometrial junction (13) and in certain pathological conditions (14). On the other hand, fibroblastlike cells of the endometrial stromal layer are also considered to be derived from undifferentiated mesenchymal cells in the same layer. Ultrastructurally, the undifferentiated mesenchymal cells that develop into endometrial stromal cells cannot be distinguished from the progenitors of smooth muscle cells. Previous experiments by the authors on leiomyomatosis peritonealis disseminata have shown that subperitoneal mesenchymal cells, which are considered to be embryologically identical with the undifferentiated mesenchymal cells that surround the paramesonephric ducts, proliferate and differentiate into cells of both the smooth muscle and decidual types in response to estrogen and progesterone (15). This experimental result and the observations of fetal uterine mesenchyme suggest that the undifferentiated mesenchymal cells around paramesonephric ducts have the potential to develop into both smooth muscle cells and endometrial stromal cells.

The mechanism that regulates smooth muscle differentiation in the human fetal uterus is still uncertain. However, in the fetal urinary bladder, completely differentiated smooth muscle cells occur as early as 14 weeks (9). This clearly demonstrates a difference between the two organs in the period of smooth muscle development. The slower differentiation of fetal uterine smooth muscle suggests that its development may be controlled by factors other than those of the bladder. Although the differentiation of male genital ducts is controlled by testicular androgens (16), the female ducts are said to differentiate autonomously without the need for any external regulatory factors from the gonads or elsewhere (17). However, it is well known that estrogen and progesterone increase in the maternal and fetal plasma during gestation (18, 19), and the reduction in the size of the uterus after parturition (6) or after ovariectomy (20) suggests that placental estrogens or fetal ovarian steroids may have some effect on the development of the female genitalia. Moreover, the existence of plump cells resmbling predecidual cells around blood vessels in the inner layer of the fetal uterus from 26 weeks implicates the influence of sex steroids on the human fetal uterus. Pasqualini et al. (21) have reported that estrogen and progesterone receptors become established in the fetal uterus of guinea pigs from 34 and 50 days of gestation, respectively, and that the uptake of tritiated progesterone occurs mainly in the stroma and myometrium, rather than in the luminal epithelium. Therefore, it is likely that the fetal uterus, especially its mesenchymal components of smooth muscle and endometrial stroma, is under the influence of estrogen and progesterone during pregnancy.

2.2. The myometrial smooth muscle during the reproductive period

At birth, there is a significant development of both the cervix and uterus that declines in the postnatal period, with the cervix predominating until the prepubescent growth spurt (1). Thereafter, following puberty, there is considerable development of the uterus, including the myometrial smooth muscle cells.

2.2.1. During the menstrual cycle. Myometrial smooth muscle cells in the nonpregnant state are spindle-shaped and embedded in an abundant connective tissue network. The cells are about 5 to 10 μm wide and 50 to 800 μm long, but these dimensions can be altered by hormonal and physical factors (3).

Ultrastructural studies of the rat uterus in diestrus demonstrate that smooth muscle cells contain ellipsoid nuclei and scarce cytoplasmic organelles located adjacent to the nucleus. However, at estrus, smooth muscle cells increase cytoplasmic organelles, such as rER and Golgi apparatus (22). Myometrial smooth muscle cells contain both estrogen and progesterone receptors. Following estrogen stimulation, the fine structure of the uterine smooth muscle is similar to the estrus condition (22–25). In contrast, following progesterone stimulation, smooth muscle cells appear larger and myofilaments more abundant; also they contain little rER, and few ribosomes and glycogen particles (26). Therefore, estrogen

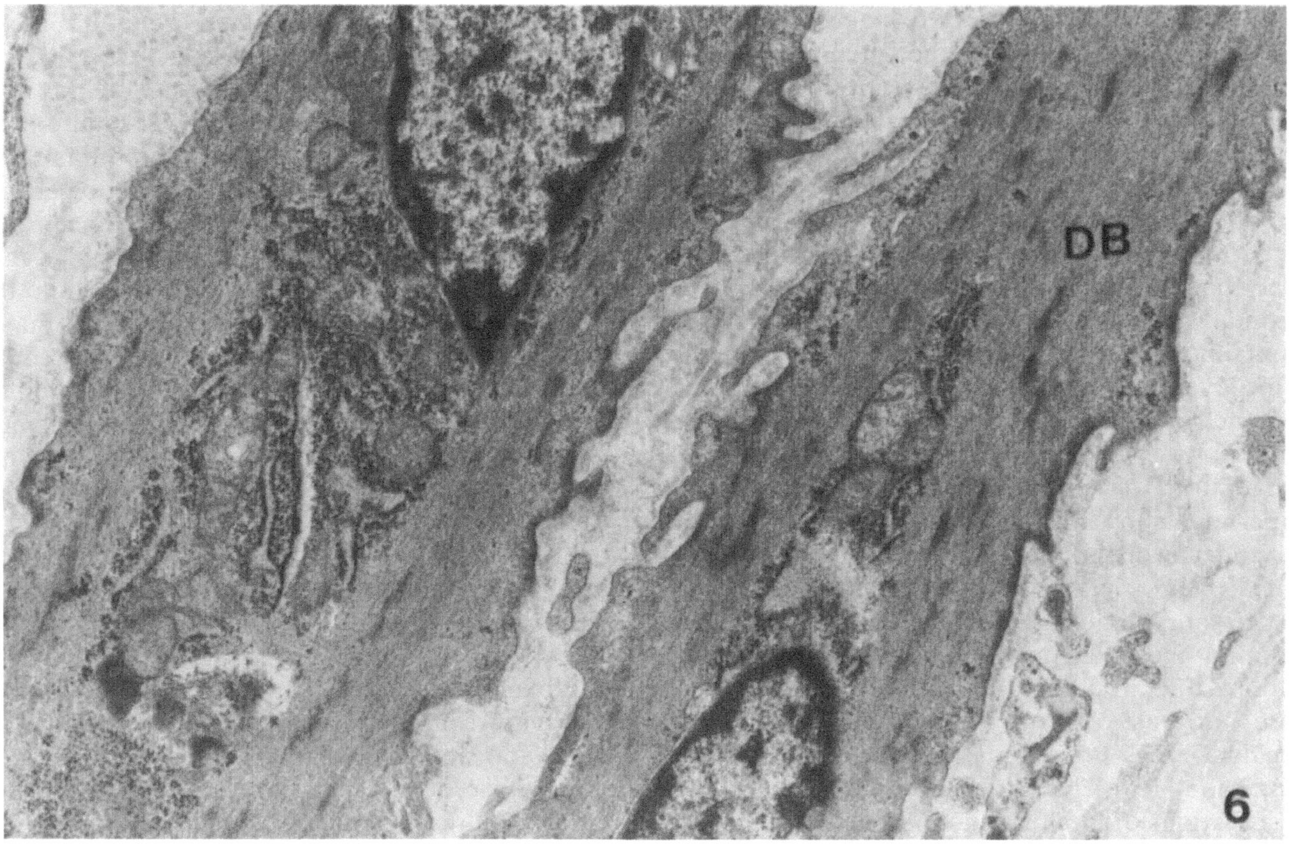

Figure 10-6. Myometrial cells in the follicular phase of the menstrual cycle contain well-developed cytoplasmic organelles, such as free ribosomes, rER, mitochondria, and Golgi apparatus. The cytoplasm is packed with filaments with dense bodies (DB). The cells are embedded in an abundant connective tissue stroma, from which they are separated by a well-defined basal lamina. X 25,000.

causes a pronounced change in the uterine smooth muscle cells, and progesterone alters the smooth muscle cells but not to the degree observed following estrogen stimulation (26).

Under the hormonal milieu of the menstrual cycle, human myometrial smooth muscle cells exhibit almost the same changes, although not as strikingly as in animals. In the follicular phase, under estrogen stimulation, myometrial smooth muscle cells appear fusiform in shape, with a centrally located nucleus (Fig. 10-6). The cytoplasmic organelles are well developed and occur around the nucleus. The rER, free ribosomes, Golgi apparatus, and mitochondria are well–developed (Fig. 10-6). Most of the cytoplasm is packed with threadlike myofilaments, oriented parallel to the long axis of the cells. Myofilaments occur in random bundles throughout the muscle cells. Besides the thick (15 nm) and thin (6 nm) myosin filaments, smooth muscle also contains a third major filament type — the intermediate filaments that form a network that links protein structures known as dense bodies (Fig. 10-6) (27). The intermediate filaments or dense bodies do not play an active part in the contractile process. Rather, they are associated with the cell membrane as well-developed cell membrane dense bodies (27). The latter often alternate with rows of surface vesicles that are apparently related to the active transport of proteins and ions, such as sodium and potassium, that are important elements in the generation of action potentials (28). The myometrial smooth muscle cells are embedded in an abundant connective tissue stroma, from which they are separated by a well-defined, but often interrupted, basal lamina.

In the luteal phase, under estrogen and progesterone stimulation, smooth muscle cells appear larger and myofilaments more abundant (Fig. 10-7). However, the rER, free ribosomes, and mito-

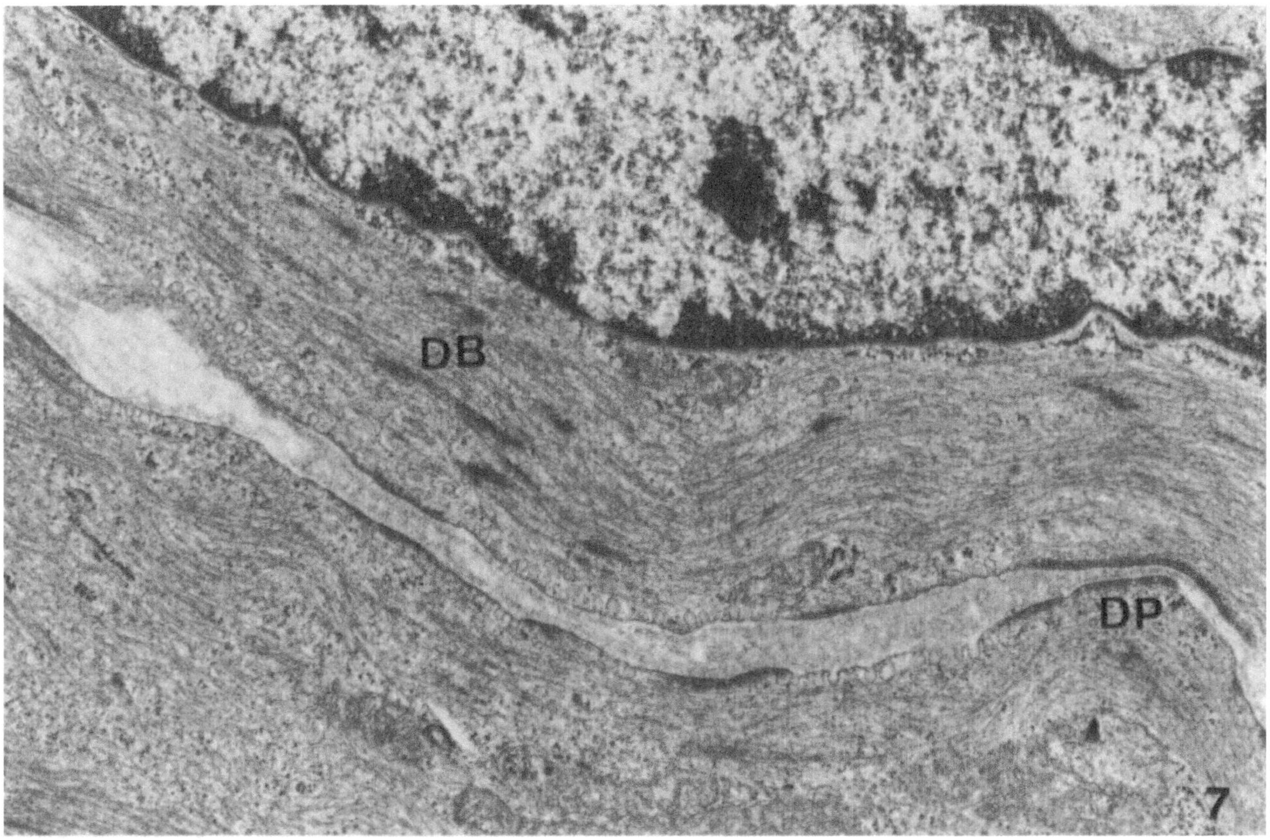

Figure 10-7. Myometrial cells in the luteal phase of the menstrual cycle contain abundant myofilaments with dense bodies (DB). The cytoplasmic organelles are scarce. Note that there are intercellular connections by closely apposed cell membrane, with or without dense plaques (DP). X 5000.

chondria are scarce and occur around the nucleus. The intercellular connection is closely apposed cell membranes (Fig. 10-7), with or without dense plaques; occasionally intermembrane gap junctions (nexuses) are observed (4).

At various stages of the menstrual cycle, gap junctions are present between the smooth muscle cells in some of the tissues from women with dysmenorrhea, during menstruation, and at other times in response to physiologic or pathologic stimuli, such as the production of prostaglandins, and their presence may result in contraction of the uterus (29, 30).

Although the uterus is innervated primarily by postganglionic adrenergic fibers from the sympathetic nervous system that originate from cell bodies in the lumbar and mesenteric ganglia and from short adrenergic fibers (31), it is generally believed that uterine contractility is controlled by myogenic and hormonal mechanisms and that modulation by nerve is not important. Nerve fibers with one to many axons exist between bundles of smooth muscle cells and around larger muscular blood vessels of the uterus; however, there is no recognizable neuromuscular contact as in skeletal muscles, and the nerves terminate in varicosities at some distance from the smooth muscle cells (32).

2.2.2. During pregnancy. While the uterus is designed to perform a variety of functions throughout the woman's reproductive life, it is during pregnancy that its major function occurs (1). Initially, the expulsive function of the myometrium has to be suppressed in order to allow implantation and the subsequent development of the embryo and growth of the fetus in the uterine cavity. At the end of a fixed period of time, the myometrium performs its considerable expulsive effort through the cervix and the vagina in order to achieve par-

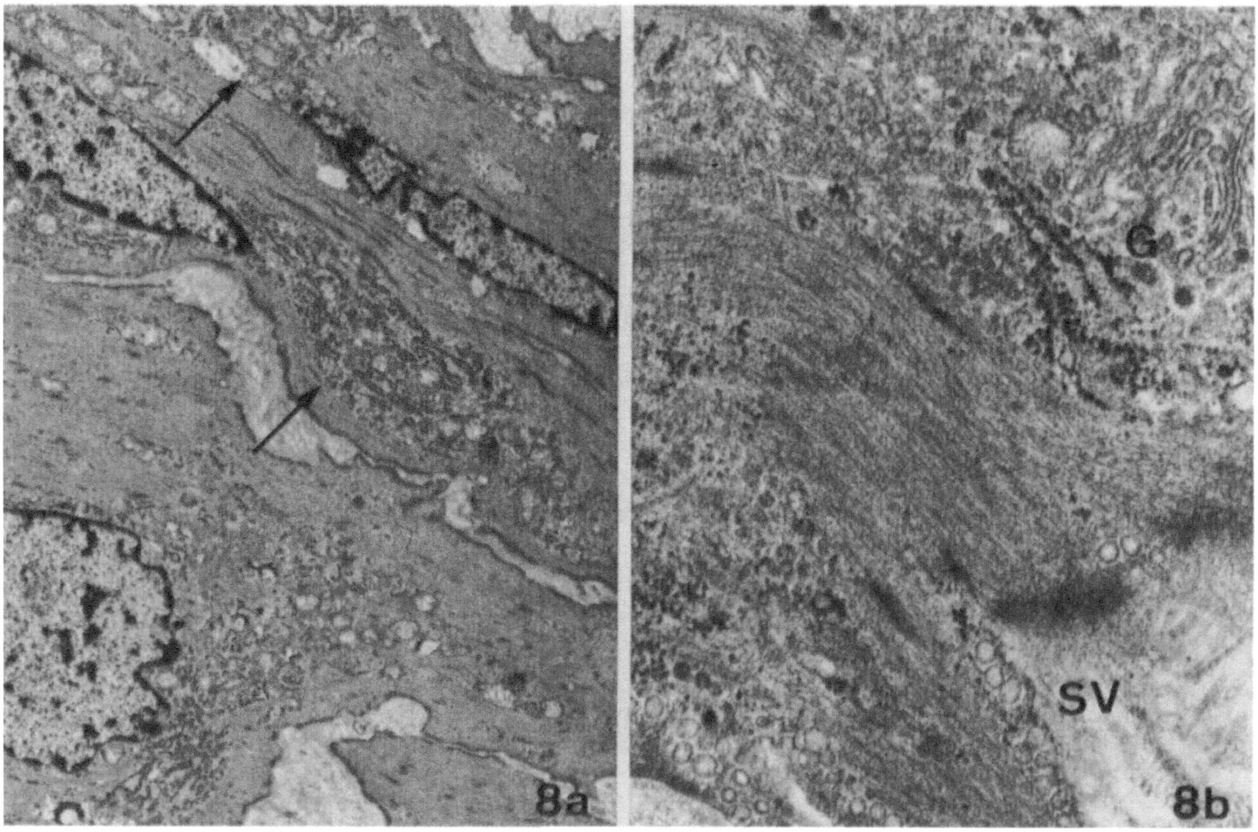

Figure 10-8. (a) Myometrial cells at 14 weeks of gestation have abundant myofilaments with dense bodies and prominent cytoplasmic organelles (arrows), such as endoplasmic reticulum, mitochondria, free ribosomes, and Golgi apparatus. Contacts between adjacent cells are frequent. X 7500. (b) Higher magnification of the myometrial cells at 14 weeks of gestation. The Golgi apparatus (G) is greatly hypertrophied, and a clear distinction between endoplasmic reticulum and Golgi cisternae is difficult to make. Numerous surface vesicles (SV) are present along the cell membrane. X 37,500.

turition. Thus, initially, the contractile nature of the myometrium is inhibited during the majority of pregnancy, and then a series of mechanisms occur at labor that initiate and sustain the highly coordinated uterine contractility (1). Accordingly, the smooth muscle cells of the uterus are arranged in bundles separated by connective tissue comprising collagen and elastic fibers, which serves not only as a support for the muscular fibers but also as a network to orient the tensile forces exerted by the contractility of this smooth muscle (1).

During early gestation, the myometrial smooth muscle cells increase in cellular size, and the most striking modifications occur at the level of the cytoplasmic organelles under the hormonal milieu during pregnancy (33–37).

The endoplasmic reticulum increases in size and appears as greatly dilated rough- and smooth-surfaced vesicles and cisternae that occur in the perinuclear area, scattered among the myofilaments or below the cell membrane (Figs. 10-8a, 10-8b) (33). The mitochondria are increased in number. The Golgi apparatus is greatly hypertrophied, and a clear distinction between endoplasmic reticulum and Golgi cisternae is at times difficult to make (Fig. 10-8b). Due to a relative increase of the ground substance, the myofilaments can be more easily observed as individual units. In some cells the myofilaments are scarce, appearing as clear cells. The cell membrane shows an increase in surface vesicles (Fig. 10-8b) (33).

Contact between adjacent cells is frequent (Fig. 10-8a). However, gap junctions are absent, or present in low frequencies, throughout pregnancy (38, 39).

At term pregnancy, the general picture of the uterine smooth muscle is similar to that of midpregnancy, but there is a further increase in the number and size of the cytoplasmic organelles and dense bodies (33). Due to the marked hypertrophy of the Golgi apparatus and endoplasmic reticulum, the muscle cells show a spongy appearance. The mitochondria are even more abundant than in midpregnancy and have a similar structure.

The dense bodies dispersed among the myofilaments appear greatly increase in size and number as compared with the uterus at midpregnancy. The fine structure of the myofilaments, cell membrane thickenings, and cellular contacts is similar to that of midpregnancy (33).

Cells believed to be modified smooth muscle cells occupy the myoendometrial junction and the decidua basalis (34). They are irregular in shape, poor in myofilament content, and rich in other cytoplasmic organelles, and form a loosely arranged layer of cells between the myometrium and the trophoblast. Modified smooth muscle cells in the basal decidua constitute a network of large cells that are capable of contraction, since they contain a small number of loosely arranged myofilaments. In this location, they form a buffer zone between the strongly contracting myometrium and the noncontracting decidua and placenta (34).

During contractions, it is believed that the smooth muscle cells become darker, decrease in volume, and exhibit changes in diameter (34). This is accompanied by a widening of the interspaces and a decrease in the areas of cellular contact. Between contractions, there are more light cells that become arranged closer to each other and exhibit large areas of interdigitation (34). The propagation of electrical activity along the cell surface is thought to occur by a local circuit mechanism and involves the flow of ions (ionic current) between cells through channels that connect the cell interiors (32). Gap junctions are believed to be the sites of continuity between cells as well as the loci of electrical coupling between cells (32, 40). A gap junction is a structure composed of identical portions of plasma membranes from two closely apposed cells with a distance of approximately 2 nm to form a seven-lined structure (32, 40). Functional studies have shown that gap junctions form pathways between coupled cells to allow the passage of current (electrical or ionic coupling) and the exchange of small metabolities (metabolic coupling) (32, 40). Studies of rats, guinea pigs, sheep, and humans (32, 38–43) demonstrate that 1) myometrial gap junctions are absent, or present in low frequency, throughout pregnancy; 2) at term, gap junction frequency increases; 3) the junctions are present in high frequency, and the sizes are increased, during delivery of the fetus; 4) the gap junctions begin to disappear within 24 hours after delivery. The junctions are also present in increased numbers in tissues from animals induced to deliver prematurely (43) and in human myometrium from women in premature labor (41).

The fact that the presence of gap junctions between uterine smooth muscle cells is exclusively limited to the period just before, during, and immediately following normal and premature parturition has significant implications for the maintenance and termination of pregnancy (32). The absence of gap junctions between smooth muscle cells throughout gestation may maintain pregnancy by limiting the electrical or metabolic communication between cells, thereby preventing coordinated contractions of the uterus (32). The rapid formation and appearance of gap junctions may initiate or allow the initiation of parturition and terminate pregnancy by providing large areas of low resistance between cells, allowing the spread of electrical information (32).

2.2.3. Postpartum (involution of the uterus). During pregnancy, the uterine mass increases greatly by the hypertrophy of myometrial smooth muscle cells and by an increase in the amounts of intercellular collagen and ground substances. In the few days immediately following parturition, the uterus regresses rapidly, and in a few weeks, it returns to its nongravid dimensions.

Studies of the guinea pig uterus (44) demonstrate that early after parturition (during the first two days), the smooth muscle cells contain an abundance of cytoplasmic organelles, and numerous surface vesicles are arranged on their surfaces. These cells differ from those at term pregnancy in several respects: an increase in the number of small surface vesicles and free polyribosomes, membrane-bound bodies (that resemble lysosomes) of various electron densities, and collagenous fibrils within the cytoplasm. Mostly these fibrils are enclosed within cytoplasmic mem-

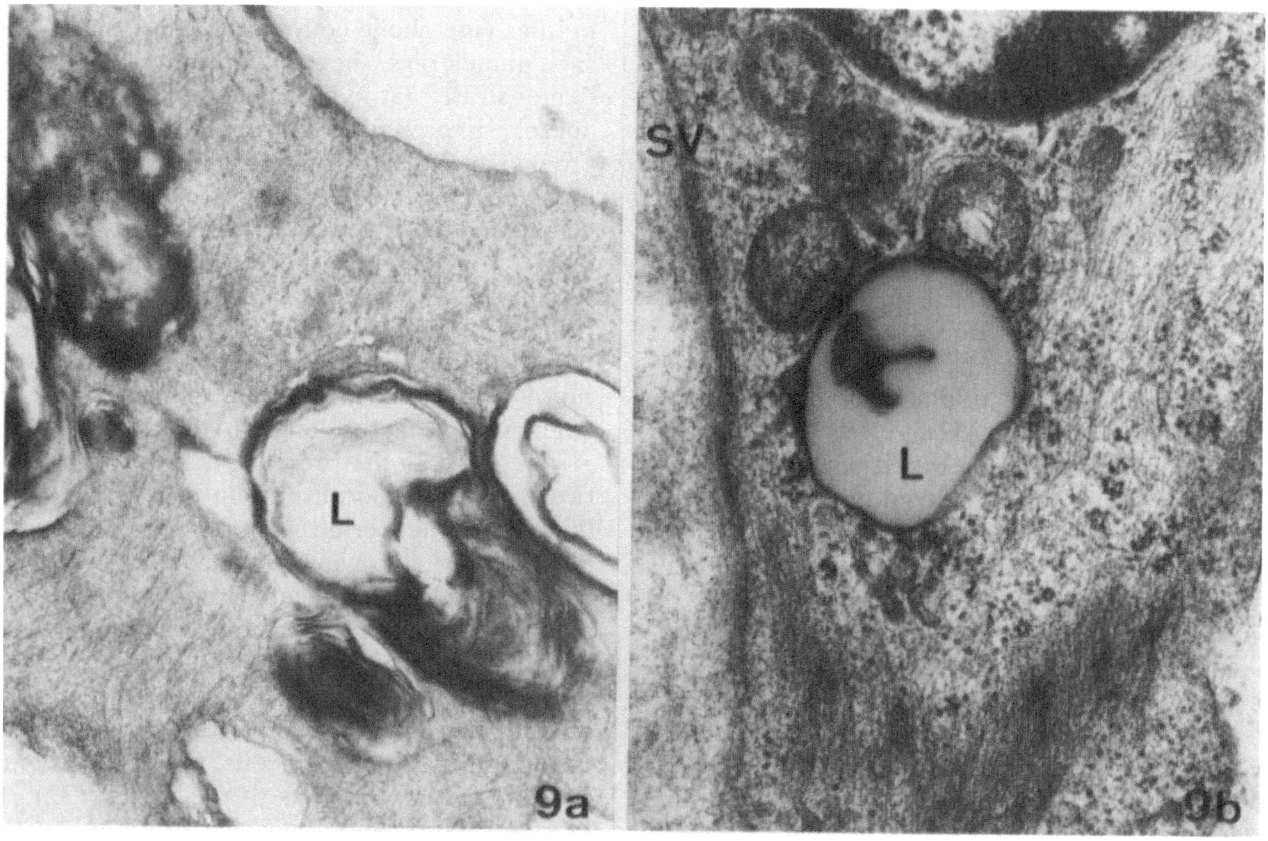

Figure 10-9. (a) Part of a smooth muscle cell from the uterus on the fourth postpartum day shows numerous lysosomal structures (L) of membranous type (phagolysosomes) in the cytoplasm. Pinocytotic vesicles are also observed. X 15,000. (b) Myometrial cells after menopause contain few cytoplasmic filaments and scarce intracytoplasmic organelles. Lipid droplet engulfed in a lysosomelike membrane-bound structure (L) are present in the cytoplasm, and a few surface vesicles (SV) are present along the cell membrane. X 37,500.

branes. After the second postpartum day, there is a gradual decrease in the amount of recognizable collagen fibrils and gradual increase in the number and size of lysosomal and phagolysosomal bodies. A reduction in the number of cytoplasmic organelles and myofilaments occurs as in the pregnant state (44).

Studies of rats (45) and humans (46, 47) also demonstrate that lysosomes in smooth muscle cells are involved in the intracytoplasmic degradation of myofilaments and collagen in the postpartum uterus (Fig. 10-9a). In addition, immunohistochemical staining of collagenase in sections of rat uterus shows the enzyme to be present in the perinuclear region of the smooth muscle cells only of the involuting myometrium (48). These observations indicate that smooth muscle cells are capable of producing collagenase, and are consistent with the hypothesis that this enzyme presides over the massive collagen degradation seen in postpartum uterine involution.

2.3. Myometrial smooth muscle cells after menopause

After menopause, with the waning of hormonal support, the uterus becomes atrophic with a concomitant loss of smooth muscle cytoplasm. As a consequence, the myometrium appears hypercellular. The nuclei are less elongated than those found in the premenopausal uterus, and they more closely resemble those of the endometrial stroma (49).

Ultrastructurally, postmenopausal myometrial smooth muscle cells contain few cytoplasmic filaments and scarce intracytoplasmic organelles (Fig. 10-9b). The nucleocytoplasmic ratio is increased. In the cytoplasm, lipid droplets engulfed in a lysosomelike membrane-bound structure are often observed. The cell membrane shows a decrease in surface vesicles (Fig. 10-9b). Ultrastructural features of the postmenopausal myometrium resemble those of the fetal uterine smooth muscle cells at 14 weeks of gestation or myofibroblast. Therefore, with the waning of ovarian hormonal support, myometrial smooth muscle cells show dedifferentiation.

2.4. *Myometrial smooth muscle cells in culture*

It has been demonstrated that uterine smooth muscle cells can be successfully isolated by enzymatic methods and cultured in vitro for many generations (50, 51). The fine structural studies of rat and human uterine smooth muscle cells during the first few days in primary culture demonstrate that they go through a transition from contractile to synthetic phenotypes (52). This process involves the loss of myofilaments, formation of a widespread rER and a prominent Golgi apparatus, and initiation of synthetic processes. As a result, the smooth muscle cells acquire a fibroblastlike appearance. In vivo, the smooth muscle of the myometrium is modified structurally and functionally during estrus and after treatment with estrogen (22–25) in a manner resembling smooth muscle cells during cultivation in vitro. This modification is also comparable to the phenotypic modulation that occurs in primary cultures of arterial smooth muscle cells (53). Uterine and vascular smooth muscle cells are both able to respond to the stimuli that bring about the transition from contractile to synthetic phenotypes. However, uterine smooth muscle cells grow markedly in size but proliferate slowly, whereas vascular smooth muscle cells respond strongly to mitogenic stimulation and then enter a stage of partly autonomous growth (53). This

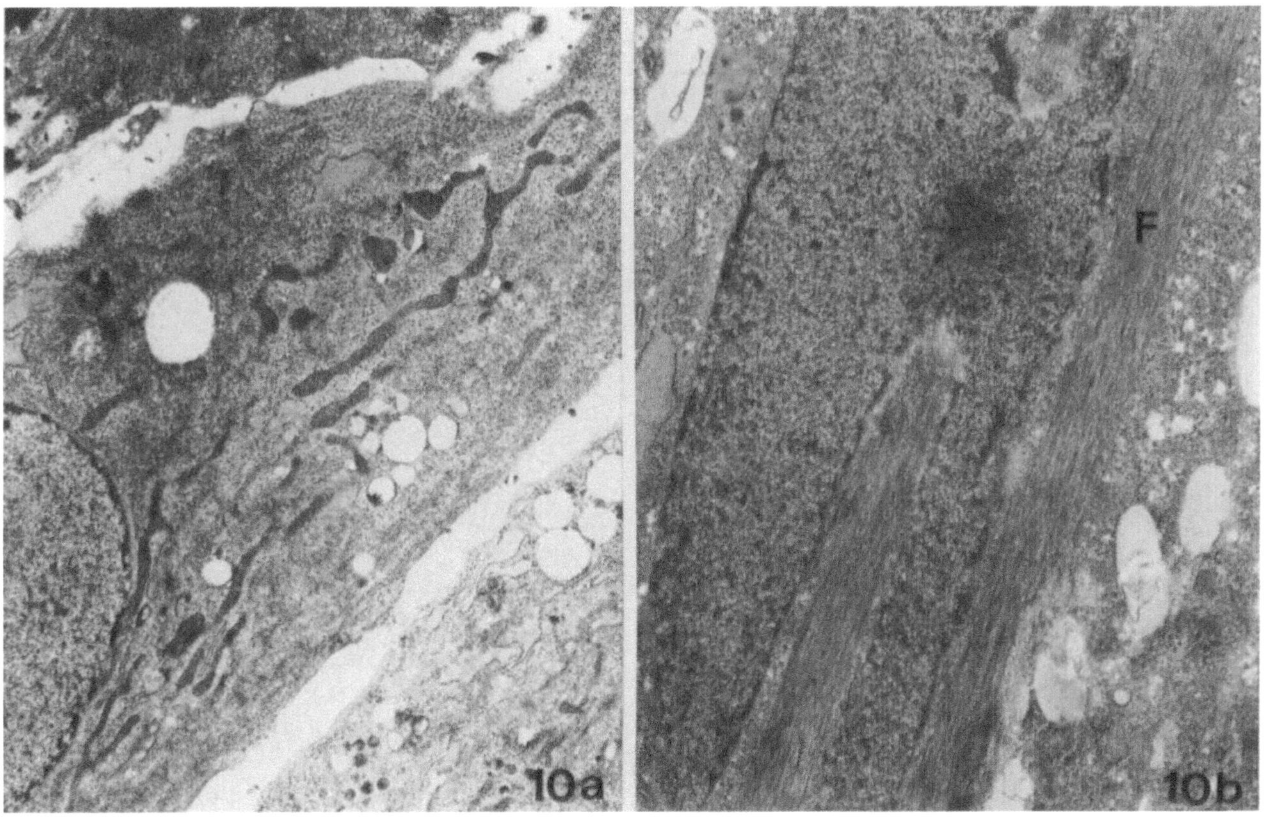

Figure 10-10. Cultured smooth muscle cells grown from the explants of normal myometrium at the 14th day (a) and 21st day (b) in control medium. At the 14th day (a), organelles such as free ribosomes, rER, and mitochondria are well developed, whereas cytoplasmic filaments are scarce. X 4000. At the 21st day (b), a moderate number of cytoplasmic filaments (F) with dense bodies are present in the cytoplasm. X 10,200.

suggests that uterine and vascular smooth muscle cells represent separate differentiation pathways and that the transition to a synthetic phenotype is a necessary but not sufficient requirement of the initiation of DNA synthesis and cellular proliferation (52).

The study of cells from myometrium explants under the influence of sex steroids (54) demonstrates that without sex steroids in the medium at the 14th day of culture, the cells are analogous to the dedifferentiational stage (synthetic phenotype) of smooth muscle cells in vitro (Fig. 10-10a), and at the 21st day of culture to the redifferentiated stage (contractile phenotype) (Fig. 10-10b). The same morphological changes are observed in culture cells of myometrial explants with estrogen-added medium. This implies that estrogen itself does not significantly affect the differentiation of cultured smooth muscle cells from myometrium in vitro, although its effect on proliferation remains to be studied (54). However, estradiol is a mitogen in the immature rat uterus and was shown to cause a 55-fold increase in the mitotic index of the epithelium and a six fold increase in the stroma and myometrium (55). In addition, the study of leiomyoma, which is also composed of smooth muscle cells, demonstrates that the mitotic index is significantly higher in the luteal phase than in the follicular phase (56) — a fact that implies that, although leiomyoma does not represent uterine smooth muscle cells, proliferation of the smooth muscle cells in the uterus may be controlled by sex steroids in a slightly different way from the epithelium.

Cultured smooth muscle cells from myometrium in estrogen- and progesterone-added medium contain more abundant filaments with dense bodies at any stage of culture examined than cells in either the control or estrogen-added medium (Fig. 10-11a, b) (54). Therefore, smooth muscle cells cultured with both estrogen and progesterone do not show their dedifferentiated phase in vitro. Progesterone with the assistance of estrogen may have its effect on differentiation

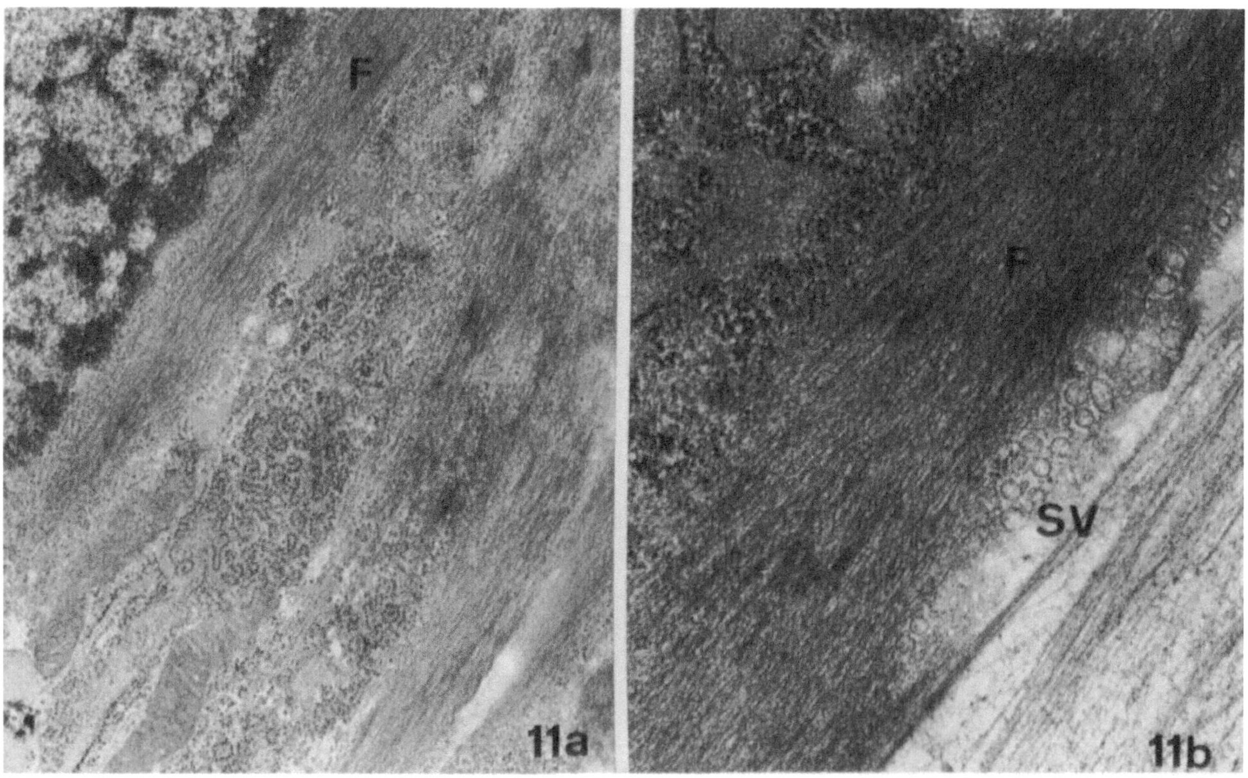

Figure 10-11. Cultured smooth muscle cells from normal myometrium at 14th day (a) and 21st day (b) in both estradiol and progesterone-added medium, showing abundant cytoplasmic filaments (F) with dense bodies and well-developed surface vesicles (SV). (a) X 15,600; (b) X 32,000.

into smooth muscle cells or maintenance of their characteristics not only in vivo (26) but also in vitro.

Consequently, in the study of the differentiation or proliferation of smooth muscle cells in the uterus, the part played by progesterone should be taken into account in addition to that played by estrogen.

3. Smooth muscle of the cervix

The cervix is the lower part of the uterus, and is divided from the upper part, or corpus, by a fibromuscular junction, usually referred to as the internal os, which makes the junction between the muscular corpus and the fibrous cervix (57). During pregnancy the cervix aids in the retention of the conceptus, but during labor it dilates in response to the contractions of the corpus and permits delivery of the fetus and placenta (58). These functions are shared by the lower uterine segment in later pregnancy and labor (58). The cervix is lined by squamous and columnar epithelial membranes, supported by an admixture of fibrovascular, muscular, and elastic tissue. The predominant stromal component is the fibrous connective tissue (59).

3.1. Development of smooth muscle in the human fetal cervix

Hunter (6) refers to the fused paramesonephric ducts as the uterus in the female embryo at nine weeks of gestation, and identifies the body and the cervix by the construction between them. According to Hunter (6), the smooth muscle differentiation begins in the periphery, and the seat of its greatest activity is at first in the region of the cervix. In another study (60), however, smooth muscle was found well differentiated in the corpus at 21 weeks of gestation, although it was absent from the wall of the cervix.

Ultrastructurally, at 15 weeks of gestation, the mesenchymal cells of the cervix are undifferentiated, as are those observed in the fetal uterine wall. At 18 weeks of gestation, the mesenchymal cells are even more elongated than those at 15 weeks. However, the cells having some ultrastructural characteristics of smooth muscle are not identified at this stage. At 22 weeks of gestation, the elongated cells having intracytoplasmic filaments with dense bodies are distributed sparsely in the cervical mesenchymal cells. Intracytoplasmic organelles such as mitochondria, rER, and Golgi apparatus are well developed. Surface vesicles and dense plaques along the cell membrane are well developed. External lamina are identified along the cell membrane. At 31 weeks of gestation, the cells exhibiting more distinct smooth muscle characteristics than those at 22 weeks are distributed sparsely or in bundles in the cervical mesenchymal cells. Smooth muscle cells observed in the fetal cervix are completely differentiated at this stage.

Therefore, the development of smooth muscle in the fetal cervix is considerably more rapid than that in the fetal uterine wall and almost the same as that in the fetal oviducts (1, 4).

3.2. The cervical smooth muscle during the reproductive period

The cervix consists mainly of fibrous tissue with varying quantities of smooth muscle. The proportion of smooth muscle ranges from 2% to 40%, with an average of 10% (59). The fibrous nature of the cervix has been suggested to be the reason that the cervix is refractory to those stimuli that elsewhere in the uterus give rise to growth and contractile responses, and also as the reason why the cervix is able to act as a barrier to retain the products of conception (59). However, some investigators (61, 62) believe that the smooth muscle in the cervix has a definite architecture, and they ascribe contractile properties to it in pregnancy. Hughesdon (61) has described an outer longitudinal layer in the corpus, which transmits a longitudinal pull to the cervix. He calls it the extrinsic muscle of the cervix (61). The inner part of the cervix is mainly collagenous with some scattered nonfunctional muscle fibers. A histological cell count in different parts of the uterus on cut sections from 40 uteri has shown that the proportion of smooth muscle in the corpus is 28%, in the isthmus 15%, and in the cervix 8% (63). In pregnancy, the amount of smooth muscle in the corpus increases to 42%, but there is a negligible increase in the cervix (63). The histological study of different levels of the cervix, comparing them with the smooth muscle content of the uterus, has alternatively shown that the lower cervix contains 6.4% muscle, the middle cervix 18.0%, the upper cervix 28.8%, and the corpus 68.8% (64).

There are a few ultrastructural studies of the smooth muscle in the cervix. Ferenczy (65) has described scattered smooth muscle cells with few organelles but abundant intracytoplasmic myofilaments, surface vesicles, and dense plaques along the cell membrane that compose about 15% of the cervical stroma with increasing numbers towards the isthmus, the portio vaginalis being virtually devoid of smooth muscle cells. Smooth muscle cells, unlike fibroblasts, produce a well-developed basal lamina. Myelinated and nonmyelinated nerve fibers, comparatively more numerous in the endocervical than portio stroma, may be encountered running parallel to smooth muscle bundles.

Nevertheless, not only the morphological features but also the functional significance of the smooth muscle in the cervix has not yet been clarified.

4. Smooth muscle of the oviduct (the myosalpinx)

The oviducts are paired hollow organs extending from the sides of the uterine fundus to the ovaries. Each tube consists of a hollow core of smooth muscle, the myosalpinx, with an inner lining of mucosa, the endosalpinx. The tube is sheathed within and supported by a portion of the broad ligament, the mesosalpinx (2).

4.1. Development of smooth muscle in the human fetal oviducts

During the early stages of development of the female genital tract, the paired paramesonephric ducts give rise to the oviducts. Differentiation

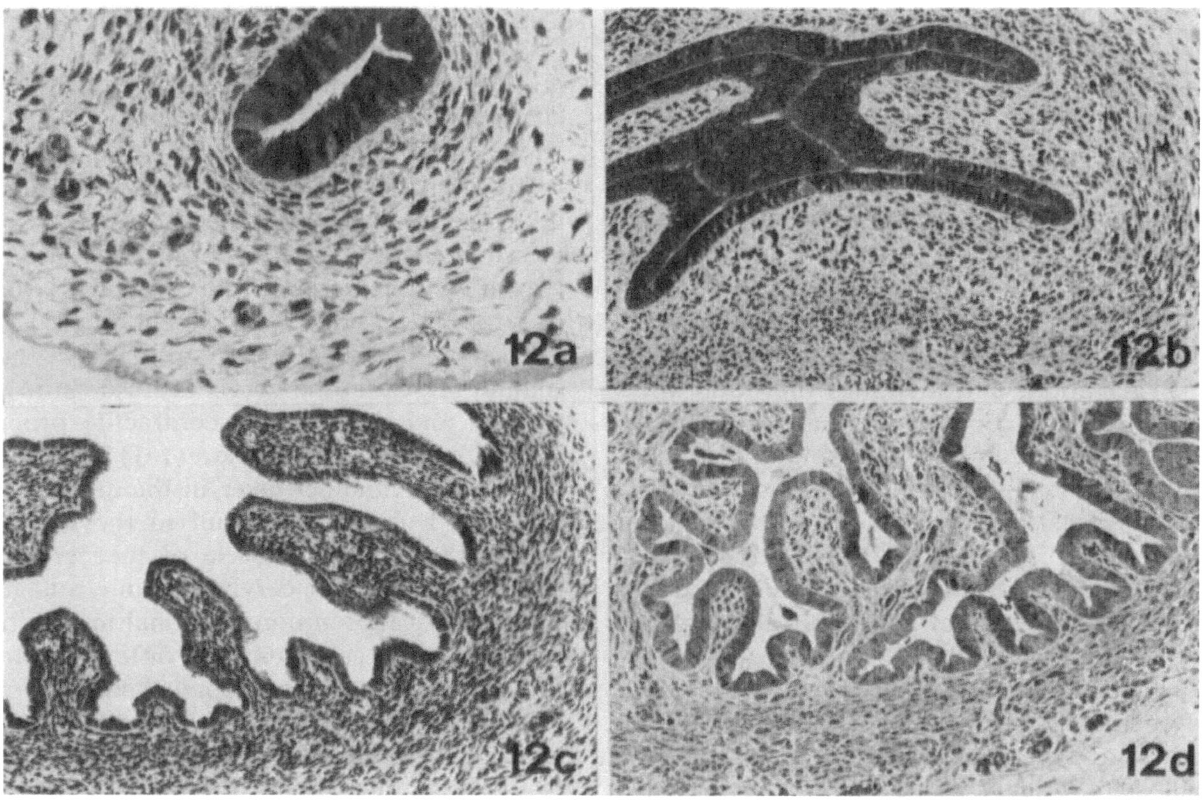

Figure 10-12. Transverse sections of the ampullary portion of fetal oviduct at 12 weeks (a), 18 weeks (b), 21 weeks (c), and 31 weeks (d) of gestation. Mesenchymal cells surrounding oviductal epithelium are condensed and develop into smooth muscle from the 21st week. (a), (c): X 200; (b), (d): X 100. (Reproduced by permission of Konishi et al.: *Anat Rec* 219: 60–68, 1987).

of the mesenchymal cells accompanied by the paramesonephric ducts also results in the formation of the myosalpinx of the oviducts as well as the myometrium of the uterus (Fig. 10-12a).

At 18 weeks of gestation (Fig. 10-12b), the mesenchymal cells are distributed sparsely in the oviductal mesenchyme. They are round or stellate, and contain large nuclei (Fig. 10-13). Nuclear chromatin is condensed near the nuclear membrane. Mitochondria, rER, and free ribosomes are well developed. Intracytoplasmic filaments are not observed (Fig. 10-13). There are negligible intercellular junctions between the cells. Collagen fibrils are sparse in the matrix. Therefore, the mesenchymal cells remain undifferentiated at this stage. In contrast, in the fetal uterine wall, the mesenchymal cells already have some characteristics of smooth muscle at this stage.

At 21 weeks of gestation (Fig. 10-12c), the cells are more elongated than those at 18 weeks, and the nucleocytoplasmic ratio is reduced. The nucleus is ellipsoid and the nuclear chromatin is dispersed within the nuclear matrix. Intracytoplasmic organelles such as mitochondria, rER, and Golgi apparatus are well developed. Intracytoplasmic filaments with dense bodies are observed (Fig. 10-14). Surface vesicles and dense plaques along the cell membrane are well developed. External laminae are identified along the cell membrane (Fig. 10-14). There are more intercellular contacts and a few desmosomelike junctions. In the fetal oviducts, well-developed smooth muscle cells are already observed at this stage.

At 31 weeks of gestation (Fig. 10-12d), the cells exhibit more distinct smooth muscle characteristics than those at 21 weeks (Fig. 10-15). The nucleus shows indentation (Fig. 10-15). Smooth muscle cells observed in the fetal ovi-

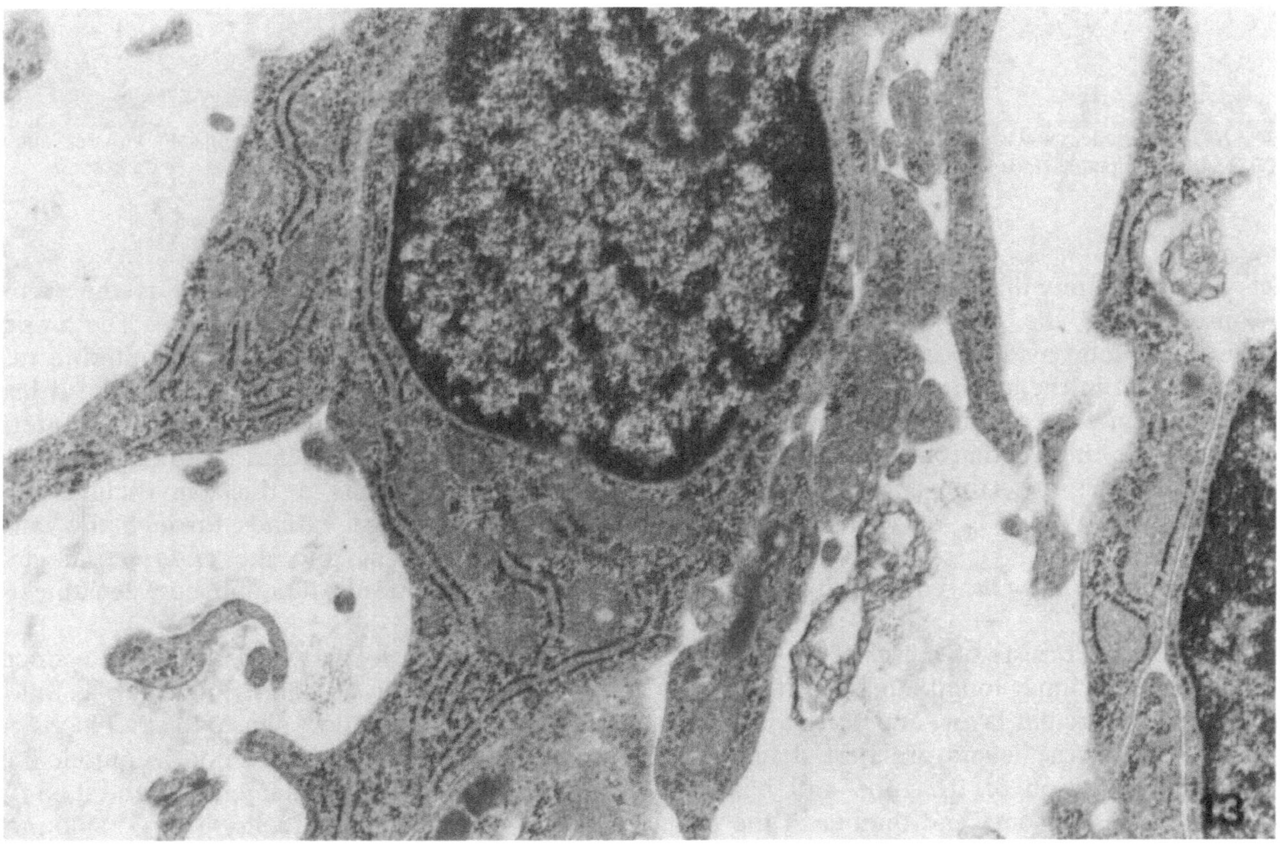

Figure 10-13. Mesenchymal cells of the fetal oviduct at 18 weeks of gestation are round or stellate. The cells contain large nuclei and well-developed cytoplasmic organelles, such as free ribosomes, rER, and mitochondria. Intracytoplasmic filaments are not present. X 25,000.

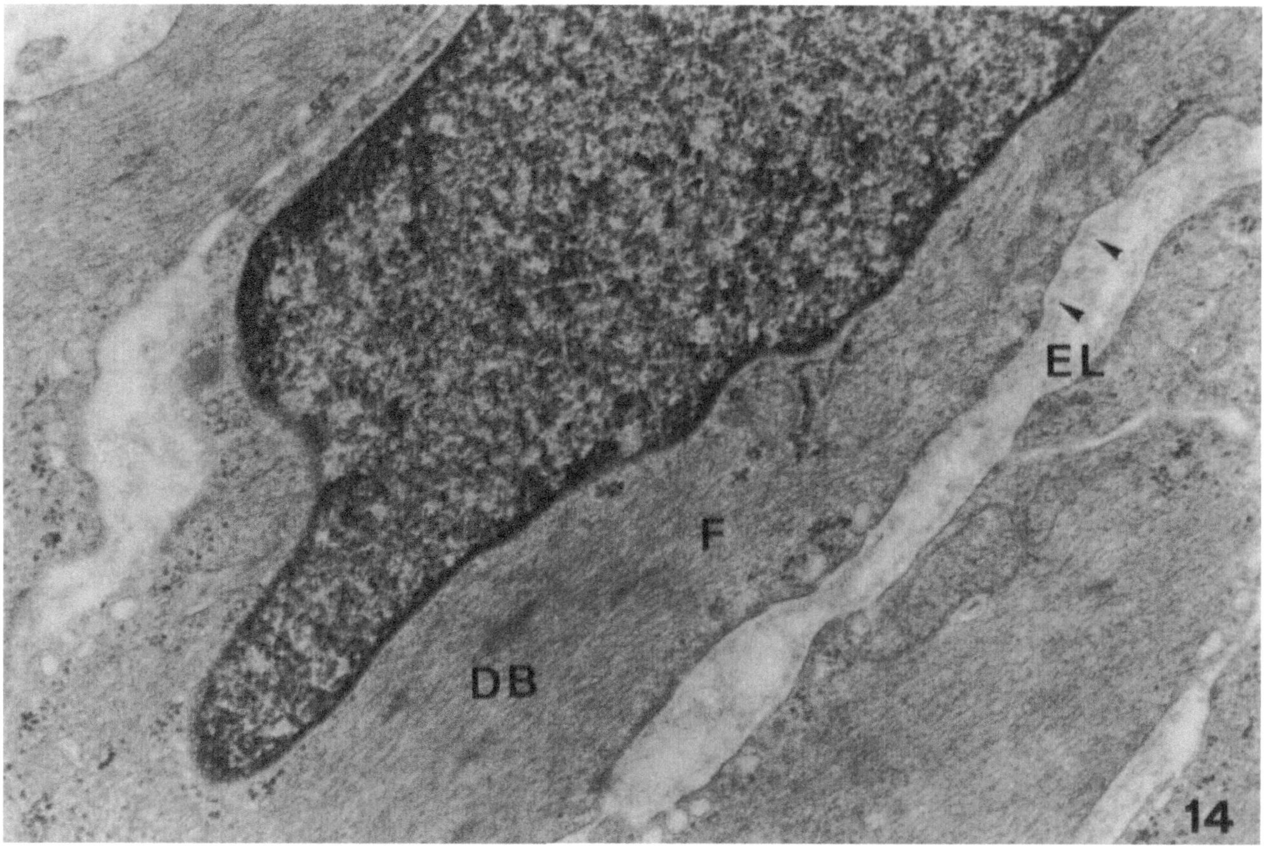

Figure 10-14. Mesenchymal cells of the fetal oviduct at 21 weeks of gestation have intracytoplasmic filaments (F) with dense bodies (DB), well-developed surface vesicles, and external lamina (EL) along the cell membrane. X 37,500.

ducts are completely differentiated at this stage.

Consequently, the development of smooth muscle in the fetal oviducts is considerably more rapid than that in the uterine wall. Nevertheless, the mechanism that results in the difference of smooth muscle differentiation between the uterus and oviduct is uncertain and remains to be verified.

4.2. Myosalpinx during the reproductive period

The myosalpinx consists of muscle fiber bundles arranged into an inner longitudinal layer, a prominent middle circular layer, and an outer longitudinal layer. These layers are best defined in the proximal portion of the tube and become progressively less distinct and thinner in the distal tube (2).

The tube may be divided into the infundibulum, ampulla, isthmus, and the intramural segment (2). The infundibulum is the funnel-shaped distal segment of the tube. The ampulla is the longest segment of the extrauterine tube, constituting two thirds of its length. The isthmus constitutes the remainder of the extrauterine tube (2). The wall of the ampulla is thin, but the isthmus exhibits a thick myosalpinx. The intramural segment extends through the lateral wall of the uterus into the endometrial cavity and is the functional junction between the tube and uterus (2).

Ultrastructural characteristics of the smooth muscle cells of the human oviducts are as follows (66). In the follicular phase of the menstrual cycle (Fig. 10-16a), the smooth muscle cells possess threadlike myofilaments oriented parallel to the long axis of the cells, a large amount of both smooth and rough endoplasmic reticulum, often associated with extensive collections of glycogen granules, well-developed Golgi appar-

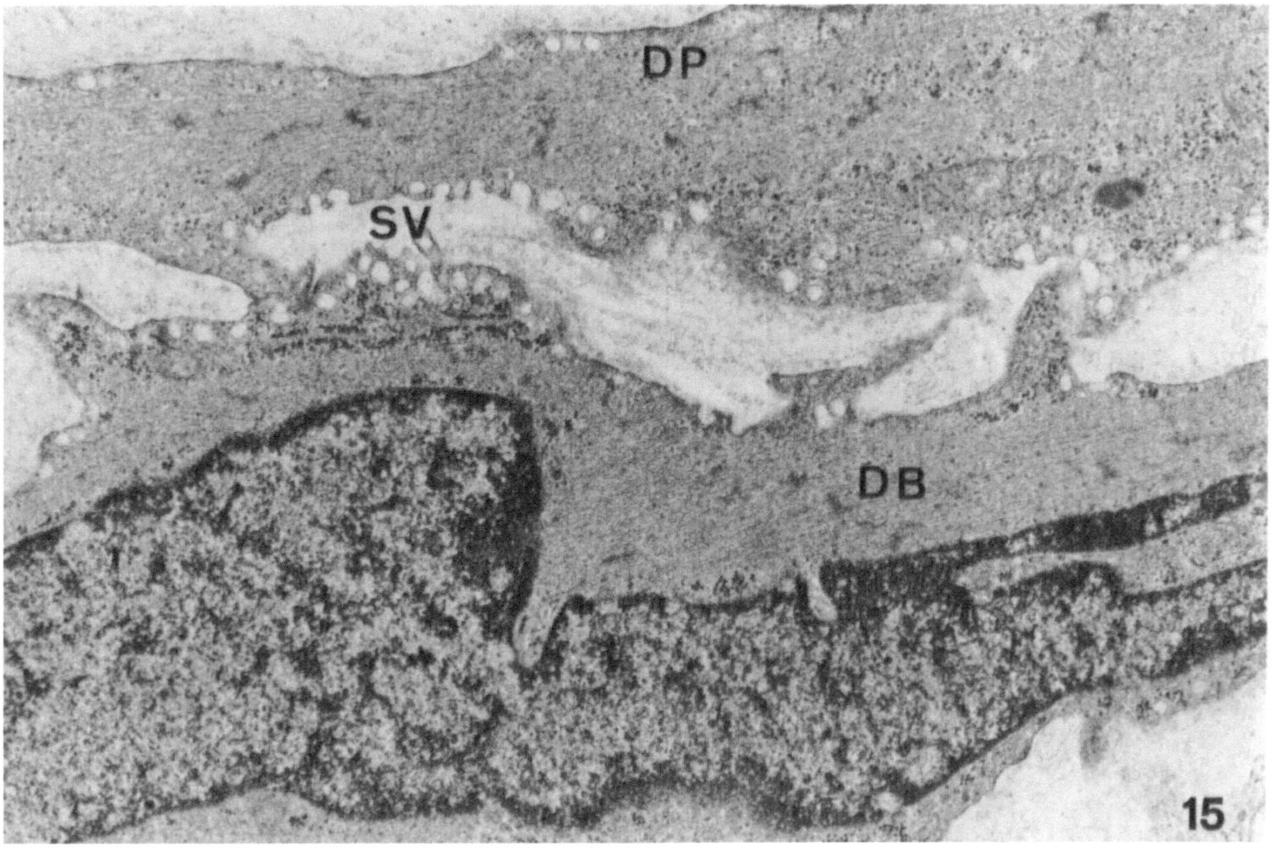

Figure 10-15. Mesenchymal cells of the fetal oviduct at 31 weeks of gestation have abundant myofilaments with dense bodies (DB), numerous surface vesicles (SV), dense plaques (DP), and external lamina along the cell membrane. Nucleus shows indentation. X 25,000.

atus, numerous surface vesicles, large lobulated nuclei, strange dense plaques, and very large amount of collagen between cells. In the luteal phase of the menstrual cycle (Fig. 10-16b), the smooth muscle cells of the oviducts contain a few intracytoplasmic organelles and often begin to contain relatively electron-lucent and/or electron-dense, membrane-bounded, lysosomelike bodies in the cytoplasm resembling the features observed in the postpartum uterus (Fig. 10-9a).

In the ampulla, there is usually a group of longitudinal muscle cells just outside of each mucosal fold in the lamina propria (66). A number of bundles adjacent to this are oriented circularly; more peripherally, the bundles interweave in both orientations. An arrangement in larger bundles cannot be discerned. The tissue is characterized by much collagen between muscle cell bundles. One type of cell-to-cell contact predominates in the muscle: a simple apposition of parallel cell membranes at a distance of 10 to 30 nm. No gap junctions are found; only rarely are intermediate contacts found (66).

In the isthmus, as in the ampulla, there is a great deal of collagen, but muscle cells are more densely distributed. Only simple appositions, aside from the rare intermediate contacts, are observed (66). There are many more nerves in the isthmus than in the ampulla. In the human tubal preparations, adrenergic nerves are identified both outside and within smooth muscle bundles. The adrenergic nerve terminals of the isthmus are often found to be located approximately 200 nm, and sometimes as close as 60–100 nm, from the membrane of (nonvascular) smooth muscle cells in the form of simple appositions (67). These close contacts often occupy a considerable area of the naked varicosity (67).

Since the smooth muscle cells of the tube are arranged into layers oriented in different direc-

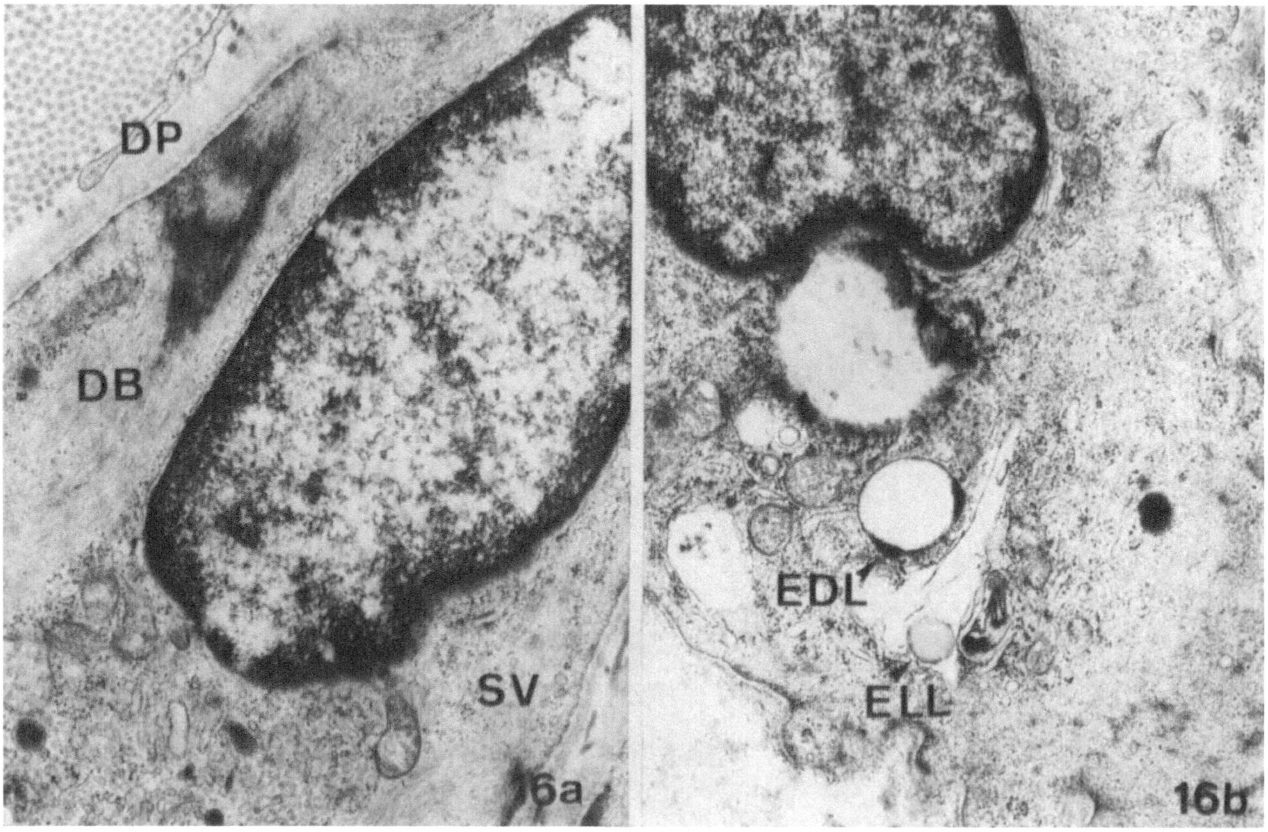

Figure 10-16. (a) Myosalpinx in the follicular phase of the menstrual cycle contains abundant myofilaments with dense bodies (DB), a large amount of both smooth and rough endoplasmic reticulum, well-developed Golgi apparatus, numerous surface vesicles (SV), and strange dense plaques (DP). X 10,000. (b) Myosalpinx in the luteal phase of the menstrual cycle contains a few intracytoplasmic organelles and relatively electron-lucent (ELL) and/or electron-dense (EDL) lysosomelike bodies in the cytoplasm. X 10,000.

tions, they are capable of generating a variety of contractile patterns. No anatomic basis for peristaltic contractile activity exists. Smooth muscle cells are in close cell-to-cell contact through the simple apposition of parallel cell membranes, which establish electrical coupling between cells (2). Thus, it is probable that action potentials originating in one area of the tube are capable of spreading throughout a given segment in longitudinally oriented fibers as well as circularly and spirally oriented fibers (66). Instead of regular peristaltic contractions, the oviduct is believed to undergo segmental contractions that originate within an area of the tube and propagate on a symmetrical basis in either direction along the tube at similar velocities (2). Consequently, it is assumed that the transport of ova or embryos may be a discontinuous pattern of backward and forward movements from areas of active contraction into quiescent regions (2). Nevertheless, the human fallopian tube, particularly the isthmic portion, is densely innervated by adrenergic nerves (67). In addition, the electrical field stimulation of adrenergic nerves in the isthmic smooth muscle preparations in vitro induces an alpha-receptor-mediated, frequency-dependent contractile response (67). It implies that the sympathetic nerves in the human oviducts are able to exert motor control over its smooth musculature, and may thus be involved in local functions essential for the normal fertilization process (67). Cyclic variations have been demonstrated in the amount of neurotransmitter present in the tube (68), which is regulated by changes in ovarian steroid production. Among the ovarian steroids, estrogen is associated with increased tubal contractility while progesterone exerts an inhibitory effect (2). There are two

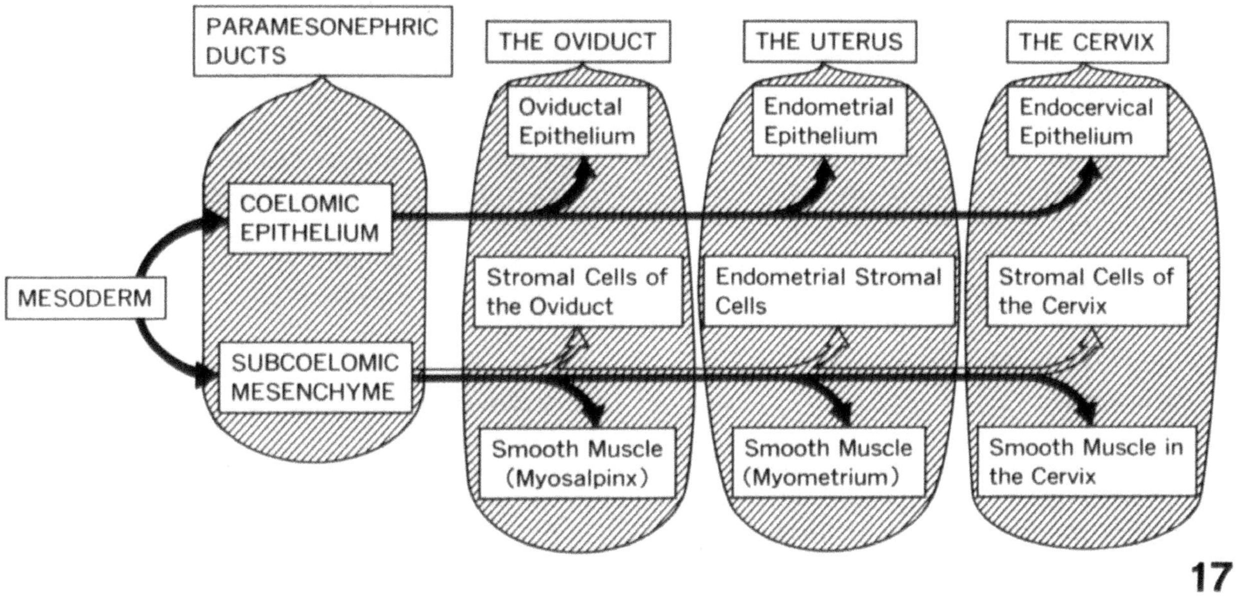

Figure 10-17. Development of epithelium and mesenchymal cells in the female genital tract.

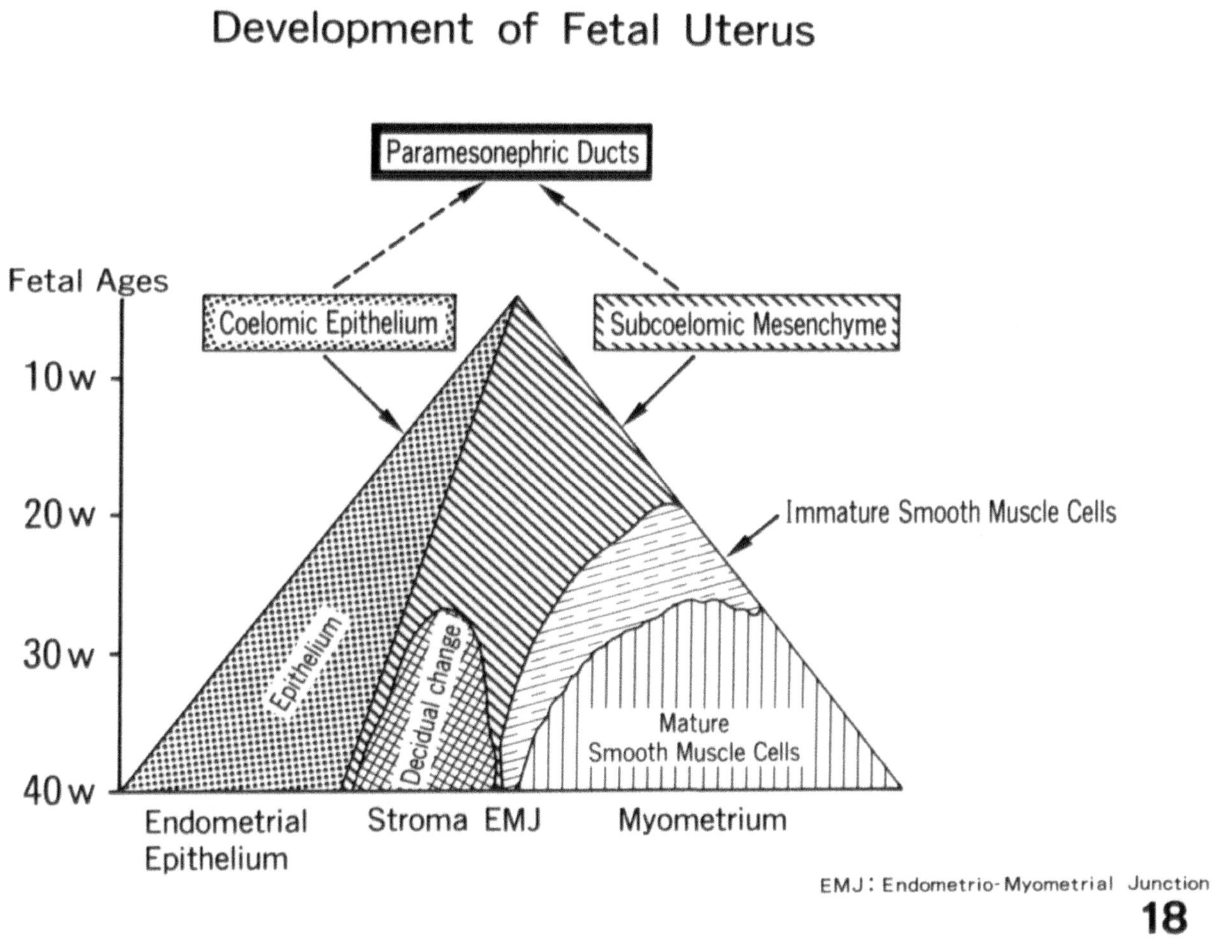

Figure 10-18. Development of fetal uterus.

peaks of contractile activity: one at the time of ovulation following the preovulatory peak in estrogen production; the other during menstruation, when progesterone levels are low, estrogen is beginning to rise, and endometrial prostaglandins are being released (2). The oviduct is not completely quiescent. Even in pregnancy with its sustained elevation of progesterone, the oviducts exhibit spontaneous activity (2).

5. Conclusions

During the fetal period, differentiation of the mesenchymal cells accompanied by the paramesonephric ducts results in the formation of the tubular muscular structure of the uterus and oviduct (Fig. 10-17). In the human fetal uterus, smooth muscle differentiation begins at about 18 weeks, and myometrium is formed in the outer layer of the uterine wall by 31 weeks gestation (Fig. 10-18). In the inner layer of the uterus that corresponds to the endometrial stroma, cells resembling those of predecidual cells appear around blood vessels by 26 weeks (Fig. 10-18), and this suggests the influence of sex steroids on the human fetal uterus. In the human fetal cervix and oviducts, smooth muscle differentiation begins about 20 weeks and is considerably more rapid by 31 weeks than that of the fetal uterine wall. Nevertheless, the mechanism that results in the difference of smooth muscle differentiation between the myometrium and the cervix or oviduct is uncertain. Compare to the development of smooth muscle cells in the fetal urinary bladder, the development of the paramesonephric ducts is very slow. Therefore, smooth muscle tissues in the female genital tract, although similar in structure to smooth muscle cells of extragenital origin, have unique developmental processes in the fetal period. In addition, during the reproductive period they show the unique ability to respond to ovarian and placental hormonal stimuli. After menopause, with the waning of ovarian hormonal support, they show atrophy. Morphological changes under the influences of ovarian steroids suggest that progesterone with the assistance of estrogen may have an effect on differentiation into smooth muscle cells of the female genital tract or on maintenance of their characteristics not only in vivo but also in vitro. Therefore, in the study of the differentiation or proliferation of smooth muscle cells in the female genital tract, the part played by progesterone should be taken into account in addition to estrogen. In conclusion, further studies are necessary in order to elucidate the enigma of smooth muscle tissues in the female genital tract.

References

1. Elstein M, Chantler EN: Functional anatomy of the cervix and uterus. In: Scientific Foundations of Obstetrics and Gynecology, 3rd ed. E Philipp, J Barnes, M Newton (eds), London: William Heinemann, p 125–144, 1986.
2. Eddy CA: The tube. In: Scientific Foundations of Obstetrics and Gynecology, 3rd ed. E Philipp, J Barnes, M Newton (eds), London: William Heinemann, p 144–153, 1986.
3. Turnbull AC, Anderson ABM: Uterine function in human pregnancy and labour. In: Scientific Basis of Obstetrics and Gynecology, 2nd ed. RR Macdonald (ed), Edinburgh: Churchill Livingstone, p 79–108, 1978.
4. Ferenczy A, Richart RM: Female Reproductive System: Dynamics of Scan and Transmission Electron Microscopy. New York: John Wiley & Son, 1974.
5. Parmley T: Embryology of the female genital tract. In: Blaustein's Pathology of the Female Genital Tract, 3rd ed. RJ Kurman (ed), New York: Springer-Verlag, p 1–14, 1987.
6. Hunter RH: Observations on the development of the human female genital tract. *Contrib Embryol* 22: 91–107, 1930.
7. O'Rahilly R: Prenatal human development. In: Biology of the Uterus. RM Wynn (ed), New York: Plenum Press, p 35–55, 1977.
8. Valdes-Dapena M: Female reproductive system. In: Histology of the Fetus and Newborn. Philadelphia: WB Saunders, p 433–499, 1979.
9. Konishi I, Fujii S, Okamura H, Mori T: Development of smooth muscle in the human fetal uterus: an ultrastructural study. *J Anat* 139: 239–252, 1984.
10. Yamamoto I: An electron microscope study on development of uterine smooth muscle. *J Electron Microsc* 10: 145–160, 1961.
11. Leeson TS, Leeson CR: The rat ureter. Fine structural changes during its development. *Acta Anat* 62: 60–79, 1965.
12. Yamauchi A, Burnstock G: Post-natal development of smooth muscle cells in the mouse vas deferens. A fine structural study. *J Anat* 104: 1–15, 1969.
13. Fujii S, Konishi I, Mori T: Smooth muscle differentiation at endometrio-myometrial junction: an ultrastructural study. *Virchows Arch [A]*, in press.
14. Bird CC, Willis RA: The production of smooth muscle by

the endometrial stroma of the adult human uterus. *J Pathol Bacteriol* 90: 75–81, 1965.
15. Fujii S, Nakashima N, Okamura H, et al.: Progesterone-induced smooth muscle-like cells in the subperitoneal nodules produced by estrogen. Experimental approach to leiomyomatosis peritonealis disseminata. *Am J Obstet Gynecol* 139: 164–172, 1981.
16. Jost A: The role of fetal hormones in prenatal development. *Harvey Lect* 55: 201–226, 1961.
17. Pelliniemi LJ, Dym M: The fetal gonad and sexual differentiation. In: Maternal – Fetal Endocrinology. D Tulchinsky, KJ Ryan (ed), Philadelphia: WB Saunders, p 252–280, 1980.
18. Tulchinsky D, Hobel C, Yeager E, Marshall JR: Plasma estrone, estradiol, estriol, progesterone, and 17-hydroxyprogesterone in human pregnancy. *Am J Obstet Gynecol* 112: 1095–1100, 1972.
19. Tulchinsky D: Placental secretion of unconjugate estrone, estradiol and estriol into the maternal and the fetal circulation. *J Clin Endocrinol Metab* 36: 1079–1087, 1973.
20. Jost A: Problems of fetal endocrinology: the gonadal and hypophyseal hormones. *Recent Prog Horm Res* 8: 379–418, 1953.
21. Pasqualini JR, Sumida C, Gulino A, et al.: Progesterone receptor during fetal development. In: Progesterone and Progestins. CW Bardin, E Milgrom, P Mauvais-Jarvis (eds), New York: Raven Press, p 77–90, 1983.
22. Ross R, Klebanoff SJ: Fine structural changes in uterine smooth muscle and fibroblasts in response to estrogen. *J Cell Biol* 32: 155–167, 1967.
23. Bo WJ, Odor DL, Rothrock M: The fine structure of uterine smooth muscle of the rat uterus at various time intervals following a single injection of estrogen. *Am J Anat* 123: 369–384, 1968.
24. Friederici HHR, DeCloux RJ: The early responses of immature rat myometrium to estrogen stimulation. *J Ultrastruct Res* 22: 402–412, 1968.
25. Bergman RA: Uterine smooth muscle fibers in castrate and estrogen treated rats. *Cell Biol* 36: 639–648, 1968.
26. Bo WJ, Odor DL, Rothrock ML: Ultrastructure of uterine smooth muscle following progesterone or progesterone–estrogen treatment. *Anat Rec* 163: 121–132, 1969.
27. Huszar G, Roberts JM: Biochemistry and pharmacology of the myometrium and labor: Regulation at the cellular and molecular levels. *Am J Obstet Gynecol* 142: 225–237, 1982.
28. Kao CY: Electrophysiological properties of the uterine smooth muscle. In: Biology of the Uterus. RM Wynn (ed), New York: Plenum Press, p 423–496, 1977.
29. Garfield RE, Hayashi RH: Presence of gap junctions in the myometrium of women during various stages of menstruation. *Am J Obstet Gynecol* 138: 569–574, 1980.
30. Garfield RE, Kannan MS, Daniel EE: Gap junction formation in myometrium: control by estrogens, progesterone, and prostaglandins. *Am J Physiol* 238: c81–c89, 1980.
31. Marshall JM: Effects of ovarian steroids and pregnancy on adrenergic nerves of uterus and oviduct. *Am J Physiol* 240: c165–c174, 1981.
32. Garfield RE: Control of myometrial function in preterm versus term labor. *Clin Obstet Gynecol* 27: 572–591, 1984.
33. Laguens R, Lagrutta J: Fine structure of human uterine muscle in pregnancy. *Am J Obstet Gynecol* 89: 1040–1048, 1964.
34. Dessouky DA: Ultrastructural observations of the human uterine smooth muscle cells during gestation. *Am J Obstet Gynecol* 125: 1099–1107, 1976.
35. Dessouky DA: Electron microscopic studies of the myometrium of the guinea pig. *Am J Obstet Gynecol* 100: 30–41, 1968.
36. Dessouky DA: Fine structural changes of the uterine smooth muscle cell boundary during gestation. *Am J Obstet Gynecol* 103: 1117–1124, 1969.
37. Althoff RW, Albert EN: Ultrastructural changes in mouse myometrium during pregnancy. *Am J Obstet Gynecol* 108: 1224–1233, 1970.
38. Garfield RE, Sims S, Daniel EE: Gap junctions: Their presence and necessity in myometrium during parturition. *Science* 198: 958–959, 1977.
39. Garfield RE, Rabideans, Challis JRG, Daniel EE: Ultrastructural basis for maintenance and termination of pregnancy. *Am J Obstet Gynecol* 133: 308–315, 1979.
40. Peracchia C: Structural correlates of junction permeation. *Int Rev Cytol* 66: 81–146, 1980.
41. Garfield RE, Hayashi RH: Appearance of gap junctions in the myometrium during labor. *Am J Obstet Gynecol* 140: 254–260, 1981.
42. Puri CP, Garfield RE: Changes in hormone levels and gap junctions in the rat uterus during pregnancy and parturition. *Biol Reprod* 27: 967–975, 1982.
43. Garfield RE, Puri CP, Csapo AI: Endocrine, structural and functional changes in the uterus during premature labor. *Am J Obstet Gynecol* 142: 21–27, 1982.
44. Dessouky DH: Myometrial changes in postpartum uterine involution. *Am J Obstet Gynecol* 110: 318–329, 1971.
45. Brandes D, Anton E: Lysosomes in uterine involution: Intracytoplasmic degradation of myofilaments and collagen. *J Gerontol* 24: 55–69, 1969.
46. Okamura H, Koshiba H, Yoshida Y: An ultrastructural study of collagen degradation in human involuting uterus. *Acta Obstet Gynaecol Jpn* 23: 179–184, 1976.
47. Jurukova Z, Milenkov C: Involvement of smooth muscle cells in collagen degradation in the postpartum uterus. *Virchows Arch [B]* 37: 237–244, 1981.
48. Blair HC, Teitelbaum SL, Ehlich LS, Jeffery JJ: Collagenase production by smooth muscle: correlation of immunoreactive with functional enzymes in the myometrium. *J Cell Physiol* 129: 111–123, 1986.
49. Hendrickson MR, Kempson RL: Surgical Pathology of the Uterine Corpus. Philadelphia: WB Saunders, 1980.
50. Rifas L, Fant J, Makman MH, Seifter S: The characterization of human uterine smooth muscle cells in culture. *Cell Tissue Res* 196: 385–395, 1979.
51. Casey ML, MacDonald PC, Mitchell MD, Snyder JM: Maintenance and characterization of human myometrial smooth muscle cells in monolayer culture. *In Vitro* 20: 396–403, 1984.
52. Palmberg L, Thyberg J: Uterine smooth muscle in pri-

mary culture. *Cell Tissue Res* 246: 253–262, 1986.
53. Nilsson J, Sjolund M, Palmberg L, Thyberg J, Heldin C-H: Arterial smooth muscle cells in primary culture produce a platelet-derived growth factor-like protein. *Proc Natl Acad Sci USA* 82: 4418–4422, 1985.
54. Kawaguchi K, Fujii S, Konishi I, Okamura H, Mori T: Ultrastructural study of cultured smooth muscle cells from uterine leiomyoma and myometrium under the influence of sex steroids. *Gynecol Oncol* 21: 32–41, 1985.
55. Kaye AM, Sheratsky D, Linder HR: Kinetics of DNA synthesis in immature rat uterus: age dependence and estradiol stimulation. *Biochim Biophys Acta* 261: 475–486, 1972.
56. Kawaguchi K, Fujii S, Konishi I, Nanbu Y, Nonogaki H, Mori T: Mitotic activity in uterine leiomyomas during the menstrual cycle. *Am J Obstet Gynecol*, in press.
57. Singer A, Jordan JA: The anatomy of the cervix. In: The Cervix. TA Jordan, A Singer (ed), London: WB Saunders, p 13–36, 1979.
58. Philpott RH: Biodynamics of the cervix. In: The Cervix. TA Jordan, A Singer (ed), London: WB Saunders, p 217–226, 1979.
59. Danforth DN: The distribution and functional activity of the cervical musculature. *Am J Obstet Gynecol* 68: 1261–1271, 1954.
60. Davies J, Kusama H: Developmental aspects of the human cervix. *Ann NY Acad Sci* 97: 534–550, 1962.
61. Hughesdon MB: The fibromuscular structure of the cervix and its changes during pregnancy and labour. *J Obstet Gynaecol Br Commonwealth* 59: 763–776, 1952.
62. Wendell-Smith CP: The lower uterine segment. *J Obstet Gynaecol Br Commonwealth* 61: 87–93, 1954.
63. Schwalm H, Dubrauszky V: The structure of the musculature of the human uterus — muscles and connective tissue. *Am J Obstet Gynecol* 94: 391–404, 1966.
64. Rorie DK, Newton N: Histologic and chemical studies of the smooth muscle in the human cervix and uterus. *Am J Obstet Gynecol* 99: 466–469, 1967.
65. Ferenczy A: The ultrastructure of the human cervix. In: Dilatation of the Uterine Cervix. F Naftolin, PG Stubblefield (ed), New York: Raven Press, p 27–44, 1980.
66. Daniel EE, Posey VA, Paton DM: A structural analysis of the myogenic control system of the human Fallopian tube. *Am J Obstet Gynecol* 121: 1054–1066, 1975.
67. Sporrong B, Helm G, Owman C, Sjoberg N-O, Walles B: Electron microscopic and pharmacologic evidence for a functional adrenergic innervation of smooth musculature in the human fallopian tube. *Brain Res Bull* 9: 695–699, 1982.
68. Owman C, Falck B, Johansson EDB, et al.: Autonomic nerves and related amine receptors mediating motor activity in the oviduct of monkey and human. A histochemical and pharmacologic study. In: Ovum Transport and Fertility Regulation. MJK Harper, CJ Pauerstein, CE Adams, et al. (eds), Copenhagen: Scriptor, p 256–275, 1976.

Author's address:
Prof. Hitoshi Okamura
Department of Obstetrics & Gynecology
Kumamoto University Medical School
Kumamoto City 860
Japan

CHAPTER 11

The smooth muscle cells in the ovary

U. MUGLIA, E. VIZZA, G. FAMILIARI, & P.M. MOTTA

1. Introduction

The role of a contractile component in the ovary of mammals, and particularly the role of smooth muscle cells (SMCs) — and their actual presence — have been argued for more than a century, since von Kölliker's first observation in 1849 (1). The reason for this controversy is to be found in both the diversity of appropriate techniques and in the specific and functional variability of contractile elements and their wide distribution throughout the ovary.

The introduction of transmission electron microscopy (TEM) and its application to the study of SMCs in the ovary definitively settled the debate. In fact, since Fumagalli and Motta (2) first described SMCs under TEM in the theca externa of ovarian follicles in some mammals, the presence of such cells in various regions of the ovary in numerous animals has been reported by many other authors.

The interest in understanding the function and influence of SMC contraction in some important ovarian phenomena, such as ovulation and atresia, comes from the perspective of pharmacological control on ovulation and thereby on reproduction (3). TEM techniques, although they play a very important role in the identification of these elements, do not alone provide a comprehensive view of the dynamic phenomena involved in ovarian physiology.

Probably only the combination of TEM with other techniques — for example, direct in vitro observation — can clarify the role and mechanism of SMC contraction in these ovarian phenomena.

The purpose of this chapter is to review the literature on the fine structure of SMCs in the different mammalian species and to compare the latter with data on humans, in order to indicate the role, if any, that SMCs might have in the physiological events of the ovary.

2. Ultrastructural features, distribution, and shape of smooth muscle cells

2.1. *Ultrastructure*

Ovarian SMCs show ultrastructural features peculiar to mature myocytes (Fig. 11-1) and very similar, when not superimposable, to those of cells forming the muscular wall of viscera cava (4). Such features are the same in all mammalian species studied so far.

Within a given organ system — for example, in the hamster (5) — comparative observations pointed out a quantitative rather than ultrastructural difference between the SMCs of the ovary and oviduct.

As first reported by Fumagalli and Motta (2), under TEM ovarian SMCs contain several cytoplasmic filaments (60–80 Å), sometimes gathered in bundles and often anchored to the plasma membrane by means of dense bodies; these are also frequently found among the filaments as well. Generally, mitochondria are not numerous and show long cristae. The Golgi complex is always present, and the associated centriole is occasionally involved in ciliogenesis.

The rough endoplasmic reticulum (RER) is moderately developed and sometimes forms wide perinuclear cisternae. However, free ribosomes are frequently found in the cytosol. Glycogen particles (20–25 nm) are also present. The plasma membrane sometimes shows areas of close contact, micropinocytotic vesicles (caveolae), and frequently a dense basal membrane covering the cell surface (6, 7).

2.2. Distribution and shape (see Table 11-1)

SMCs in the mammalian ovary can appear either isolated or arranged in bundles in the theca externa of developing (Fig. 11-1), mature (Fig. 11-2), and atretic follicles (Fig. 11-3), in the stroma surrounding the corpus luteum (CL) (Fig. 11-4), in the stroma of the tunica albuginea, and irregularly dispersed among the interstitial endocrine cells. The muscular component in the ovary is less represented than in other organs, such as the viscera cava, and closely depends on both the maturity and functional stage of the ovary, as well as on the developmental stage of the follicle. All the above factors affect the number, maturational stage, and topographical distribution of ovarian SMCs. Furthermore, many observations suggest a great variability in the number and distribution of SMCs among the different species.

2.2.1. Comparative features in the mammalian species (see Table 11-1). Okamura et al. (8) described rare SMCs in the theca externa of the rabbit ovary and in its cortical stroma. In other studies of different mammals, including the rabbit (7), SMCs were found primarily in the theca externa, arranged in two or three irregular layers, and were also present in the stroma surrounding the atretic follicles and CL. In these areas they were in close proximity to both the capillary vessels and endocrine cells. On the other hand, few isolated elements have been reported in the interfollicular and cortical stroma by these authors, who describe SMCs as mainly spindle-shaped elements sometimes showing two or more elongated branches that contain myofilaments (7).

In the cat ovary, few SMCs are detectable in the theca externa of various developing follicles, in the interfollicular stroma, among stromal cells of the CL, in the interstitial gland, and in the atretic follicles (7, 8). However, Burden (9) reported many SMCs in antral follicles.

In the mouse ovary, on the other hand, SMCs are well represented in the following areas: interfollicular stroma, CL, interstitial cells, and the theca externa of growing follicles. A few cells spread among fibroblasts and fibrocytes are reported in the tunica albuginea and in the primary follicles and subcortical areas (7).

In the theca externa of mouse antral follicles showing clear signs of atresia (Fig. 11-3), the smooth muscle component forms a capsule having an irregular outline due to elements fixed in contraction (10).

In both the rat and monkey, the SMCs delimit lobules of interstitial tissue, while in the medullar stroma they are organized in thick bundles running along nerves and large blood and lymphatic vessels (11). SMCs are occasionally seen in the theca of growing follicles at early stages of antrum formation, whereas they form multiple layers in mature follicles (12). They appear elongated, flattened, and spindle-shaped; intermediate elements are also observed among them.

In the rat ovarian stroma around the CL, where SMCs are more abundant than in the follicle, they form a multiple-layered surface cover (7, 12) (Fig. 11-1C). In the CL at advanced stages of growth, it is possible to observe SMCs undergoing degeneration.

The topographic and quantitative distribution of myocytes is comparable in the monkey and the rat, except for two slight differences concerning their distribution in the perifollicular and cortical stroma. In fact, SMCs are relatively more abundant in the cortical stroma of the monkey, where they appear isolated and show a rounded lateral extrusion of the cell body containing no filaments. Moreover, triangular-shaped aggregates of SMCs with the apex directed towards the ovarian surface have been observed near the basal membrane of small follicles in the perifollicular stroma of the monkey (11).

In the hamster and in the gerbil, the amount, shape, and distribution of SMCs are definitely comparable. SMCs appear as spindle-shaped ele-

Table 11-1. Comparative features of smooth muscle cells in the mammalian species

Author(s)	Species	Location	Type of cells	Technique and function
Motta G. (1929) (23)	Human		Myocytes	Light microscopy (LM); musculature was responsible for contraction of the entire ovary and, indirectly, for ovulation
Fumagalli and Motta (1969) (2)	Rabbit Cat Mouse	Stroma and perifollicular areas	Myocytes	Transmission electron microscopy (TEM)
O'Shea (1970) (12)	Rat	Theca externa of small and large antral follicle and corpora lutea (CL)	Smooth muscle cells (SMCs), fibroblasts with few filaments, and intermediate cells	TEM; SMCs are involved in ovulation as well as in collapse of postovulatory follicles
Osvaldo-Decima (1970) (11)	Monkey Rat	Theca externa of developing, mature and atretic follicles (AFs); around lobules of interstitial tissue and around endocrine cells of theca externa	SMCs	TEM; SMCs form an irregular layer around follicles that cannot be sufficient by itself to increase pressure and cause ovulation
Coutinho and Maia (1971) (21)	Human	Stroma	Fibromuscular cells	LM; contractile response of fibromuscular tissue to intravenous administration of prostaglandins recorded by introducing a catheter into the stroma
Fink and Schofield (1971) (36)	Cat	Theca externa and stroma of the cortex	Myocytes without intracellular caveolae and a continuous basal lamina	LM and TEM
Fumagalli et al. (1971) (6)	Cat Mouse Rabbit	Various areas	SMCs	TEM; cause follicular dehiscence and atresia
Motta et al. (1971) (37)	Mouse Rabbit	Unable to establish whether in vascular wall or theca externa	Isolated few myocytes	TEM
O'Shea (1971) (38)	Sheep	Theca externa	SMCs Intermediate cells	TEM; the contractile cells play a role in follicle rupture and persist around the functional CL and undergo degeneration
Burden (1972) (39)	Cat Guinea pig Rabbit	Theca externa of large vesicular follicles	SMCs Intermediate cells	TEM; the thecal SMCs are under neural control; their coordinated contraction in the theca externa causes extrusion of the ovum
Okamura et al. (1972) (8)	Human Cat Rabbit	Theca externa and cortex	SMCs	TEM and histochemistry; contraction of the SMCs induces complete dissociation of the apex
Palti and Freund (1972) (22)	Human		SMCs	LM observation of ovarian contractility in vitro; leads to ovulation and empting of follicle cavity

Table 11-1. (Continued)

Author(s)	Species	Location	Type of cells	Technique and function
Virutamasen et al. (1972) (32)	Rabbit	Perifollicular areas	Myocytes	LM in vivo observation of ovarian contractility; the recognition of myocytes and autonomic nerves suggests that they are involved in ovulation, which is under control of local neuromuscular factors
Burden (1973) (9)	Cat	Mesovarium, hilar, medullary, and cortex; in the theca externa, an incomplete sphere of perifollicular muscle; SMCs around CL	SMCs	TEM and histochemistry; under neuronal control, contraction of SMCs may cause detachment of the cumulus oophorus, lift the stigma from the apex and expell ovum from the follicle
McReynolds et al. (1973) (13)	Gerbil Hamster	Theca externa; stroma surrounding CL and interstitial tissue	SMCs Fibroblasts Intermediate cells	TEM; as stigma becomes thinner, the thecal SMCs show a substantial state of contraction; a constant intrafollicular pressure is thus maintained and follicular rupture occurs; SMCs are involved also in follicular contraction or collapse after ovulation and during artresia.
O'Shea (1973) (17)	Sheep	Theca externa	SMCs Myoid cells Fibroblasts	TEM
Walles et al. (1974) (34)	Cat Guinea pig	Theca externa	SMCs in close contact with adrenergic termination	TEM and cytochemical demonstration of spontaneous ovarian contraction
Bjersing and Cajander (1974) (40)	Rabbit	Theca externa, apex of ovulatory follicles	SMCs	TEM; contractile elements of apex may facilitate focal disruption and follicle rupture
Walles et al. (1975) (16)	Cow	Theca externa, apex of ovulatory follicles	Smooth muscle-like cells are reached by nerve terminals (as closely as 50–100 nm from the cell membrane) that are likely to be both adrenergic and cholinergic; intermediate cells	TEM and fluorescence correlated to in vitro LM observations; induction of SMC contraction using sympathomimetic agents
Walles et al. (1978) (41)	Rat	Theca externa around CL stroma	SMCs in close relationship with adrenergic nerve terminals in several layers around theca externa, isolated or branching bundles in the ovarian stroma	Histochemistry; SMC capsule of follicular and CL wall exhibits motor activity under sympathomimetic influence
Amenta et al. (1979) (7)	Cat Mouse Rabbit Rat	Cells isolated in the stroma or forming a capsule around theca externa of developing, mature and AFs, CL, and interstitial glands	SMCs Myoid cells	TEM; contraction of SMCs is incapable by itself of rupturing the follicular wall

Table 11-1. (Continued)

Author(s)	Species	Location	Type of cells	Technique and function
Pendergrass and Talbot (1979) (42)	Hamster	Theca externa, apex of preovulatory follicles	SMCs arranged in layers of 4–6 cells, intermediate cells, contractile forms of cells of surface epithelium (SEC)	TEM; the authors suggest that SMCs cause extrusion of the oocytes while SEC may assist stigma formation and rupture subsequent to enzymatic action or inflammation
DiDio et al. (1980) (35)	Mouse Rabbit Rat	Various areas, including Perifollicular areas	SMCs Intermediate cells Fibroblasts	TEM; SMC contraction is involved as an auxiliary factor in the detachment of the cumulus, opening of the apex, collapse of postovulatory follicles
Pendergrass (1980) (5)	Hamster	Perifollicular areas	Smoothmuscle-like and intermediate cells	TEM; brief contraction during ovulation
Motta and Familiari (1981) (10)	Mouse	Perifollicular stroma of developing and AFs	SMCs arranged around AFs in irregular outline due to their contraction	LM, freeze-fracture, and TEM; contraction of SMCs may contribute to the collapse and consequent involution of the follicular complex
Martin and Talbot (1981) (14)	Hamster	Theca externa in basal hemisphere of preovulatory follicles	SMCs organized in one or three layers	In vitro, by LM and TEM; SMC contraction causes apical movement of the V-shaped basal pole, change in height and diameter, and collapse of follicular wall after rupture
Martin and Talbot (1981) (33)	Hamster	Theca externa in basal hemisphere of preovulatory follicles	SMCs	LM and TEM; several drugs that inhibit SMC contraction prevent ovulation; SMC action is involved in the rupture of the follicle
Schroeder and Talbot (1982) (43)	Hamster	Preovulatory follicle	SMCs	In vitro ovulation measurement of intrafollicular pressure, and scanning electron microscopy; SMC action keeps the pressure constant, stretches cells at the apex, and enlarges holes in the developing rupture site
Talbot and Chacon (1982) (44)	Hamster	Theca externa of basal hemisphere of follicles	SMCs	LM and TEM; SMC contraction can be caused by stretching induced by increase of liquor folliculi or by stimulation of adrenergic and cholinergic nerve terminals of follicle wall or by 5-HT
Talbot and Schroeder (1982) (45)	Hamster	Basal pole of theca externa of pre-ovulatory follicles	SMCs	LM, TEM, and intrafollicular pressure measurement; contraction force is not sufficient to cause follicle rupture if the apex is not enzymatically weakened
Martin et al. (1983) (15)	Hamster	Postovulatory follicle and CL	SMCs	TEM; description of the SMC fate after ovulation and during all the CL lifespan
Doss et al. (1984) (46)	Rat	Stroma, theca externa of large follicle and CL	SMCs	Histochemistry

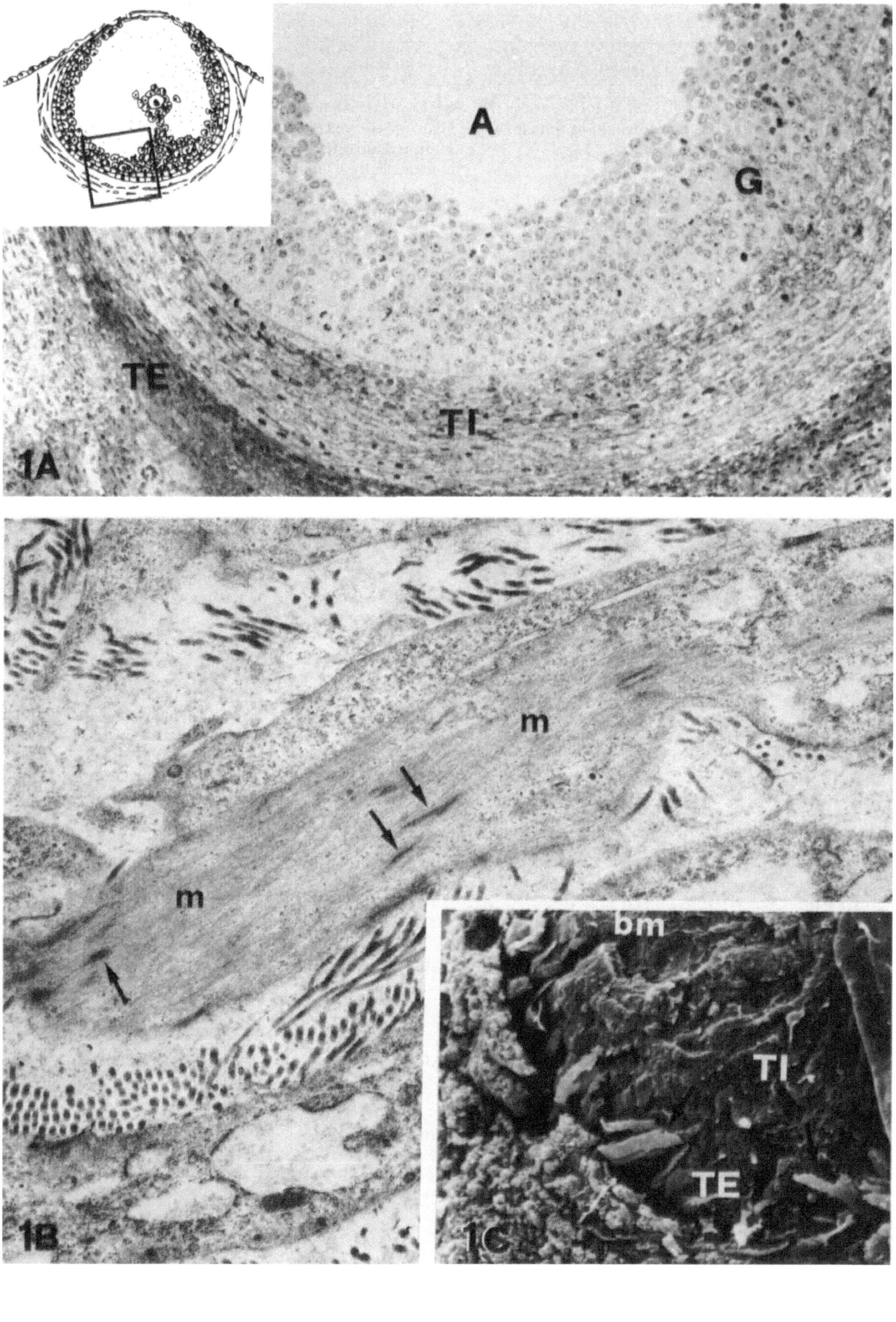
A
G
TE
TI
1A
m
m
1B
bm
TI
TE
1C

ments present in the interstitial tissue, CL, and theca externa (13, 14). In the follicular external theca of the hamster, spindle-shaped SMCs forming up to four layers have been observed together with intermediate elements; such SMCs project long, ribbonlike cytoplasmic processes from both extremities of their cellular body. Gap junctions and few desmosomes are also detected in SMCs fixed in contraction and having an indented nucleus. Such figures are visible under TEM in preovulatory follicles in which the simultaneous contraction of the whole follicle wall can be demonstrated by direct in vitro observation (14). According to Martin and Talbot (14), the SMCs are mainly located at the basal pole of the preovulatory follicle (basal hemisphere, opposite the stigma), whereas they occasionally occur at the apex (stigma), which is formed mainly by fibroblasts.

Martin et al. (15) described the following cytological pictures in the theca externa of growing CL in the hamster. In particular, SMCs fixed in contraction and showing an indented nucleus were observed at the early stages of CL growth, whereas in the last stages of the lifespan of the CL, few SMCs, fibroblast-like cells, and regressing figures occurred. In addition, these SMCs, isolated or in clusters, showed a cytoplasm with a reduced number of filaments.

In the cow, the stigma of the preovulatory follicle has been studied. Spindle-shaped SMCs are present in this region as well as cells showing intermediate features between myocytes and fibroblasts. Axonal varicosities showing no membrane specializations have been detected as close as 50–100 nm from such intermediate elements (16).

No smooth muscle-like cells have been observed in primary follicles of the sheep, not even in the perifollicular stroma (17–20).

In secondary follicles at early stages of thecal differentiation, elongated cells immersed in a poor connective matrix rich in fibers start to appear between fibroblasts and fibrocytes. Such cells contain a fair amount of cytoplasmic filaments and are linked to each other by desmosomes. In antral follicles (Fig. 11-1A–B), swollen spindle-shaped smooth muscle-like cells can be easily detected, separated by a connective matrix containing few collagen fibers. Furthermore, a fairly good amount of intermediate elements, some of which are at very advanced developmental stages, are found (20). In preovulatory follicles (Fig. 11-2), the long SMCs appear flattened rather than spindle-shaped, and their number varies greatly. A conspicuous amyelinic component can be observed close to vessels rather than close to SMCs (20). Smooth muscle-like cells containing lipid droplets are visible in the CL; such lipid droplets, together with other cell features, indicate cellular degeneration. The degenerative process might depend upon a steroidogenic secretion of closely related endocrine cells (7).

2.2.2. SMCs in the human ovary. The available data on the muscular component of human ovary are scanty, and the majority deal with ovarian contractility as a whole, both in vivo and in vitro (21, 22). Further knowledge comes to us from classical histological studies (light microscopy) (23, 24).

Okamura et al. (8) demonstrated that SMCs in the follicular theca externa and cortical stroma are rather abundant compared with other species, such as the cat and the rabbit. Myocytes appear elongated and spindle-shaped and, in some cases, show an indented plasmalemma. Intermediate forms between fibroblasts and SMCs occur as well.

2.2.3. General remarks about quantity and shape of ovarian SMCs.

←

Figure 11-1. Growing graafian follicle (sheep). (A) LM. At this stage of follicular growth, SMCs and intermediate forms begin to appear in the theca externa among fibroblasts, forming a sort of capsule around the follicle. A: Antrum; G: granulosa; TI: theca interna; TE: theca externa. X 100. (B) A fusiform SMC observed in the theca externa of the same follicle. The cytoplasm contains numerous myofilaments (m) arranged in parallel and associated with dense bodies (arrows). X 22,000. (C) SEM. The wall of a growing graafian follicle of a rat after KOH digestion and ultrasonication. Correlative SEM and extracellular matrix digestion show the three-dimensional surface arrangement of fibroblasts and SMCs (arrows) in the theca externa (TE). bm: basal membrane of the follicle; TI: theca interna. X 3,000.

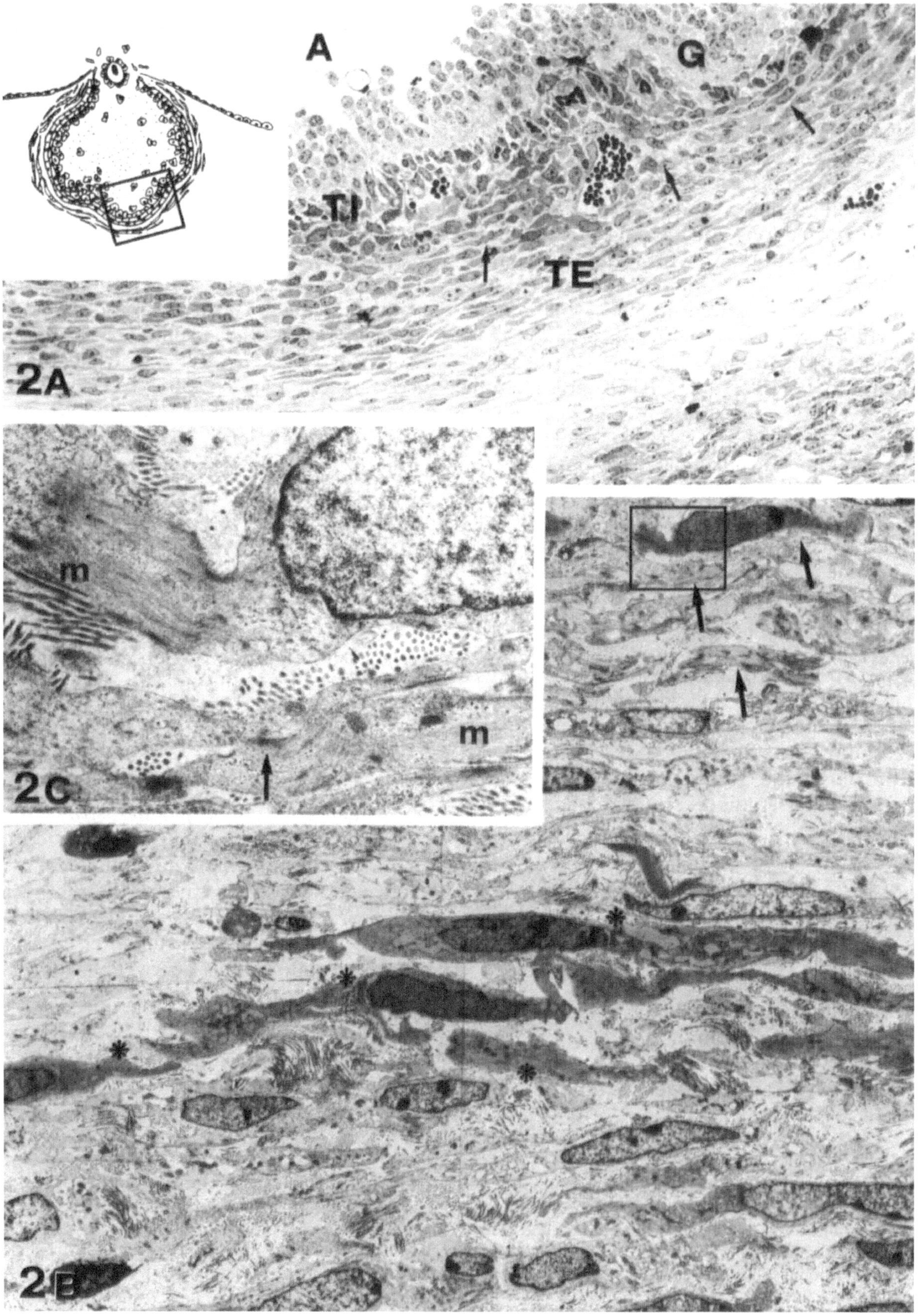
A
G
TI
TE
2A
m
m
2C
2B

Quantity. Since the number of SMCs is directly related to their total contractile power, this datum is very important. However, it should be pointed out that any quantitative evaluation of SMCs in the ovary that depends on the functional stage of the ovary at the moment of observation is greatly subject to the extreme physiological variability of the organ. Consequently, the quantitative evaluations expressed by the authors, who had to cope with such a difficult matter, cannot be objective, since they are not supported by reliable statistical data.

A comparison between different species on the basis of the available literature is therefore unreliable, except when the smooth muscle component is organized in a well-defined structure, such as a capsula.

Shape. As a rule, SMCs appear elongated and spindle-shaped, even if it is sometimes possible to observe myocytes showing two or more projections containing myofilaments (rabbit, cat, rat, mouse). However, it should be considered that the above-described cell figures derive from observations by TEM that obviously give bidimensional images; a spatial reconstruction from serial sections or observations by SEM would undoubtedly be more reliable.

3. Intermediate cell types

Intermediate forms between fibroblasts and myocytes are frequently observed, particularly in the theca externa. O'Shea (12) described in the rat the following cell types, which are detectable in all the mammalian species so far studied:

Fibroblast-like cells. These show a marked development of RER, which forms wide cisternae containing pale flocculent material. A well-developed Golgi apparatus is frequently present; few filaments are visible in the peripheral cytoplasm. Such filaments, also detectable in fibroblasts, are not likely to have a contractile role (25).

Intermediate forms between fibroblast-like and smooth-muscle-like cells (Fig. 11-2B). These are characterized by thicker, wider longitudinal filaments arranged in parallel bundles running in a large part of the central cytoplasm. They also show all features of fibroblast-like cells and sometimes dense bodies, caveolae, and a basal lamina, all of which are typical of myocytes.

The significance of such intermediate forms is still unclear, even if many authors have suggested various theories, all of which, however, lack experimental evidence. According to O'Shea (12), myoid cells of the external theca are not pre-existent and steadily organized in the follicular theca, but rather develop dynamically and cyclically from fibroblasts. It is therefore suggested that local hormonal factors or a change in the blood flow might control such a process. This hypothesis is supported by other findings (7) of intermediate forms containing lipid droplets — in close contact with steroidogenic cells — in the rabbit, cat, rat, and mouse. It has been suggested that such lipid inclusions would herald further cell degeneration. O'Shea (17) detected immature myoid cells in the ovine theca externa showing lipid droplets and other signs of degeneration and suggested that, contrary to what happens in the rat (12), such cellular forms would be able to regress even before producing mature forms (myocytes). Motta and Familiari (10) consider the immature forms occurring in developing or atretic follicles of the external theca in the mouse to be directly related to the differentiative stage of the follicular wall.

According to Martin et al. (15), myocytes would be able to turn into fibroblasts during luteolysis in the hamster by gradually losing their myofilaments. This hypothesis is supported by in vitro observations of SMCs turning into fibroblasts.

Therefore, the significance of intermediate

←

Figure 11-2. Ovulatory follicle (sheep). (A) LM. The basal pole (opposite the stigma) appears wrinkled by the contraction of SMCs (arrows). A: antrum; G: granulosa; TI: theca interna; TE: theca externa. X 150. (B) TEM. General view of the theca externa of the same follicle. Many SMCs (arrows) and intermediate forms (asterisks) are detectable among fibroblasts. X 2,300. (C) Higher magnification of the SMCs outlined in B. The cytoplasm shows myofilaments (m), pinocytotic vesicles (caveolae), dense bodies, and a specialized junction (arrow) connecting two SMCs laterally. X 14,000.

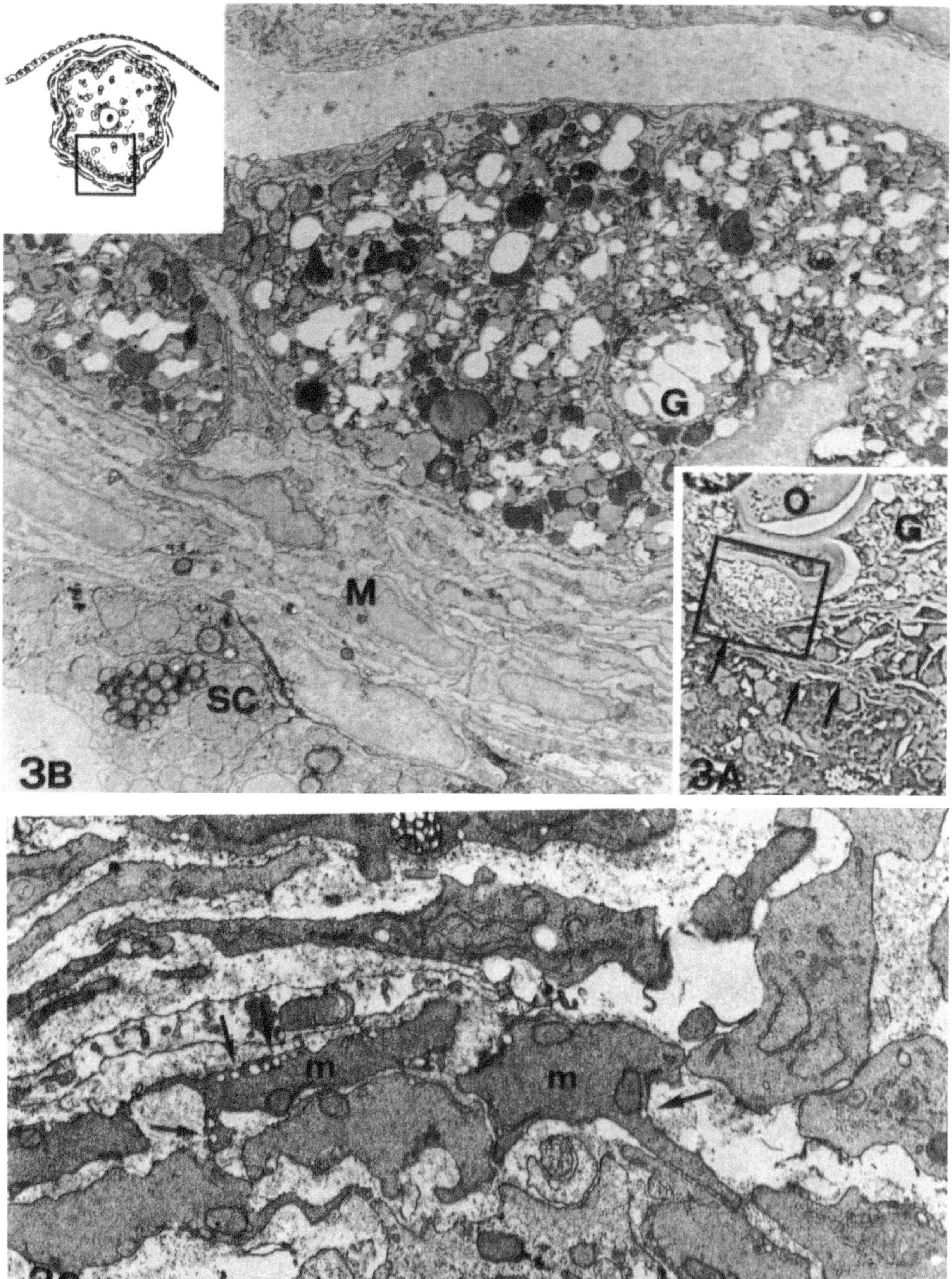
G
O
G
M
SC
3B
3A
m
m
3C

forms is still to be clarified. Perhaps the actual role and fate of such cells could finally be revealed by using specific (cellular) markers.

4. Origin and role of ovarian SMCs

The definitive demonstration of myocytes or myoid cells in the ovary has given rise to the problem of their origin and role.

The hypothesis that SMCs originate from fibroblasts is most favoured, even if not yet supported by experimental evidence. According to this hypothesis, the fibroblasts of the theca externa would turn into myocytes after producing the connective tissue, not unlike what happens to the fibroblasts of the aortic tunica media, which have been shown (26–28) to turn into myocytes forming the vessels' muscular wall after producing the collagen fibers.

The demonstration of several forms that are intermediate between fibroblasts and fibrocytes strongly supports such a hypothesis.

The differentiation of fibroblasts into myocytes would proceed parallel to that of the theca externa, following the development and regression of the latter (2, 6); once having reached full maturity, myocytes would then be able to regress to fibroblasts by losing their myofilaments, as shown in the CL of the hamster (15), or else they would undergo cyclic degeneration (7).

However, immature myoid forms showing signs of regression have been detected in the sheep (17–20).

Several researchers have speculated about the possible contraction and the role played by those cells known as smooth muscle-like, myoid cells, or myocytes. The frequent detection by TEM of forms fixed in contraction in both preovulatory and atretic follicles and in the CL has clearly shown their capability to contract. It is not unreasonable to assume, on the other hand, that the ovarian SMCs, although scanty in number if compared with SMCs of viscera cava, can nevertheless be involved in the contraction of the theca externa of the follicle.

The demonstration of a constant intrafollicular pressure before ovulation (29–33) suggests that a well-developed muscular component is not necessary for ovulation. Therefore, this component likely plays a complementary role. In fact, according to recent descriptions (14), SMCs of the follicular theca externa would stretch the stigma wall in preovulatory follicles, widening the narrows caused by enzymatic digestion. The decrease of inner follicular pressure, caused by liquor bleeding, would be balanced by the contraction of SMCs. Moreover, contraction of SMCs would push both liquor and cumulus towards the digested stigma, just prior to expulsion.

The possible control of contraction might take place through a specific innervation whose terminals have been detected by TEM in the theca externa of some species, close to SMCs, having the appearance of varicosities (7, 34). After follicular dehiscence, SMCs might continue to exert their contractile action on the collapsed wall of the postovulatory follicle and subsequently on that of the remnant CL. The same contractile forms might play a role in the formation of atretic follicles. Motta and Familiari (10) suggest that the muscular component of the external theca in the preovulatory follicle may follow the fate of the follicle itself by contracting its own concentric layers, favouring, in this way, both follicular dehiscence and folding of the follicular wall. Such a mechanism, based on ultrastructural findings in the mouse, would favour the complete collapse and emptying of the preovulatory follicle. The same mechanism might act in the formation of

←

Figure 11-3. Atretic graafian follicle (mouse). (A) LM. At low magnification, the atretic follicle appears surrounded by a sort of capsule (arrows) having an irregular outline; granulosa (G) and theca interna (TI) show a variable degree of compression. O: oocyte. X 100. (B) TEM. At higher magnification (closer view of (A), a continuous layer of shortened and contracted SMCs (M) can be easily observed. G: degenerating granulosa cells showing signs of luteinization; SC: thecal layers with some steroidogenic cells. X 15,000. (C) TEM. Contracted SMCs in the capsula surrounding the same follicle. An abundance of filaments (m) may be seen within the cytoplasm, and the plasma membrane shows numerous pinocytotic vesicles (arrows). The plane of the section is parallel to the long axis of the cells; the myofilaments appear arranged in parallel longitudinal bundles. X 50,000. (From PM Motta and G Familiari, 1981 (10).)

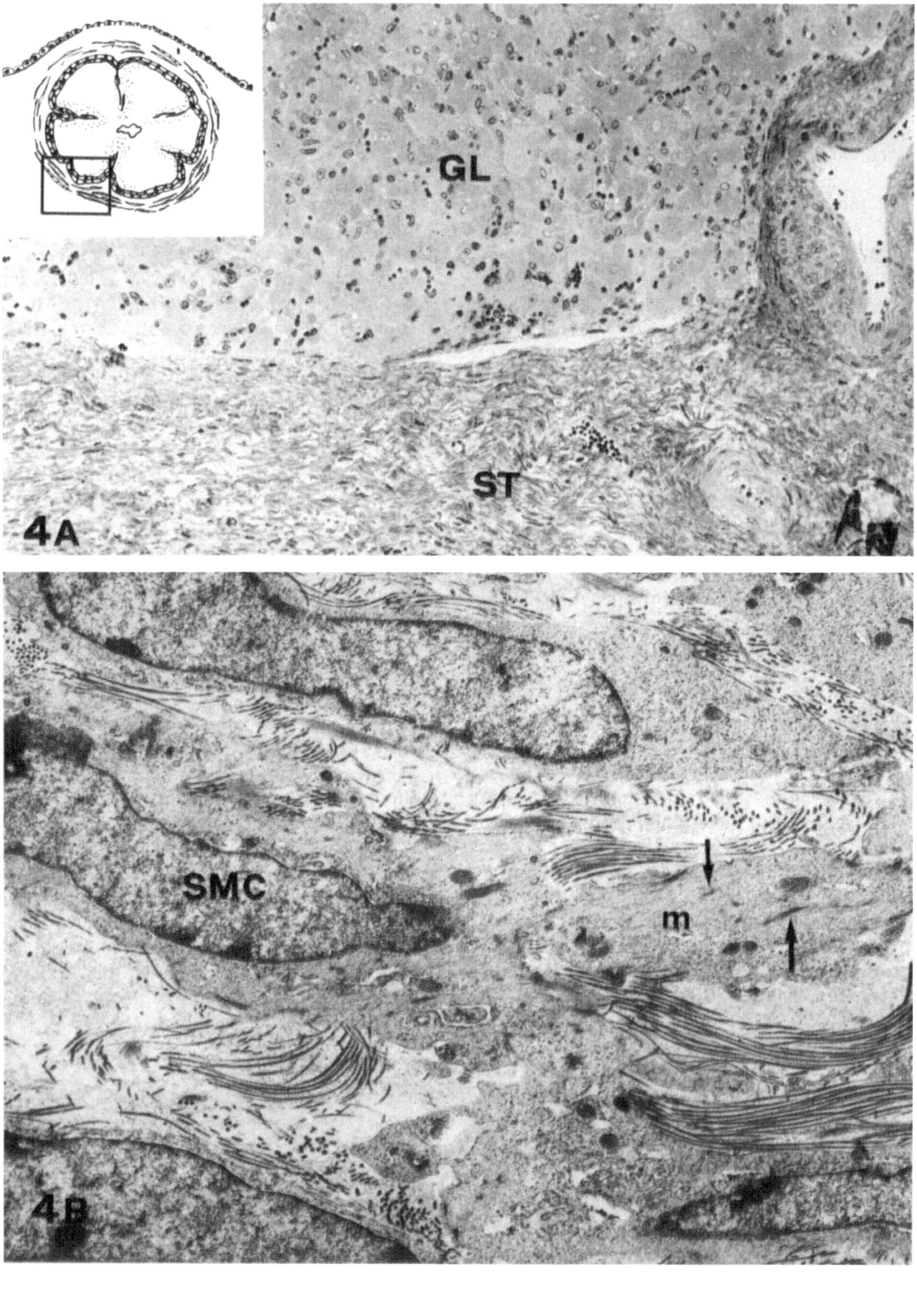
GL
ST
4A
SMC
m
4B

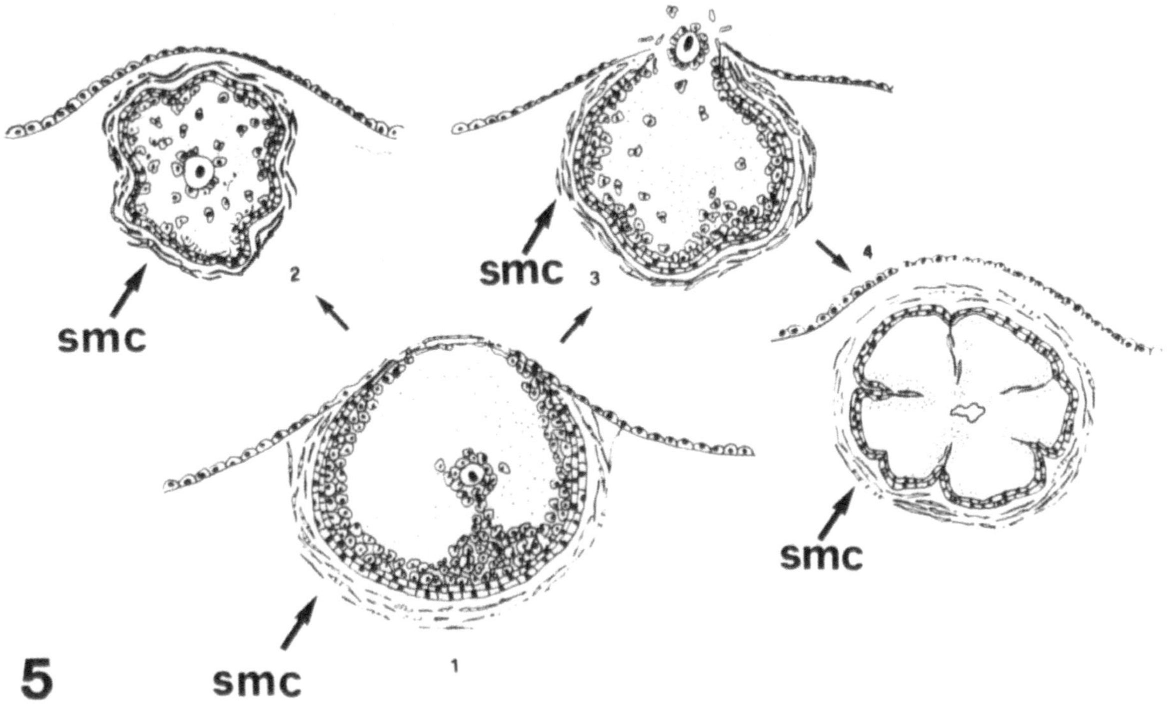

Figure 11-5. Diagramatic synthesis of the role that SMCs may play at different stages of follicular development in some mammals. The contraction of SMCs in the theca of the growing follicle (1) may favour the collapse and alteration of the follicular complex, and then the formation of an atretic follicle (2). Alternatively, SMCs may assist in the rupture of the follicle and in the dehiscence of the oocyte when other factors (nerves, enzymes, hormones) simultaneously intervene to cause ovulation (3). Finally, after ovulation, the contractile elements compacting the follicular residuals may favour the transformation of the postovulatory follicle into a corpus luteum (4). (Modified from PM Motta and G Familiari, 1981 (10).)

atretic follicles (10). Martin et al. (15) supported this hypothesis, further suggesting that, in the hamster, contraction of SMCs might be involved in the formation of CL by compacting follicular remnants (Fig. 11-5).

SMCs occur not only in the theca externa of the ovarian follicle but are widely distributed throughout the ovary. Myocytes might occur in the medullary stroma as contractile elements remaining in the perifollicular areas after the transformation of the follicular complex towards CL or atretic follicle (7).

However, the possibility cannot be excluded that a peripheral irregular layer of contractile elements, radiating from the hilus and mesovarium, and capable of compressing the whole ovary during ovulation, occurs in some mammals (23). Such a hypothesis has not been ruled out by recent investigations on the contractile power of the ovary as a whole, both in vivo and in vitro (21, 22, 32). Moreover, the presence of myocytes might affect the blood flow, by varying the contraction of the entire ovary, converting in this way ischemia and anemia into hyperemia, or vice versa, in order to help the follicle during ovulation (35).

5. Conclusions

In conclusion, according to the most recent theoiies, the contraction of ovarian myocytes, cyclic-

←

Figure 11-4. Corpus luteum (sheep). (A) LM. Segment of the wall of a mature corpus luteum. In the abundant stroma (ST) surrounding the gland (GL), close to the endocrine cells, both SMCs and intermediate forms have been observed. X 100. (B) TEM. Spindle-shaped SMCs (SMC) in the stroma surrounding an area of the same corpus luteum. Note myofilaments (m) and characteristic dense bodies (arrows). X 20,000.

ally maturing in the theca externa from fibroblasts, is likely to be involved in the following events:

-Ovulation, with detachment of the cumulus oophorus and expulsion of follicular contents following dehiscence

-Compacting of follicular residuals, and their conversion into CL or atretic follicle

-Control of ovarian vascular tone

Although recent investigations have shed some light upon several aspects of the problem, many other areas need further elucidation. It is still unclear to what extent the ovarian smooth muscle component is involved in both ovulation and evolution of the postovulatory follicle. The use of in vitro culture techniques in addition to electron microscopy has overcome the static limitations imposed by the observation of fixed material, providing us with an adequate, though not complete, dynamic picture of the phenomenon.

Nervous mediation of the ovarian smooth muscle component is still poorly understood; therefore, experimental models involving the use of drugs are not reliable, since they do not naturally stimulate this component.

Furthermore, the significance of intermediate forms is still unclear; cellular markers could provide an important aid in following each developing cell form.

Finally, the role that such contractile elements as a whole can play in the ovary needs further elucidation, in light of their wide distribution.

References

1. Kölliker A: Beitrage zur Kenntniss der glattern Muskeln. *f f Abhandl Wiss Zool* 1: 48–87, 1849.
2. Fumagalli Z, Motta PM: Sulla presenza al microscopio elettronico di cellule muscolari lisce nell'ovaio di alcuni mammiferi. 28th Congr. Soc. Ital. Anat. (abstract book). Naples, September 24-28, 1969, p 59.
3. Mossman HW, Duke KL: Comparative morphology of the mammalian ovary. Madison: University of Wisconsin Press, 1973.
4. Gabella G: Fine structure of smooth muscle. *Philos Trans R Soc Lond B* 265: 7–16, 1973.
5. Pendergrass PB: Ultrastructural comparison of smooth muscle from ovarian follicle and oviduct of the golden hamster. *Cell Tissue Res* 209: 43–48, 1980.
6. Fumagalli Z, Motta PM, Calvieri S: The presence of smooth muscular cells in the ovary of several mammals as seen under the electron microscope. *Experientia* 27: 682–683, 1971.
7. Amenta F, Allen DJ, DiDio LJA, Motta PM: A transmission electron microscopic study of smooth muscle cells in the ovary of rabbits, cats, rats and mice. *J Submicrosc Cytol* 11(1): 39–51, 1979.
8. Okamura H, Virutamasen P, Wright KH, and Wallach EE: Ovarian smooth muscle in the human being, rabbit and cat. *Am J Obstet Gynecol* 112: 183–191, 1972.
9. Burden HW: The distribution of smooth muscle in the cat ovary with a note on its adrenergic innervation. *J Morphol* 140: 467–476, 1973.
10. Motta PM, Familiari G: Occurrence of a contractile tissue in the theca externa of atretic follicles in the mouse ovary. *Acta Anat* 109: 103–114, 1981.
11. Osvaldo-Decima L: Smooth muscle in the ovary of the rat and monkey. *J Ultrastruct Res* 29: 218–237, 1970.
12. O'Shea JD: An ultrastructural study of smooth muscle-like cells in the theca externa of ovarian follicles in the rat. *Anat Rec* 167: 127–140, 1970.
13. McReynolds HD, Siraki CM, Bramson PH, Pollak RJ: Smooth muscle-like cells in the ovaries of the hamster and gerbil. *Z Zellforsch* 140: 1–8, 1973.
14. Martin GG, Talbot P: The role of follicular smooth muscle cells in hamster ovulation. *J Exp Zool* 216: 469–482, 1981.
15. Martin GG, Van Steenwyk G, Walker CM: The fate of thecal smooth muscle cells in the postovulatory hamster follicles. *Anat Rec* 207: 267–277, 1983.
16. Walles B, Edvinsson L, Falck B, Owman C, Sjoberg NO, Svensson KG: Evidence for a neuromuscular mechanism involved in the contractility of the ovarian follicular wall: fluorescence and electron microscopy and effects of tyramine on follicle strips. *Biol Reprod* 12: 239–248, 1975.
17. O'Shea JD: The ultrastructure, origin and fate of the theca externa of ovarian follicles in the sheep. *Res Vet Sci* 14: 273–278, 1973.
18. Muglia U, Germanà G, Ciriaco E, Correr S: Osservazioni ultrastrutturali sulla componente muscolare liscia del follicolo di ovaio di ovino. 42nd Congr. Soc. Ital. Anat. (abstract book). Siena: September 27–30, 1987, p 262.
19. Muglia U, Vizza E, Germanà G, Ciriaco E: Smooth muscle component in the developing ovarian follicle of the sheep. Abstracts VIII International Symposium on Morphological Science. *Quaderni di Anatomia Pratica* 44: 280, 1988.
20. Muglia U, Vizza E, Germanà G, Ciriaco E: Smooth muscle component in the developing ovarian follicle of the sheep and other mammals. In: Developments in Ultrastructure of Reproduction. PM Motta (ed), New York: Alan R. Liss Inc., p. 103–109, 1989.
21. Coutinho EM, Maia HS: The contractile response of the human uterus, fallopian tubes and ovary to prostaglandins in vivo. *Fertil Steril* 22: 539–544, 1971.
22. Palti T, Freund M: Spontaneous contractions of the human ovary in vitro. *J Reprod Fertil* 28: 113–115, 1972.
23. Motta G: Sull'importanza delle cellule muscolari dell'ovaio e sul meccanismo della deiescenza del follicolo. *Riv Ital Ginec* 10: 269–423, 1929.

24. Jacobowitz D, Wallach EE: Histochemical and chemical studies of the autonomic innervation of the ovary. *Endocrinol* 81: 1132–1139, 1967.
25. Chapman JA: Fibroblasts and collagen. *Br Med Bull* 18: 233–237, 1962.
26. Karrer HE, Cox J: An electron microscope study of the aorta in young and in aging mouse. *J Ultrastruct Res* 5: 1–27, 1961.
27. Cliff WJ: The aortic tunica media in growing rats studied with the electron microscope. *Lab Invest* 17: 599–615, 1967.
28. Ross MH: The fine structure and development of the peritubular contractile cell component in the seminiferous tubules of the mouse. *Am J Anat* 121: 523–558, 1967.
29. Blandau RJ, Rumery RE: Measurements of intrafollicular pressure in ovulatory and preovulatory follicles of the rat. *Fertil Steril* 14: 330–341, 1963.
30. Espey LL, Lipner H: Measurements of intrafollicular pressures in the rabbit ovary. *Am J Physiol* 205: 1067–1072, 1963.
31. *Rondell P*: Biophysical aspects of ovulation. *Biol Reprod* 2 (Suppl): 64–89, 1970.
32. Virutamasen P, Wright KH, Wallach EE: Effects of catecholamines on ovarian contractility in the rabbit. *Obstet Gynecol* 39: 225–236, 1972.
33. Martin G, Talbot P: Drugs that block smooth muscle contraction inhibit in vivo ovulation in hamsters. *J Exp Zoo* 216: 483–491, 1981.
34. Walles B, Edvinsson L, Nybell G, Owman C, Sjoberg NO: Modifications of ovarian motility by amines: a mechanism involved in ovulation? *Eur J Obstet Gynecol Reprod Biol* 4: 103–107, 1974.
35. DiDio LJA, Allen DJ, Correr S, Motta PM: Smooth musculature in the ovary. In: Biology of the Ovary. PM Motta, ESE Hafez (eds), The Hague / Boston / London: M Nijhoff, p 106–118, 1980.
36. Fink G, Schofield GC: Experimental studies on the innervation of the ovary in cats. *J Anat* 109: 115–126, 1971.
37. Motta PM, Cherney DD, DiDio LJA: Scanning and transmission microscopy of the ovarian surface in mammals with special reference to ovulation. *J Submicrosc Cytol* 3: 85–100, 1971.
38. O'Shea JD: Smooth muscle-like cells in the walls of ovarian follicles and corpora lutea in sheep. *J Reprod Fertil* 24: 283–285, 1971.
39. Burden HW: Ultrastructural observation on ovarian perifollicular smooth muscle in the cat, guinea pig, and rabbit. *Am J Anat* 133: 125–142, 1972.
40. Bjersing L, Cajander S: Ovulation and the mechanism of follicle rupture. *Cell Tissue Res* 153: 15–30, 1974.
41. Walles B, Groschel-Stewart U, Owman C, Sjoberg NO, Unsicker K: Fluorescence histochemical demonstration of a relationship between adrenergic nerves and cells containing actin and miosin in the rat ovary, with special reference to the follicle wall. *J Reprod Fertil* 52: 175–178, 1978.
42. Pendergrass BP, Talbot P: The distribution of contractile cells in the apex of the preovulatory hamster follicle. *Biol Reprod* 20: 205–213, 1979.
43. Schroeder PC, Talbot P: Intrafollicular pressure decrease in hamster preovulatory follicles during smooth muscle cell contraction in vitro. *J Exp Zool* 224: 417–426, 1982.
44. Talbot P, Chacon RS: In vitro ovulation of hamster oocytes depends on contraction of follicular smooth muscle cells. *J Exp Zool* 224: 409–415, 1982.
45. Talbot P, Schroeder PC: 5-hydroxytryptamine causes contraction of smooth muscle cells in preovulatory hamster follicles. *J Exp Zool* 224: 427–436, 1982.
46. Doss DN, Boulos IK, Fredens K: The presence of smooth muscle cells in the rat ovary. *Histochemistry* 81: 205–206, 1984.

Author's address:
Prof. U. Muglia
Department of Veterinary Anatomy
Faculty of Veterinary Medicine
University of Messina
Via S. Cecilia 30
98100 Messina
Italy

CHAPTER 12

Morphology of vascular smooth muscle fibers and pericytes: scanning electron microscopic studies

YASUO UEHARA, TAKASHI FUJIWARA, & TOSHIYUKI KAIDOH

1. Introduction

Blood vessels are not simply passive conduits, but rather a system in which structure and function change gradually along the length of the vessels, from the arterial origin at the heart to the periphery, and also from the periphery to the venous end.

Vascular smooth muscles, in particular, exhibit significant functional variation in their electrophysiological and mechanical properties and in their sensitivity to various vasoactive substances (1–4). Although recent studies with transmission electron microscopy have elucidated in great detail the structural features of smooth muscle fibers (for review, see 5–8), these studies have not provided sufficient information to interpret the functional variability of the smooth muscle fibers. Rhodin (9) published an excellent article on the vascular wall architecture, illustrating, on the basis of his careful examination of serial histological and ultrathin sections, the structure and principal arrangement of the smooth muscle fibers in various portions of the vascular tree.

Capillary vessels are associated with stellate cells, known as pericytes. Since there are always transitional forms between pericytes and smooth muscle fibers at both arterial and venular sides of microvessels (10), these two types of cells are often collectively termed *periendothelial cells*. Several important reviews describing the structure and function of pericytes (11–13) have appeared. Accumulating evidence suggests that they are contractile, containing smooth-muscle-like molecules such as actin (14–17), myosin (15, 18–20), tropomyosin (21), desmin (22), and GMP-dependent protein kinase (23). Zimmermann (10) considered pericytes as modified smooth muscle fibers, and Meyrick and Reid (24) suggested that they were resting stem cells capable of differentiating into smooth muscle fibers.

The shape and arrangement of pericytes have been studied by a number of investigators, using various light microscopic techniques such as methylene-blue (25) and Janus-green-B vital staining (26), silver impregnation (10, 27–29), histochemical staining for DPN-diaphorase (30), in vivo observation with Nomarski's interference microscopy (31), and the fluorescent phallacidin method to localize filamentous actin (32). Among these procedures, Zimmermann's Golgi-Kopsch silver impregnation (10) has been so far the most successful in visualizing these cells. However, the method is so capricious that many investigators are reluctant to use it. Light microscopic techniques and the vessels previously examined are listed in Table 12-1.

At the ultrastructural level, vascular smooth muscle fibers and pericytes have been directly visualized with scanning electron microscopy (SEM), using various procedures to selectively remove extracellular connective tissue components. The histological background and practical information relative to the procedures widely used to study various tissues and cells have been reviewed in the Chapter 6 of this book. Most of the procedures applied to the examination of vascular wall cells are modifications of the

Table 12-1. Light Microscopic Methods for Visualizing Vascular Smooth Muscle Fibers and Pericytes

Methods	Cells	Tissues	References
HCl tissue maceration	M	Various tissues of mammals	(56)
Silver impregnation	P	Frog hyaloid membrane	(27, 28)
	P & M	Various tissues of animals	(10)
Vital staining	P	Human lung	(29)
Methylene blue	P	Mouse intestine	(25)
Janus green B	P & M	Frog nictitating membrane	(26)
Histochemistry DPN-diaphorase	P	Human retina	(30)
Nomarski's microscopy	P & M	Rat mesocecum	(31)
Fluorescent phallacidin	M	Mouse mammary gland	(32)

M: smooth muscle fibers; P: pericytes.

method introduced by Evan et al. (33, 34), which consists of hydrochloric acid hydrolysis and collagenase digestion of collagen fibrils, elastic fibers, and basal laminae. Apart from these chemical digestion methods, Castenholz (35) has developed a unique method to isolate cerebral vessels with ultrasonic treatment, and has demonstrated the SEM images of the muscle fibers and pericytes. Shiraishi et al. (36) also isolated brain vessels by ultrasonification and treated them with hydrochloric acid. Microcorrosive resin casting of blood vessels (37) often produces *plastic strips* around the vascular casts that exhibit morphological features of periendothelial cells (38, 39). The mechanism of the strip formation is not clear at present, but Castenholz (39) suggested that the plastic spreads within the tissue space that the originally occupied monocytes and pericytes. The cells are squeezed and move into different sites of the space for unknown reasons. These SEM studies have depicted the three-dimensional cellular morphology in greater detail than was hitherto possible, confirming and extending Zimmermann's results at the ultrastructural level. Table 12-2 summarizes currently available SEM methods and the vessels investigated.

This chapter concerns itself primarily with the morphological diversity of vascular smooth muscle fibers and pericytes in various portions of the vascular tree as examined with SEM, and also deals with the three-dimensional morphological changes undergone by arterial and arteriolar smooth muscle fibers upon vasoconstriction, adding new information to the previous studies (40–43).

The SEM procedures used in this study were either enzymatic digestion (with collagenase, hyaluronidase, or trypsin, singly or in combination) followed by glutaraldehyde fixation and hydrochloric acid hydrolysis (44, 45), or hydrochloric acid hydrolysis alone of fixed specimens (46).

2. Morphology of vascular smooth muscle fibers and pericytes

The morphological features of vascular smooth muscle fibers and pericytes are clearly recognized when examined with SEM. Despite drastic acid treatment, there appear to be no obvious artifactual alterations, except for some degree of cellular shrinkage. This chapter describes large vessels, such as elastic and muscular arteries and small veins, and small vessels, e.g., microvessels, including muscular, terminal, and precapillary arterioles, arterial, true, and venous capillaries, and postcapillary, collecting, and muscular venules. Microvascular segments are identified according to their vascular diameters, their wall structure and thickness, and the relationship of the vessel to the vascular system as a whole (47–49). The SEM images of wall cytoarchitecture offer another criterion for segmental identification (45).

2.1. *Elastic arteries*

Elastic arteries have a thick media consisting of alternating elastic and muscular laminae. In the rat thoracic aorta, the media contains at least

Table 12-2. Scanning Electron Microscopic Methods for Visualizing Vascular Smooth Muscle Fibers and Pericytes

Methods	Cells	Tissues	References
HCl and/or collagenase	P & M	Hamster muscle	(65)
Collagenase-trypsin	M	Rat retina	(77)
HCl-collagenase	M	Hamster muscle	(77)
	P	Rabbit retina	(78)
	P	Monkey thyroid gland	(79)
KOH-collagenase	M	Rat intestine	(80)
HCl	M	Monkey mesentery	(46, 75)
	M	Mouse muscle	(81)
	P & M	Rabbit kidney	(82)
Trypsin-OsO4 maceration	P	Rat muscle	(66)
Collagenase and hyaluronidase-HCl	P & M	Rat mammary gland	(45)
Ultrasonification	P & M	Rat brain	(35)
Ultrasonification-HCl	M	Dog brain	(36)
Corrosion cast	P & M*	Rat brain	(38, 39)

M: smooth muscle fibers; P: pericytes;
P & M*: plastic strips of the cells.

seven or eight muscular laminae. Removal of connective tissue components often causes exfoliation of the muscular laminae, enabling us to examine all laminae in succession. The outermost lamina assumes a tattered appearance consisting of irregular and randomly oriented muscle fiber groups (Fig. 12-1). In the deeper laminae, the muscle fibers are organized into broader, more

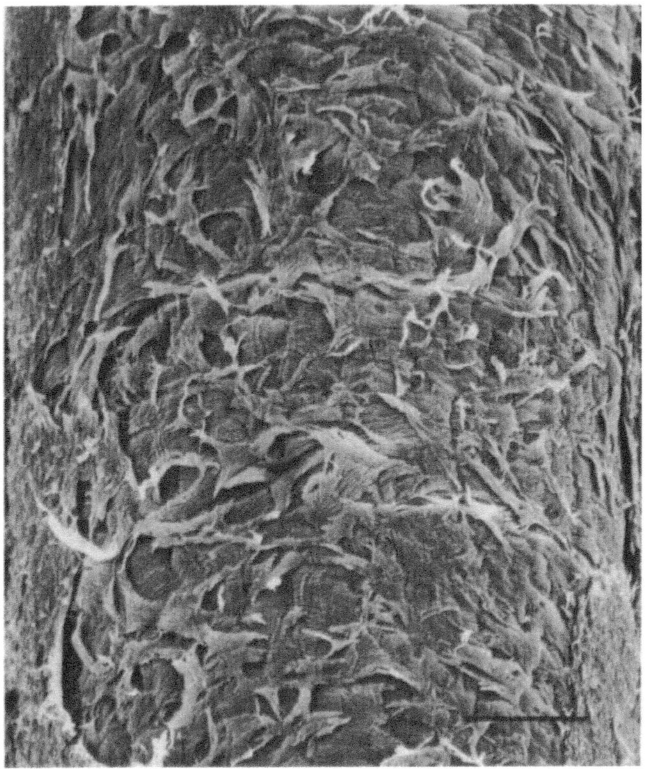

Figure 12-1. Adventitial aspect of the media of the rat thoracic aorta. Muscle fiber sheets assume a tattered appearence. Bar: 200 μm.

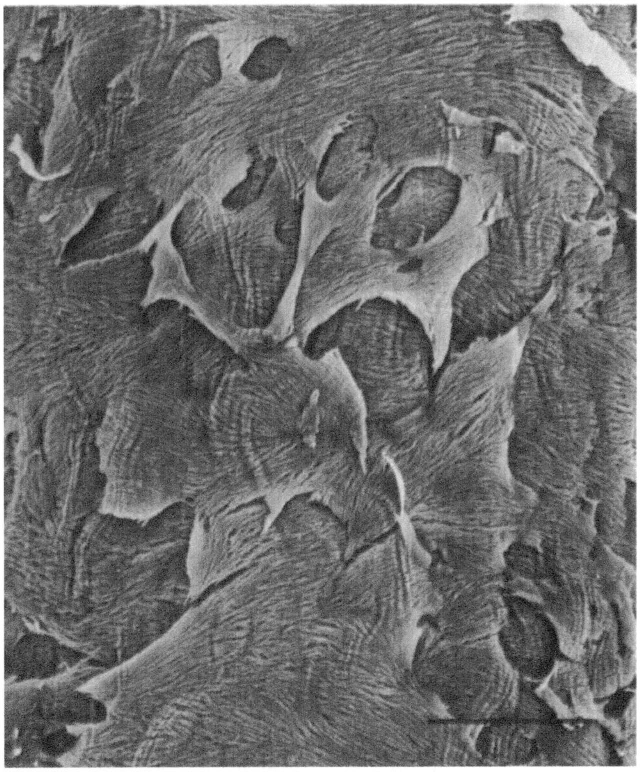

Figure 12-2. Outer muscle laminae of the rat thoracic aorta contain perforating muscular sheets. Fiber groups run rather randomly. Bar: 200 μm.

or less continuous sheets, in which the fibers are arranged in almost parallel groups. In and between the sheets are perforations of various diameters (Fig. 12-2). The disposition of muscle fiber groups varies in different sheets or in different areas of the same sheet. In the deepest lamina, the muscular sheets consist of almost continuous and parallel muscle fibers that are oriented circularly, although occasionally slightly diagnoal fiber groups occur (Fig. 12-3). Longitudinal muscle bundles may be present in the subendothelial layer.

The arrangement of aortic smooth muscle fibers has been variously interpreted in previous studies on sections. Pease (50) reported that muscle fibers in the rat were arranged diagnoally

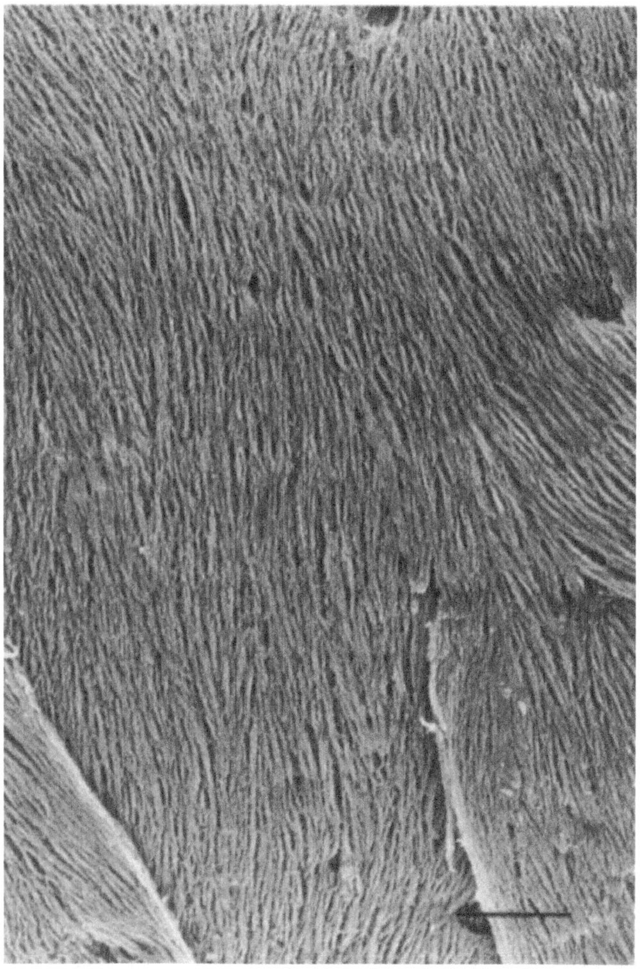

Figure 12-3. Deeper muscular laminae of the rat thoracic aorta. The broad muscular sheets contain a parallel array of muscle fibers that are slightly diagonally oriented. Bar: 50 μm.

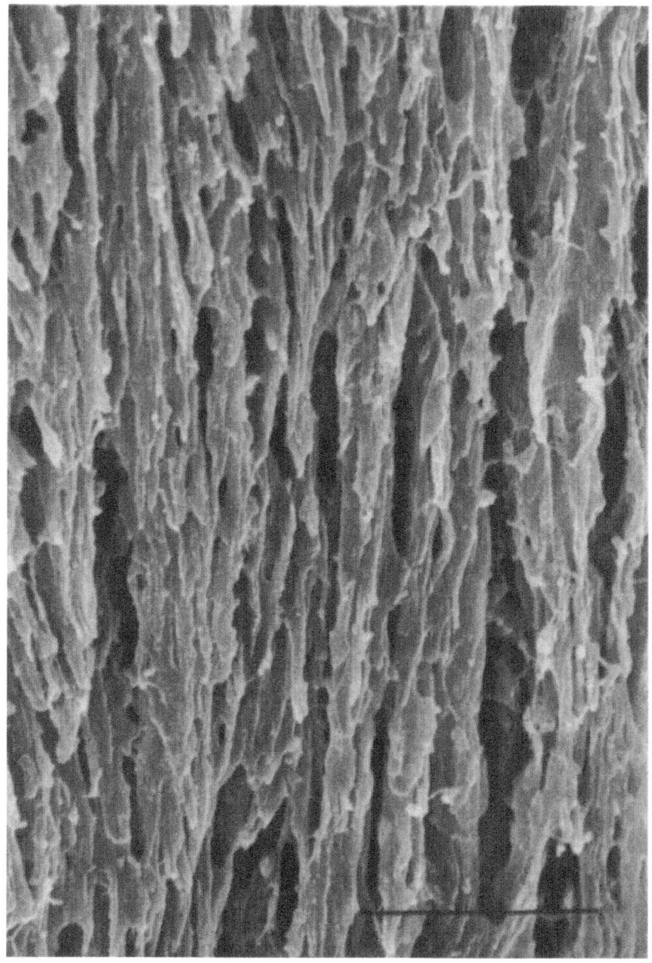

Figure 12-4. Smooth muscle fibers in the rat thoracic aorta. Fibers are elongated and possess a number of lateral processes with undefined boundaries. Bar: 5 μm.

in parallel array, and that successive layers were oriented in different directions, providing a basis for complex balanced forces. Bunce (51) found muscle fibers in the inner part of the media in the dog; these were directed both longitudinally and circularly and were arranged in herringbone fashion in the central part of the media. Rhodin (9) reported that the majority of muscle fibers in the resting part of the media in the squirrel monkey were oriented slightly diagonally. The angle between the fiber axis and the longitudinal vessel axis was reported to be 20° to 40° (52, 53). The arrangement of muscle fibers may vary among different portions of the aorta and from species to species.

Aortic smooth muscle fibers were described

as being elongated but angular, and irregularly shaped, with multiple cellular processes attaching the cells to collagen fibrils and elastic laminae (9, 54).

By SEM, smooth muscle fibers appear elongated and highly irregular in shape with branched fiber ends. They are 3–5 μm in their widest diameter. The surface of muscle fibers is highly ragged, with a number of longitudinal ridges and fingerlike or nodular processes (Fig. 12-4). The adjacent fibers are interconnected repeatedly in end-to-end or side-by-side fashion. Since the cell boundaries are poorly defined, the cell length is therefore hardly measurable.

The muscle sheets often exhibit alternating cross-ridges and gutters in some places (Fig. 12-5). The ridges are formed by interdigitating fingerlike projections and tapered ends of adjacent fibers. We have reported similar features in the innermost aspect of the media of the monkey mesenteric arteries (46), and suggested that they may provide attachment devices of muscle fibers to the elastic laminae.

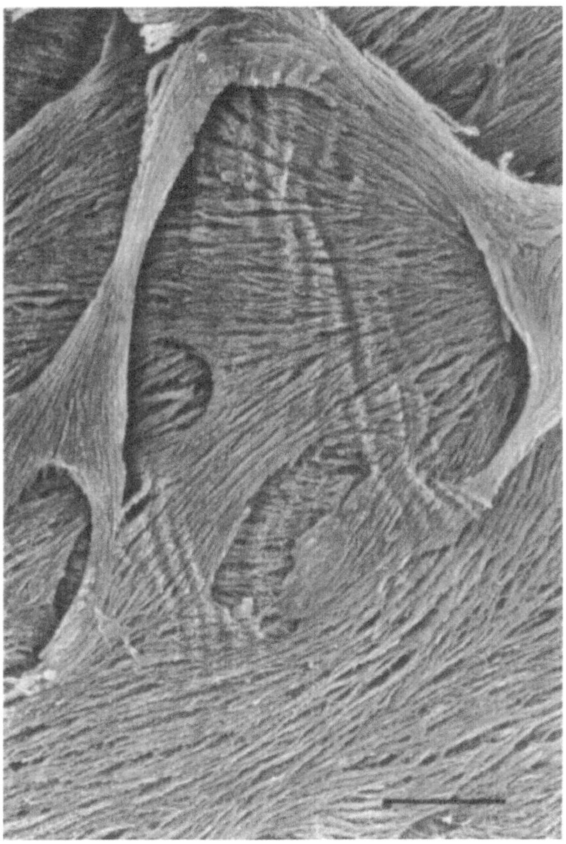

Figure 12-5. Parallel ridges and gutters found on the mscular sheet of the rat thoracic aorta. Bar: 50 μm.

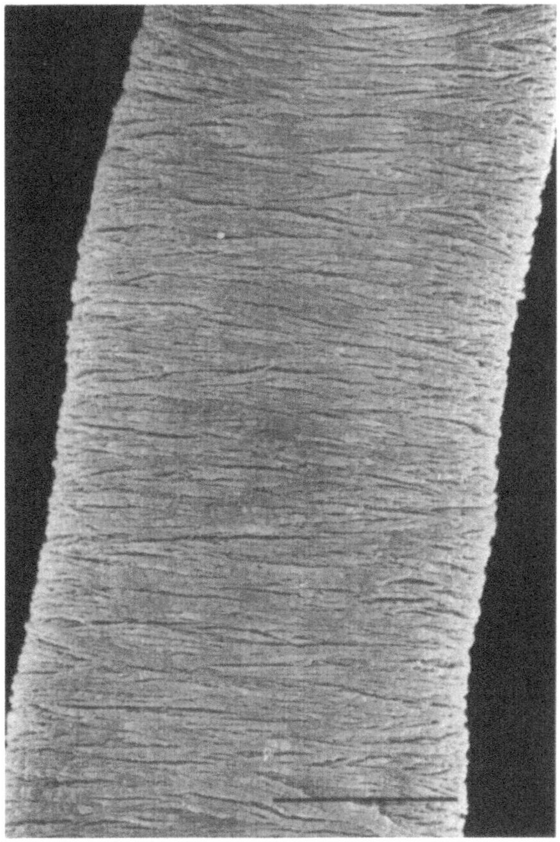

Figure 12-6. Guinea pig muscular artery about 100 μm in diameter. The media consists of a parallel array of circular muscle fibers. Bar: 50 μm.

2.2. Muscular arteries

The following results were obtained from vessels that were dilated by perfusing fixative at about twice the physiological blood pressure.

Muscular arteries range in diameter approximately from 100 μm to 300 μm in small rodents and from 100 μm to 1000 μm in larger animals such as the monkey. In general, the vessels have a well-developed compact media consisting of concentric layers of muscle fibers mostly circularly oriented in a highly regular fashion (Fig. 12-6). Muscle fiber groups that are slightly obliquely oriented occur occasionally, with a pitch lower than 10° (36).

The medial architecture of muscular arteries has been studied with light microscopy by

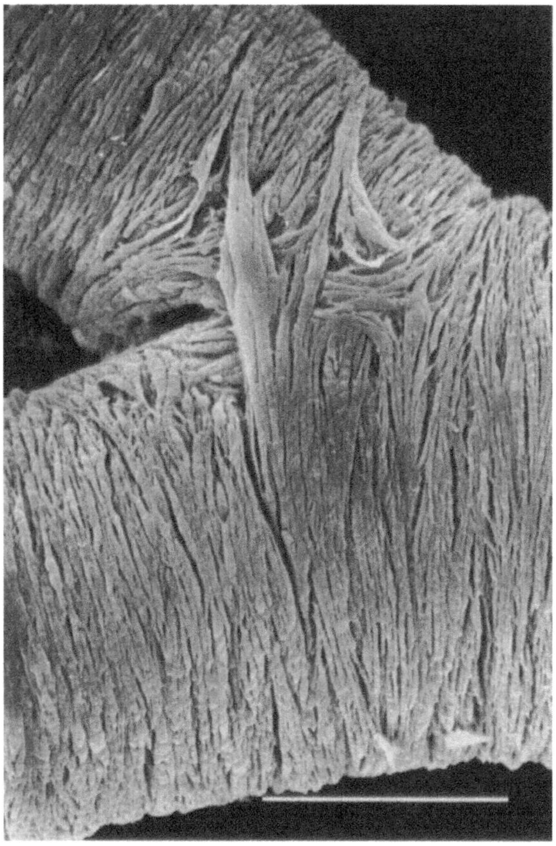

Figure 12-7. Branching point of the guinea pig mesenteric artery. Note the disordered arrangement of smooth muscle fibers. Bar: 50 μm.

several investigators. Some authors confirmed the circular orientation of the muscle fibers (42, 55), whereas others suggested a helical or spiral orientation (56, 57).

Individual muscle fibers are elongated and fusiform, ranging from 4–5 μm in their widest diameter, and from 50–70 μm in length. They usually have simply tapered fibers ends. On the adventitial surface of the outermost muscle fibers, nodular protrusions less than 4 μm in diameter occasionally occur. These may form attachment sites of the cells to the internal elastic lamina (46).

Longitudinal muscle bundles have often been found by SEM in the medio-adventitial border of the mesenteric arteries of the monkey (46) and in the brain arteries of the dog (36). These muscle bundles have already been noted in previous histological studies on the arterial intima in various organs such as the heart, lung, ovary, uterus, and penis (9). Those in the medio-adventitial border have also been described in the mesenteric arteries of the turkey and chicken (58) and in the coronary (59) and renal arteries (60) of the rat. Intimal longitudinal muscle fibers may widen the vessel lumen or, upon constriction, may block the blood flow either partly or completely. They may be involved in strengthening the vascular wall against the passive stretch of the vessel (50).

The regular circular orientation of the muscle fibers is largely disturbed at bifurcation points of the vessels (36). Extensions of circular muscle bundles of the parent vessel stretch over and lie between two branches (Fig. 12-7). This disorderly arrangement may be related to the mechanical reinforcement of the branching point.

2.3. Muscular and terminal arterioles

Muscular arterioles are generally defined as having two or three layers of fusiform muscle fibers,

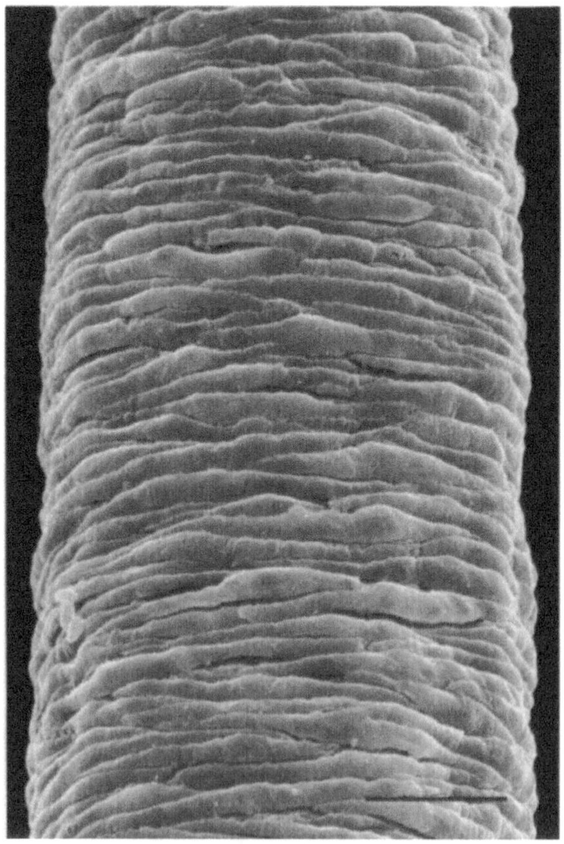

Figure 12-8. Subarachnoidal muscular arteriole of the rat. Muscle fibers are fusiform with tapered ends. They are tightly apposed to each other and are circularly oriented. Bar: 20 μm.

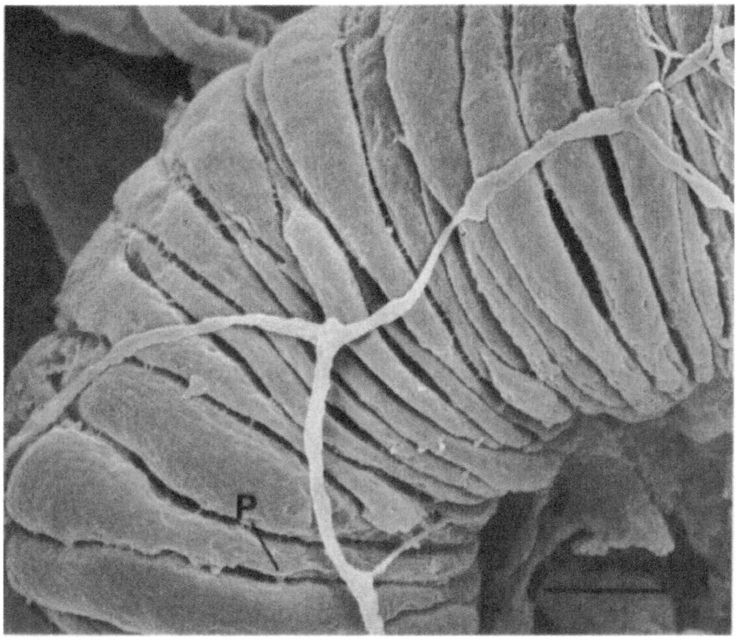

Figure 12-9. Terminal arteriole about 20 μm in diameter with a compact layer of spindle-shaped smooth muscle fibers. Each muscle fiber has a central bulge and unbranched tapered ends. A few slender side projections (P) connect the adjacent cells. Bar: 5 μm.

ranging from about 30 μm to less than 100 μm in diameter. They have a media essentially resembling that of the small arteries mentioned earlier. Smooth muscle fibers are arranged in regular circular fashion and have generally unbranched tapered ends. Figure 12-8 shows the SEM image of a rat subarachnoidal arteriole about 75 μm in diameter. Here, the muscle fibers are 3 μm to 5.5 μm in diameter, and 50 μm to 70 μm in length.

The circular orientation appears to be a common feature of muscular arterioles (5, 61), though a slight diagonal arrangement has been occasionally noted (43, 62, 63).

Smaller arterioles less than 30 μm in diameter with a single muscle layer are defined as terminal arterioles. Muscle fibers resemble in shape and arrangement those in the muscular arterioles. Individual muscle fibers are 50–60 μm long and have a central bulge of 5–6 μm in diamter. They are closely associated with each other and encircle the vessel in about one turn. The number of turns is dependent upon the vascular diameter (Fig. 12-9). In the medio-adventitial border of the terminal arterioles of the dog brain, asteroid cells that are considered to be modified smooth muscle fibers (36) occur. Their functional significance and origin are still unknown.

2.4. *Precapillary arterioles*

Further distally, terminal arterioles branch and taper to produce precapillary arterioles 6–12 μm in diameter. The muscle fibers gradually come to be branched. In the initial portion of the precapillary arteriole, muscle fibers have only longitudinal bifurcations on one or both sides of the bulging cell body (Fig. 12-10). As the vessels ramify and taper, the branches increase in number and begin to possess thinner secondary processes that connect the adjacent muscle fibers and processes (Fig. 12-11). The primary processes are all arranged circularly around the vessel, while the secondary processes are more or less longitudinally oriented. The branched muscle fibers average about 4–6 μm in width at their thickest bulges and about 20–30 μm in length. We have previously reconstructed arteriolar smooth muscle fibers in the guinea pig and rat (64), demonstrating that branched muscle fibers contained contractile filaments and other cell organelles that are typical of smooth muscle

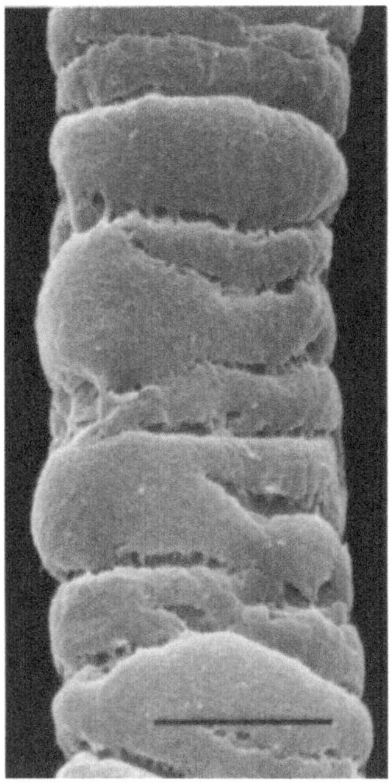

Figure 12-10. Subarachnoidal precapillary arteriole of the rat. Smooth muscle fibers split longitudinally on both sides of cell body. Bar: 5 μm.

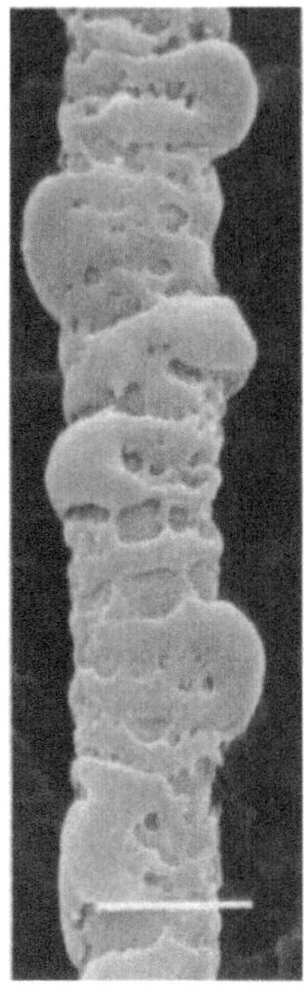

Figure 12-11. Thinner precapillary arteriole about 5 μm in diameter with branched smooth muscle fibers. Bar: 5 μm.

fibers. The reconstructed shape and size of the fusiform and branched muscle fibers coincide well with the intact ones examined with SEM.

Precapillary sphincters are generally known to occur as ring structures at the orifices of capillaries, but they have not so far been detected in any published SEM studies of microvessels.

2.5. Capillaries

Highly branched spidery cells with bulging cell bodies and ramifying processes occur in the subsequent smaller vessels about 4–7 μm in diameter, e.g., arterial capillaries. They represent the pericytes originally described by Zimmermann (10). The cellular processes are mostly circularly oriented with respect to the vessel axis. The gaps between the cells and cell processes are further increased with the increased free stromal surface area. The exposed area of endothelium is proportional to the degree of exchange of substances (13). True capillaries are identified by their diameter, which is smaller than the size of red blood cells, being less than about 5 μm in laboratory rodents. The appearance of the pericytes of true capillaries varies considerably in different organs. For example, those in the skeletal muscles have longitudinal processes on both sides of the cell body that give rise to numerous circularly oriented secondary processes. The cells assume, as a whole, a configuration resembling a snake skeleton, as was described by Zimmermann (10; see also 65, 66). The pericytes in the rat mammary and thyroid glands and in the mouse large intestine, on the other hand, have short primary processes with fewer secondary processes (Fig. 12-12). They are scattered along the vessel length with a center-to-center distance of 10–30 μm in the rat mammary gland, about 30 μm in the rat thyroid gland, and 30–50 μm in the mouse large intestine. The distribution of capillary pericytes is different from organ to organ and from species to species (67).

Next to the true capillaries are venous capillaries about 5–8 μm in diameter, possessing pericytes that basically resemble those in arterial capillaries.

2.6. Postcapillary venules

Postcapillary venules range from 10–40 μm in diameter and exhibit the most elaborate cytoar-

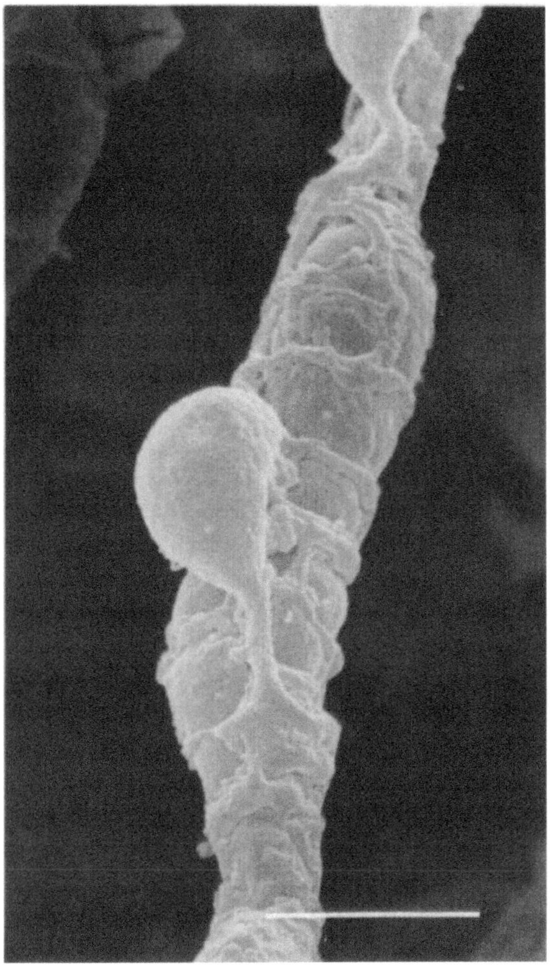

Figure 12-12. True capillary of the rat mammary gland. The pericytes possess primary longitudinal processes and several secondary circular processes. A large area of the adventitial surface of the vessel lacks pericytic investment. Bar: 5 μm.

chitecture of all the microvascular segments. They are invested by a dense lacework of spidery pericytes. The segment has been considered to be involved in the defense mechanism and in the extravasation of fluid and migration of blood cells during inflammatory phenomena (11, 68–73). Figure 12-13 shows what appears to be a blood cell passing through the vascular wall. Venular pericytes may trap the migrating blood cells. Pericytes of postcapillary venules have been reported to detach and eventually develop into macrophages when they are stimulated (72). However, pericytes and endothelial cells appear to attach firmly to each other by their processes.

2.7. *Collecting venules*

With the repeated confluence of capillaries and postcapillary venules, the diameter of the vessels rapidly increases to more than 30 μm to form collecting venules. Periendothelial cells of such venules are stellate and possess fewer attenuated processes. Further, these cells are scattered with a center-to-center distance between adjacent cells of more than 20 μm. They have a bulging central cell body about 3–5 μm in diameter, and their ramifying processes contact each other to form a loose network. Rhodin (48) showed that pericytes of this segment contained contractile filaments and therefore considered them to be primitive smooth muscle fibers. This thin, loose cellular investment may help the vessel to dilate passively in reserving large amounts of blood (Fig. 12-14).

2.8. *Muscular venules*

Smooth muscle fibers of muscular venules, thicker than 60 μm in diameter, are arranged circularly in a discontinuous manner with varying interspace less than 4 μm wide. They are ribbonlike with a varying width along their length, being less than 5 μm wide and about 100 μm long. These smooth muscle fibers characteristically have numerous thin serrate lateral projections less than 0.5 μm wide that connect the neighboring cells. Thus they differ strikingly in shape from the arteriolar smooth muscle fibers described earlier. Transitional forms between these muscle fibers and spidery pericytes can be seen in the initial portion of this segment. Here, the cells, which are elongated and possess fewer branches, are predominantly circularly oriented.

2.9. *Small veins*

The wall structure of veins varies considerably according to their caliber, age, species, and location in the body. Even the same vein will vary markedly in structure along its length and on opposite sides of a cross section (74). Figure 12-15 shows an adventitial aspect of a monkey mesenteric vein about 200 μm in diameter. Smooth muscle fibers show a highly disordered arrangement (75). Th outer muscle fibers tend to be

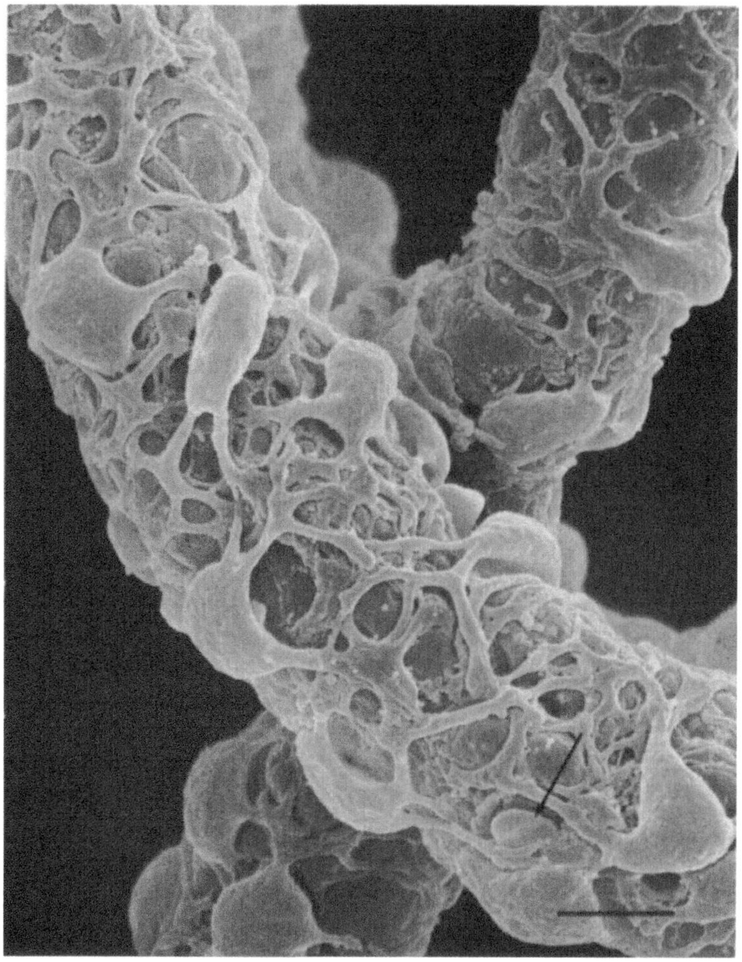

Figure 12-13. Postcapillary venule of the rat mammary gland is invested by a dense cellular lacework of spidery pericytes. What appears to be a blood cell is seen in the vascular wall (arrow). Bar: 5 μm.

oriented obliquely or longitudinally and are attached to and intermingled with the more or less circularly oriented inner muscle fibers. The outer smooth muscle fibers are occasionally flattened in the radial direction of the vessel and have a maximum width of 6–8 μm and a length of 40–100 μm. The inner smooth muscle fibers are thinner than the outer ones, being less than 5 μm in width and 60–90 μm in length.

By contrast, guinea pig mesenteric veins about 150 μm in diameter show regularly arranged circular smooth muscle fibers that are about 3 μm thick and more than 50 μm long. They are separated by a gap varying from 0.5 to 1.0 μm in width and are interconnected frequently by thin lateral projections that resemble those of muscular venules described earlier (Fig. 12-16).

3. Changes of vascular smooth muscle fibers upon vasoconstriction

Vessels can be dilated either by local application of acetylcholine or by perfusion of buffered glutaraldehyde at twice physiological pressure. In dilated arteries and arterioles, smooth muscle fibers have a generally smooth surface texture. In vessels constricted by immersion in buffered saline containing norepinephrine, the smooth muscle fibers showed drastic changes in their adventitial surface texture (76). Muscle fibers of the artery exhibit a highly ragged surface with numerous prominent transverse folds about 0.5 μm to 2 μm thick. However, the bulging central portion of the fibers, which contains the nucleus and fewer myofilaments, remains unchanged

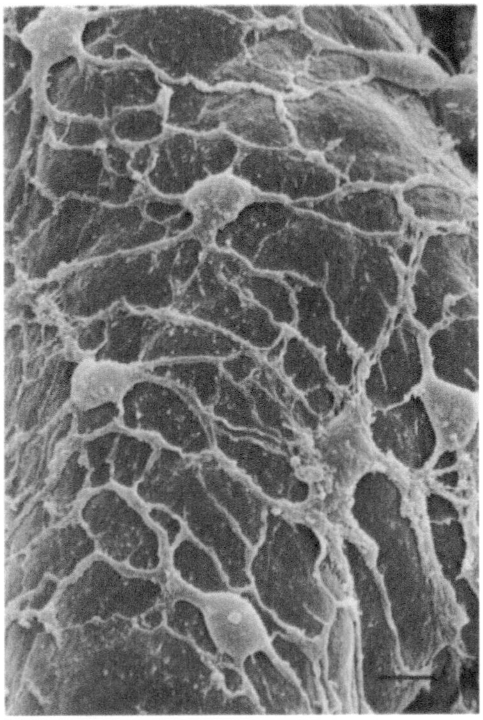

Figure 12-14. Collecting venule of the rat subarachnoid has scattered stellate periendothelial cells possessing fewer attenuated processes. Bar: 5 μm.

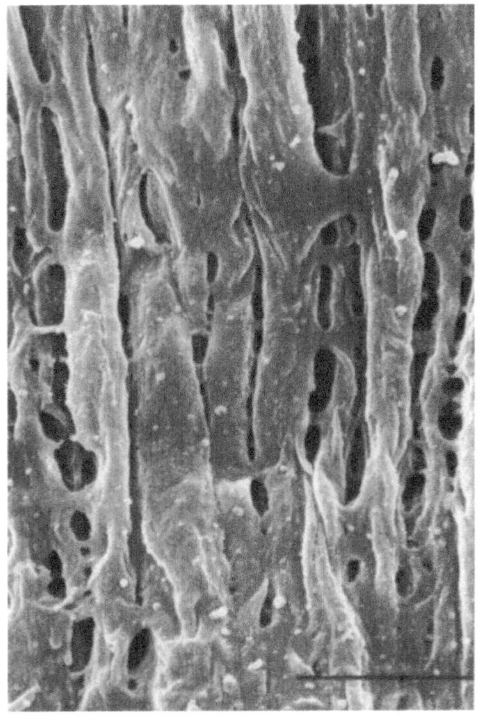

Figure 12-16. Smooth muscle fibers of the guinea pig mesenteric vein are elongated and circularly oriented. They are frequently interconnected by thin lateral projections. Bar: 5 μm.

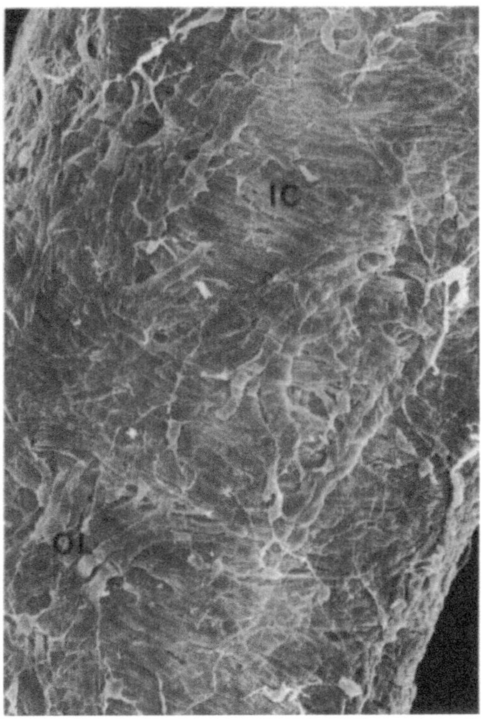

Figure 12-15. Small mesenteric vein of the monkey. Smooth muscle fibers show highly disordered arrangement, consisting of outer oblique or longitudinal (OL) and inner circular (IC) fibers. Bar: 50 μm.

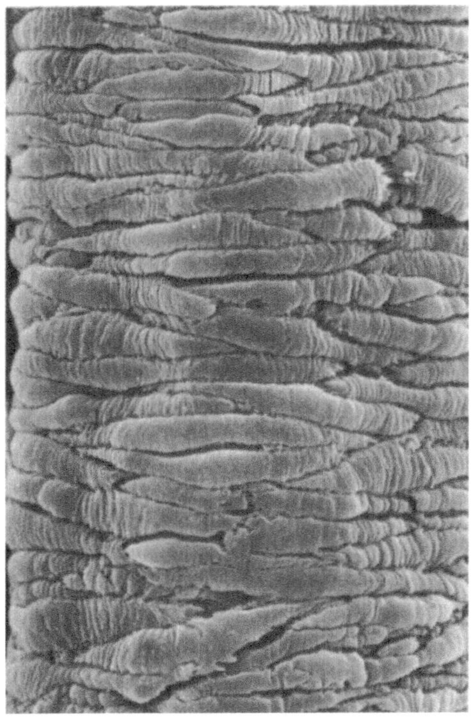

Figure 12-17. Constricted muscular artery of the rat brain. Muscle fibers exhibit a highly rugged surface texture with numerous transverse folds, except on the central cell bulge. Bar: 20 μm.

(Fig. 12-17). In constricted monkey mesenteric arteries, a group of bulbous structures also occurs intermingled with transverse folds (Fig. 12-18).

Figure 12-19 shows a constricted precapillary arteriole in which branched muscle fibers also undergo significant changes; they give rise to focal collections of folds and small nodules. The differences in the surface texture may be related to the myofilamentous organization and also to the amount and arrangement of associated extracellular connective tissues. When vessels constrict, the length of the muscle fiber must shorten, as one would expect. We are undertaking a systematic measurement of smooth muscle fibers so as to correlate vascular diameter and fiber length. In one of our experiments, when the diameter of the rat cerebral artery reduced from 90 μm to 60 μm, the muscle fibers shortened by about 40%. Hayek (40), Lang (42), and Rhodin (9) have suggested that arterial muscle fibers in relaxed vessels were transversely oriented and became diagonally oriented upon contraction. However, in a SEM observation, the circular orientation was unaltered irrespective of the functional state of the vessels. So far, according to SEM results, capillary and venular pericytes exhibit no recognizable changes under vasoconstriction. The contractility of pericytes may be much weaker, if present at all, than that of arterial smooth muscle fibers.

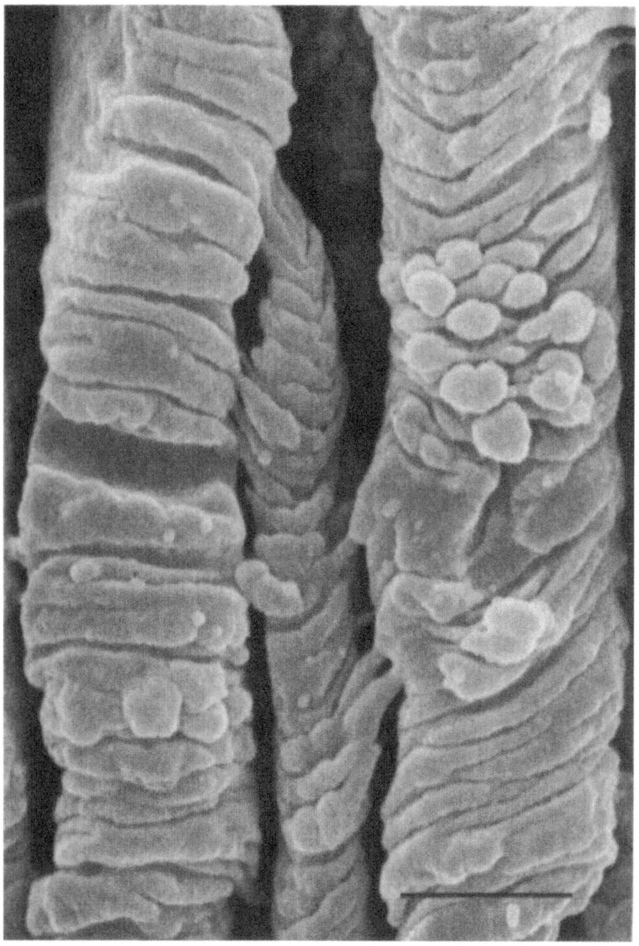

Figure 12-18. Strongly contracted muscle fibers of the monkey mesenteric artery are endowed with bulbous protrusions together with transverse folds. Bar: 2 μm.

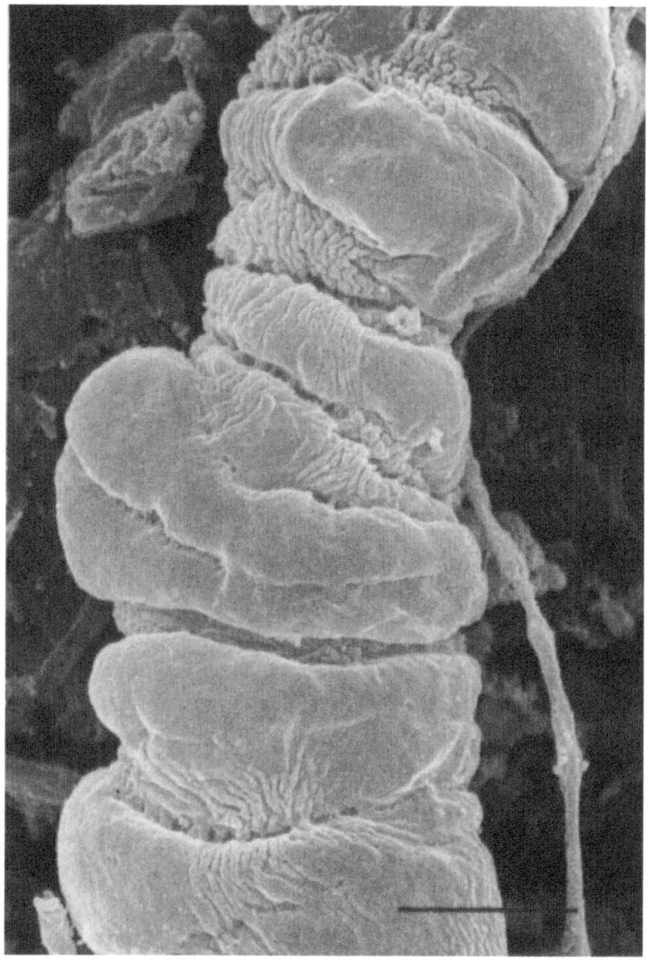

Figure 12-19. Constricted precapillary arteriole of the rat intestine. Branched smooth muscle fibers give rise to focal collections of folds and nodules. Bar: 5 μm.

References

1. Bevan JA, Ljung B: Longitudinal propagation of myogenic activity in rabbit arteries and in the rat portal vein. *Acta*

Physiol Scand 90: 703–715, 1974.
2. Altura BM: Pharmacology of venular smooth muscle: New insights. *Microvasc Res* 16: 91–117, 1978.
3. Vanhoutte PM: Heterogeneity in vascular smooth muscle. In: Microcirculation Vol 2. G Kaley, BM Altura (eds) Baltimore: University Park Press, p 181–309, 1978.
4. De Mey JG, Vanhoutte PM: Heterogeneous behavior of the canine arterial and venous wall: Importance of the endothelium. *Circ Res* 51: 439–447, 1982.
5. Rhodin JAG: Fine structure of vascular walls in mammals, with special reference to smooth muscle component. *Physiol Rev* 42 (Suppl 5): 48–81, 1962.
6. Somlyo AP, Somlyo AV: Vascular smooth muscle: I. Normal structure, pathology, biochemistry, and biophysics. *Pharmacol Rev* 20: 197–272, 1968.
7. Devine CE: Vascular smooth muscle morphology and ultrastructure. In: Microcirculation, Vol, 2. G Kaley, BM Altura (eds), Baltimore: University Park Press, p 3–39, 1978.
8. Somlyo AV: Ultrastructure of vascular smooth muscle. In: Handbook of Physiology: The Cardiovascular System 2, Vol 2: Vascular Smooth Muscle. DF Bohr, AP Somlyo, HV Sparks (eds), Bethesda, MD: American Physiological Society, p 33–67, 1980.
9. Rhodin JAG: Architecture of the vessel wall. In: Handbook of Physiology: The Cardiovascular System 2, Vol 2. DF Bohr, AP Somlyo, HV Sparks (eds), Bethesda, MD: American Physiological Society, p 1–31, 1980.
10. Zimmermann K: Die feinere Bau der Blutcapillaren. *Z Anat Entwickl* 68: 29–109, 1923.
11. Majno G: Ultrastructure of the vascular membrane. In: Handbook of Physiology: Section 2, Circulation, Vol 3. WF Hamilton, P Dow (eds), Washington, DC: American Physiological Society, p 2293–2375, 1965.
12. Wolff JR: Ultrastructure of the terminal vascular bed as related to function. In: Microcirculation, Vol 1. G Kaley, BM Altura (eds), Baltimore, MD: University Park Press, p 95–130, 1977.
13. Sims DE: The pericyte — A review. *Tissue Cell* 18: 153–174, 1986.
14. Forbes MS, Rennels ML, Nelson E: Ultrastructure of pericytes in mouse heart. *Am J Anat* 149: 47–70, 1977.
15. Le Beux YJ, Willemot J: Actin- and myosin-like filaments in rat brain pericytes. *Anat Rec* 190: 811–826, 1978.
16. Wallow IH, Burnside B: Actin filaments in retinal pericytes and endothelial cells. *Invest Ophthalmol Vis Sci* 19: 1433–1441, 1980.
17. Herman IM, D'Amore PA: Microvascular pericytes contain muscle and non-muscle actins. *J Cell Biol* 101: 43–52, 1985.
18. Groschel-Stewart U: Immunochemistry of cytoplasmic contractile proteins. *Int Rev Cytol* 65: 193–254, 1980.
19. Meyrick B, Fujiwara K, Reid L: Smooth muscle myosin in precursor and mature smooth muscle cells in normal pulmonary arteries and the effect of hypoxia. *Exp Lung Res* 2: 303–313, 1981.
20. Joyce NC, Haire MF, Palade GE: Contractile proteins in pericytes. II. Immunocytochemical evidence for the presence of two isomyosins in graded concentrations. *J Cell Biol* 100: 1387–1395, 1985.
21. Joyce NC, Haire MF, Palade GE: Contractile proteins in pericytes. I. Immunoperoxidase localization of tropomyosin. *J Cell Biol* 100: 1379–1386, 1985.
22. Fujimoto T, Singer SJ: Immunocytochemical studies of desmin and vimentin in pericapillary cells of chicken. *J Histochem Cytochem* 35: 1105–1115, 1987.
23. Joyce NC, DeCamilli P, Boyles J: Pericytes, like vascular smooth muscle cells, are immunocytochemically positive for cyclic GMP-dependent protein kinase. *Microvasc Res* 28: 206–219, 1984.
24. Meyrick B, Reid L: The effect of continued hypoxia on rat pulmonary arterial circulation. *Lab Invest* 38: 188–200, 1978.
25. Mayer S: Die Muskularisierung der capillaren Blutgefässe. Nachweis des anatomischen Substrats ihrer Kontraktilität. *Anat Anz Jena Bd* 21: 112–132, 1902.
26. Bensley RR, Vimtrup BJ: On the nature of Rouget cells of capillaries. *Anat Rec* 39: 37–55, 1928.
27. Rouget C: Mémoire sur le dévelopement, la structure et les propriétes physiologiques des capillaires sanguins et lymphatiques. *Arch Physiol Normale Pathol* 5: 603–661, 1873.
28. Rouget C: Sur la contractilité des capillaires sanguins. CR *Acad Sci* 88: 916–918, 1879.
29. Weibel ER: On pericytes, particularly their existence on lung capillaries. *Microvasc Res* 8: 218–235, 1974.
30. Kuwabara T, Cogan DG: Retinal vascular patterns. VI. Mural cells of the retinal capillaries. *Arch Ophthalmol* 69: 492–502, 1963.
31. Beacham WS, Konishi A, Hunt CC: Observations on the microcirculatory bed in rat mesocecum using differential interference contrast microscopy in vivo and electron microscopy. *Am J Anat* 146: 385–426, 1976.
32. Emerman JT, Vogl AW: Cell size and shape changes in the myoepithelium of the mammary gland during differentiation. *Anat Rec* 216: 405–415, 1986.
33. Evan AP, Dail WG, Dammrose D, Palmer C: Scanning electron microscopy of cell surfaces following removal of extracellular material. *Anat Rec* 185: 433–446, 1976.
34. Evan AP: SEM of cell surfaces following HCl and collagenase treatment. In: Scanning Electron Microscopy in Cell Biology and Medicine. K. Tanaka, T Fujita (eds), Amsterdom/Tokyo: Excerpta Med./Biomed. Res Found. p 119–124, 1981
35. Castenholz A: Visualization of periendothelial cells in arterioles and capillaries by scanning electron microscopy of ultrasound-treated and plastoid-injected brains in rats. *Scanning Electron Microsc* 1: 161–170, 1983.
36. Shiraishi T, Sakaki S, Uehara Y: Architecture of the media of the arterial vessels in the dog brain: A scanning electron-microscopic study. *Cell Tissue Res* 243: 329–335, 1986.
37. Murakami T: Application of the scanning electron microscope to the study of the fine distribution of the blood vessels. *Arch Histol Jpn* 32: 445–454, 1971.
38. Anderson BG, Anderson WD: Myocardial microvasculature studied by microcorrosion casts. *Biomed Res* 2 (Suppl): 209–217, 1981.
39. Castenholz A, Zoltzer H, Erhardt H: Structures imitating myocytes and pericytes in corrosion casts of terminal

blood vessels. A methodical approach to the phenomenon of 'plastic strips' in SEM. *Mikroskopie* 39: 95–106, 1982.
40. von Hayek H: Über die Kontraktionsfähigkeit der kleinsten Lungenarterien. *Z Anat Entwickl Gesch* 116: 373–376, 1952.
41. Van Citters RL, Wagner BM, Rushmer RF: Architecture of small arteries during vasconstriction. *Circ Res* 10: 668–675, 1962.
42. Lang J: Mikroskopische Anatomie der Arterien. *Angiologica* 2: 225–284, 1965.
43. Phelps PC, Luft JH: Electron microscopical study of relaxation and constriction in frog arterioles. *Am J Anat* 125: 399–428, 1969.
44. Fujiwara T, Uehara Y: Scanning electron microscopy of the myenteric plexus. *J Electron Microsc* 29: 397–400, 1980.
45. Fujiwara T, Uehara Y: The cytoarchitecture of the wall and the innervation pattern of the microvessels in the rat mammary gland: A scanning electron microscopic observation. *Am J Anat* 170: 39–54, 1984.
46. Fujiwara T, Uehara Y: Scanning electron microscopical study of vascular smooth muscle cells in the mesenteric vessels of the monkey: Arterial smooth muscle cells. *Biomed Res* 3: 649–658, 1982.
47. Chambers R, Zweifach BW: Topography and function of the mesenteric capillary circulation. *Am J Anat* 75: 173–205, 1944.
48. Rhodin JAG: Ultrastructure of mammalian venous capillaries, venules and small collecting veins. *J Ultrastruct Res* 25: 452–500, 1968.
49. Rhodin JAG: Ultrastructure of the microvascular bed. In: The Microcirculation in Clinical Medicine. R Wells (ed), New York: Academic Press, p 13–31, 1973.
50. Pease DC: Arterial and arteriolar systems. Microscopic and submicroscopic anatomy. In: Blood Vessels and Lymphatics. DI Abramson, (ed), New York: Academic Press, p 12–25, 1962.
51. Bunce DF, II: Atlas of Arterial Histology. St. Louis: Green, 1974.
52. Thoma R: Über die Strömung des Blutes in der Gefässbahn und die Spannung der Gefässwand. *Beitr Pathol Anat Allgem Pathol* 66: 92–158, 1920.
53. Seifert K: Elektronenmikroskopische Untersuchungen der Aorta des Hauschweines. *Z Zellforsch Microskop Anat* 58: 331–368, 1968.
54. Gabella G: Structure of smooth muscle. In: Smooth Muscle: An Assessment of Current Knowledge. E Bülbring, AF Brading, AW Jones, T Tomita (eds), London: Edward Arnold, p 1–46, 1981.
55. Staubesand J: Anatomie der Blutgefässe. I. Funktionelle Morphologie der Arterien, Venen und arterio-venösen Anastomosen. In: Angiologie. M Ratschow (ed), Stuttgart: Thieme, p 23–82, 1959.
56. Strong KC: A study of the structure of the media of the distributing arteries by the method of microdissection. *Anat Rec* 72: 151–168, 1938.
57. Fischer H: Über die funktionelle Bedeutung des Spiralverlaufes der Muskulatur in der Arterienwand. *Gegenbaurs Morphol Jahrbuch* 91: 394–445, 1951.
58. Ball RA, Sautter JH, Katter MS: Morphological characteristics of the anterior mesenteric artery of fowl. *Anat Rec* 146: 251–255, 1963.
59. Yohro T, Burnstock G: Fine structure of "intimal cushions" at branching sites in coronary arteries of vertebrates: A scanning and transmission electron microscopic study. *Z Anat Entwickl Gesch* 140: 187–202, 1973.
60. Osborne-Pellegrin MJ: Some ultrastructural characteristics of the renal artery and abdominal aorta in the rat. *J Anat* 125: 641–652, 1978.
61. Dacey RG Jr, Duling BR: A study of rat intracerebral arterioles: methods, morphology, and reactivity. *Am J Physiol* 243: H598–H606, 1982.
62. Rhodin JAG: The ultrastructure of mammalian arterioles and precapillary sphincters. *J Ultrastruct Res* 18: 181–223, 1967.
63. Hua C, Cragg B: Measurements of smooth muscle cells in arterioles of guinea pig ileum. *Acta Anat* 107: 224–230, 1980.
64. Komuro T, Desaki J, Uehara Y: Three-dimensional organization of smooth muscle cells in blood vessels of laboratory rodents. *Cell Tissue Res* 227: 429–437, 1982.
65. Uehara Y, Komuro T, Desaki J: Morphology of vascular smooth muscle cells and pericytes as revealed by transmission and scanning EM. In: Electron Microscopy, Vol II, Biology. Ninth International Congress of Electron Microscopy, p 464–465, 1978.
66. Mazanet R, Franzini-Armstrong C: Scanning electron microscopy of pericytes in rat red muscle. *Microvasc Res* 23: 361–369, 1982.
67. Tilton RG, Kilo C, Williamson JR, Murch DW: Differences in pericyte contractile function in rat cardiac and skeletal muscle microvasculatures. *Microvasc Res* 18: 336–352, 1979.
68. Marchesi VT, Florey HW: Electron microscopic observations on the emigration of leukocytes. *QJ Exp Physiol* 45: 343–348, 1960.
69. Florey HW, Grant LH: Leucocyte migration from small blood vessels stimulated with ultraviolet light, an electron microscope study. *J Pathol Bacteriol* 82: 13–17, 1961.
70. Majno G, Palade GE: Studies on inflammation. I. The effect of histamine and serotonin on vascular permeability: An electron microscopic study. *J Biophys Biochem Cytol* 11: 571–605, 1961.
71. Majno G, Palade GE, Schoefl GI: Studies on inflammation. II. The site of action of histamine and serotonin along the vascular tree: A topographic study. *J Biophys Biochem Cytol* 11: 607–626, 1961.
72. Movat HZ, Fernando NVP: The fine structure of the terminal vascular bed. IV. The venules and their perivascular cells (pericytes, adventitial cells). *Exp Mol Pathol* 3: 98–114, 1964.
73. Cotran RS: The delayed and prolonged vascular leakage in inflammation: II. An electron microscopic study of the vascular response after thermal injury. *Am J Pathol* 46: 589–620, 1965.
74. Franklin KJ: The physiology and pharmacology of veins. *Physiol Rev* 8: 346–364, 1928.
75. Fujiwara T, Ikeuchi M, Uehara Y: Scanning electron

microscope study of smooth muscle cells in the mesenteric veins of the monkey. *Biomed Res* 4: 225–230, 1983.
76. Uehara Y, Fujiwara T: The morphological changes of arterial smooth muscle cells upon vasodilation and vasoconstriction. In: Progress in Microcirculation Research II. FC Courtice, DG Garlick, MA Perry (eds), Kensington: Committee in Postgraduate Medical Education, The University of New South Wales, p 405–410, 1984.
77. Uehara Y, Suyama K: Visualization of the adventital aspect of the vascular smooth muscle cells under the scanning electron microscope. *J Electron Microsc* 27: 157–159, 1978.
78. Murakami M, Sugita A, Shimada T, Nakamura K: Surface view of pericytes on the retinal capillary in rabbits revealed by scanning electron microscopy. *Arch Histol Jpn* 42: 297–303, 1979.
79. Shimada T: Lymph and blood capillaries as studied by a new SEM technique. *Biomed Res* 2 (Suppl): 139–143, 1981.
80. Miller BG, Woods RI, Bohlen HG, Evan AP: A new morphological procedure for viewing microvessels: A scanning electron microsopic study of the vasculature of small intestine. *Anat Rec* 203: 493–503, 1982.
81. Holley JA, Fahim MA: Scanning electron microscopy of mouse muscle microvasculature. *Anat Rec* 205: 109–117, 1983.
82. Gattone VH II, Luft FC, Evan AP: Renal afferent and efferent arterioles of the rabbit. *Am J Physiol* 247: F219–F228, 1984.

Author's address:
Prof. Yasuo Uehara
Department of Anatomy
Ehime University School of Medicine
Shigenobu
791-02
Ehime
Japan

Index

GPSR Compliance

The European Union's (EU) General Product Safety Regulation (GPSR) is a set of rules that requires consumer products to be safe and our obligations to ensure this.

If you have any concerns about our products, you can contact us on ProductSafety@springernature.com

In case Publisher is established outside the EU, the EU authorized representative is:

Springer Nature Customer Service Center GmbH
Europaplatz 3
69115 Heidelberg, Germany

Batch number: 10684220

Printed by Printforce, the Netherlands